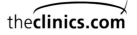

VETERINARY CLINICS

OF NORTH AMERICA

Small Animal Practice

Updates in Dermatology

GUEST EDITOR
Karen L. Campbell, DVM, MS

January 2006 • Volume 36 • Number 1

SAUNDERS

An Imprint of Elsevier, Inc.
PHILADELPHIA   LONDON   TORONTO   MONTREAL   SYDNEY   TOKYO

W.B. SAUNDERS COMPANY
A Division of Elsevier Inc.

Elsevier, Inc., 1600 John F. Kennedy Blvd., Suite 1800, Philadelphia, PA 19103-2899

http://www.vetsmall.theclinics.com

VETERINARY CLINICS OF NORTH AMERICA:	**Volume 36, Number 1**
SMALL ANIMAL PRACTICE	**ISSN 0195-5616**
January 2006	**ISBN 1-4160-3467-6**
Editor: John Vassallo	

The ideas and opinions expressed in *Veterinary Clinics of North America: Small Animal Practice* do not necessarily reflect those of the Publisher. The Publisher does not assume any responsibility for any injury and/or damage to persons or property arising out of or related to any use of the material contained in this periodical. The reader is advised to check the appropriate medical literature and the product information currently provided by the manufacturer of each drug to be administered to verify the dosage, the method and duration of administration, or contraindications. It is the responsibility of the treating physician or other health care professional, relying on independent experience and knowledge of the patient, to determine drug dosages and the best treatment for the patient. Mention of any product in this issue should not be construed as endorsement by the contributors, editors, or the Publisher of the product or manufacturers' claims.

Veterinary Clinics of North America: Small Animal Practice (ISSN 0195-5616) is published bimonthly (For Post Office use only: volume 36 issue 1 of 6) by Elsevier, Inc. Corporate and editorial offices: Elsevier, Inc., 1600 John F. Kennedy Blvd., Suite 1800, Philadelphia, PA 19103-2899. Accounting and circulation offices: 6277 Sea Harbor Drive, Orlando, FL 32887-4800. Periodicals postage paid at Orlando, FL 32862, and additional mailing offices. Subscription prices are $170.00 per year for US individuals, $275.00 per year for US institutions, $85.00 per year for US students and residents, $225.00 per year for Canadian individuals, $345.00 per year for Canadian institutions, $235.00 per year for international individuals, $345.00 per year for international institutions and $115.00 per year for Canadian and foreign students/residents. To receive student/resident rate, orders must be accompanied by name of affiliated institution, date of term, and the *signature* of program/residency coordinator on institution letterhead. Orders will be billed at individual rate until proof of status is received. Foreign air speed delivery is included in all *Clinics* subscription prices. All prices are subject to change without notice. POSTMASTER: Send address changes to *Veterinary Clinics of North America: Small Animal Practice*, Elsevier, Customer Service Department, 6277 Sea Harbor Drive, Orlando, FL 32887-4800, USA; phone: (+1)(877) 839-7126 [toll free number for US customers], or (+1)(407) 345-4020 [customers outside US]; fax: (+1)(407) 363-1354; email: usjcs@elsevier.com.

Veterinary Clinics of North America: Small Animal Practice is also published in Japanese by Gakusosha Company Ltd., 2-16-28 Nishikata, Bunkyo-ku, Tokyo 113, Japan.

Reprints: For copies of 100 or more, of articles in this publication, please contact the Commercial Reprints Department, Elsevier Inc., 360 Park Avenue South, New York, New York 10010-1710. Tel. (212) 633-3813 Fax: (212) 462-1935, email: reprints@elsevier.com

Veterinary Clinics of North America: Small Animal Practice is covered in *Current Contents/Agriculture, Biology and Environmental Sciences, Science Citation Index, ASCA, Index Medicus, Excerpta Medica,* and *BIOSIS*.

Printed in the United States of America.

Updates in Dermatology

GUEST EDITOR

KAREN L. CAMPBELL, DVM, MS, Professor and Section Head, Specialty Medicine, Department of Veterinary Clinical Medicine, College of Veterinary Medicine, University of Illinois, Urbana, Illinois

CONTRIBUTORS

PAUL B. BLOOM, DVM, Diplomate, American College of Veterinary Dermatology; Diplomate, American Board of Veterinary Practitioners (Canine and Feline Specialty); Private Practice, Allergy and Dermatology Clinic for Animals, Livonia; Assistant Adjunct Professor, Department of Small Animal Clinical Sciences, Department of Dermatology, Michigan State University, East Lansing, Michigan

STEPHANIE R. BRUNER, DVM, Diplomate, American College of Veterinary Dermatology; Staff Dermatologist, Greater Cincinnati Veterinary Specialists, Wilder, Kentucky

LOUIS-PHILIPPE DE LORIMIER, DVM, Diplomate, American College of Veterinary Internal Medicine (Oncology); Clinical Assistant Professor, Medical Oncology, Department of Veterinary Clinical Medicine, College of Veterinary Medicine, University of Illinois at Urbana-Champaign, Urbana, Illinois

DAVID DUCLOS, DVM, Diplomate, American College of Veterinary Dermatology; Clinical Veterinary Dermatology Specialist, Animal Skin and Allergy Clinic, Lynnwood, Washington

CECILIA FRIBERG, DVM, Diplomate, American College of Veterinary Dermatology; Animal Dermatology Center of Chicago, Chicago, Illinois

KINGA GORTEL, DVM, MS, Animal Dermatology Clinic, Marina del Rey, California

HILARY A. JACKSON, BVMS, DVD, MRCVS, Diplomate, American College of Veterinary Dermatology; Associate Professor, Dermatology, North Carolina State University, College of Veterinary Medicine, Raleigh, North Carolina

ROBERT A. KENNIS, DVM, MS, Diplomate, American College of Veterinary Dermatology; Department of Clinical Sciences, College of Veterinary Medicine, Auburn University, Auburn, Alabama

ROSANNA MARSELLA, DVM, Diplomate, American College of Veterinary Dermatology; Associate Professor of Veterinary Dermatology, Blanche Saunders

Dermatology Laboratory, Department of Small Animal Clinical Sciences, College of Veterinary Medicine, University of Florida, Gainesville, Florida

ALONDRA L. MARTIN, DVM, Midwest Veterinary Dermatology, Buffalo Grove, Illinois

DAVID D. MARTIN, DVM, Diplomate, American College of Veterinary Anesthesiologists; Senior Veterinary Specialist, Sedation and Pain Management Team, Companion Animal Division, Pfizer Animal Health, New York, New York

ELIZABETH R. MAY, DVM, Diplomate, American College of Veterinary Dermatology; Assistant Professor of Dermatology, Department of Veterinary Clinical Sciences, Veterinary Teaching Hospital, Iowa State University, Ames, Iowa

KAREN A. MORIELLO, DVM, Diplomate, American College of Veterinary Dermatology; Clinical Professor of Dermatology, Department of Medical Sciences, School of Veterinary Medicine, University of Wisconsin–Madison, Madison, Wisconsin

SANDRA NEWBURY, DVM, Shelter Veterinarian and Director of Animal Medical Services, Dane County Humane Society, Madison, Wisconsin

EDMUND J. ROSSER, JR, DVM, Diplomate, American College of Veterinary Dermatology; Professor and Head of Dermatology, Department of Small Animal Clinical Sciences, Michigan State University College of Veterinary Medicine, East Lansing, Michigan

CANDACE A. SOUSA, DVM, Diplomate, American Board of Veterinary Practitioners, Canine and Feline Practice; Diplomate, American College of Veterinary Dermatology; Adjunct Clinical Professor, University of California; Senior Veterinary Specialist, Veterinary Specialty Team, Pfizer Animal Health, El Dorado Hills, California

Updates in Dermatology

CONTENTS

VOLUME 36 • NUMBER 1 • JANUARY 2006

Pain management has become a rapidly growing area of veterinary medicine over the past 5 to 7 years. Dermatologic patients are a segment that may have been overlooked and present some unique challenges for sedation and pain management. This article focuses on potential pain management strategies for certain dermatologic procedures and conditions as well as on current knowledge of acceptable anesthetics for intradermal allergy testing.

The carbon dioxide (CO_2) laser has many unique uses in veterinary dermatology. It can be used for oral lesions, such as viral papillomas, gingival hyperplasia, epulis, melanomas, fibromas, and other tumors, or for reactive tissue affecting the tongue or oral mucosa. It can be used for various neoplastic conditions, such as canine or feline pigmented viral plaques, bowenoid in situ carcinoma, actinic in situ carcinoma, and certain cases of squamous cell carcinoma. It is also useful for pinnal, neoplastic, nonneoplastic, or inflammatory lesions; because of the precise control of tissue destruction, the surgeon can remove abnormal tissue and spare normal tissue and structures. Similarly, lesions on the feet can be treated with this laser. The CO_2 laser's major advantage is hemostasis and limited tissue penetration. These two factors allow the surgeon to see what is being removed and to control precisely what is removed and what is spared. With this laser, it is easy to remove tissue right along vital structures, such as blood vessels, and to remove only the abnormal tissue without cutting into the blood vessel or other similar normal structures that should be avoided. Veterinarians in various specialties, particularly dermatology, surgery, and ophthalmology, are finding the CO_2 laser to be a useful tool, are finding new ways to deal with old problems, and are learning to understand old problems in new ways because they are able to see them without the obstruction by blood.

bacterial, and parasitic), allergic diseases, autoimmune diseases, neoplastic diseases, and a miscellaneous category. Lesions often progress through several stages, and the patient may be presented at any point; thus, a basic understanding of the progression of the disorder is helpful.

Canine and Feline Eosinophilic Skin Diseases 141
Paul B. Bloom

Eosinophilic dermatosis (eosinophilic skin disease) consists of a heterogeneous group of diseases that, in most cases, are secondary to underlying antigenic stimulation (hypersensitivity reaction). Treatment options may include glucocorticoids (GCs), antifungal agents, antibiotics, food trials, allergen-specific immunotherapy, or cyclosporine. To avoid the indiscriminate administration of chronic GCs or random therapeutic trials, a systematic approach to the diagnosis of these diseases should be performed. Diagnosing and managing these diseases are discussed.

Atopy: New Targets and New Therapies 161
Rosanna Marsella

Recent research has emphasized the complexity of this disease, indicating how type I hypersensitivity is intermingled with T-cell imbalances and, possibly, abnormalities of the barrier function. New strategies for patient management are reviewed, including modulation of the lymphocytic response through the use of calcineurin inhibitors, potential inhibition of the IgE response through use of anti-IgE vaccines, and alternative modalities for immunotherapy. Decrease of allergen exposure by frequent bathing, adjunctive antihistamine therapy, and neuropeptide modulation are useful adjuvant treatments for many patients. Future strategies may include the use of probiotics, inhibitors of cytokines and chemokines, and a targeted approach based on the genetic mutations of the individual patient.

Food Allergies: Update of Pathogenesis, Diagnoses, and Management 175
Robert A. Kennis

Food allergy with dermatologic involvement is a recognized clinical entity in dogs. There is controversy regarding the true prevalence of this disease because of the difficulty encountered in achieving an accurate diagnosis. Further, the terminology in the literature is inconsistent, and it may be difficult to search for information on this topic. The pathogenesis and immune function have been elucidated better through the development of investigative models; however, there are still many unknowns. New diagnostic techniques have been investigated, but the food elimination test diet continues to remain the "gold standard." Finally, there have been many new commercially available diets to aid in the diagnosis and management of food-allergic dogs. The purpose of this article is to provide updated concepts on the pathogenesis, diagnosis, and management of food-allergic dogs with dermatologic complications.

Staphylococcus intermedius and, less commonly, *Staphylococcus aureus* have been associated with most cases of bacterial skin disease in the dog and cat. Recently published information suggests that newly reported *Staphylococcus* organisms as well as coagulase-negative *Staphylococcus* species should be considered in addition to *S intermedius* and *S aureus* in pyoderma cases. The question of zoonotic transfer and the concern surrounding methicillin-resistant *Staphylococcus* mandate a new or modified approach to bacterial skin diseases in small animals. This article focuses on the characteristics of the newly reported *Staphylococcus* species as well as on the importance of recognizing and treating emerging pathogens.

German Shepherd Dog pyoderma (GSP) is a unique recurrent or refractory deep pyoderma that is characterized by pruritus (the chief complaint), with deep pyoderma typically beginning over the lumbosacral region. The condition may progress to affect multiple regions of the body and become a generalized skin disease. The underlying disease processes that may be involved in the development of GSP include flea allergy dermatitis, atopic dermatitis, cutaneous adverse food reactions (food allergy), hypothyroidism, ehrlichiosis, and T- and B-lymphocyte and neutrophil abnormalities. The management of GSP requires a thorough and systematic approach to investigate each dog for the possible triggering disease processes. As each disease is identified, the specific treatment for that disease needs to be initiated with the objective of resolving the recurrent nature of this deep pyoderma. The initial supportive medical treatment in cases of GSP requires 8 weeks of continuous systemic antibiotic therapy and medicated baths while the clinician attempts to determine each underlying disease process involved in a given case of GSP. Finally, the combination of diseases present for a given dog with GSP varies from case to case.

Canine epitheliotropic cutaneous T-cell lymphoma (CTCL; mycosis fungoides), although an infrequent anatomic variant of lymphoma, is the most common type of cutaneous lymphoma in dogs. Challenging to treat once a definitive diagnosis has been obtained, clinical management primarily involves skin-directed therapy, disease-modifying agents, and systemic chemotherapy. Recent retrospective studies have shown the oral alkylator lomustine (CCNU) to be of value for the therapy of canine CTCL, with encouraging response rates. Additional treatment options are also discussed in this review, including future therapies and others currently undergoing investigation.

This article reviews several important updates in our understanding and treatment of canine demodicosis. New species of *Demodex* mites have been demonstrated in some dogs with canine demodicosis. Advances in clarifying the role of the immune system in the disease have also been made. The prognosis for patients with generalized disease has improved in the past decade, primarily because of the important progress that has been made in the treatment of demodicosis in dogs.

Sebaceous adenitis is a rare idiopathic dermatosis that has been described most often in dogs but has been reported to occur in other mammals. The disease seems to represent an inflammatory disorder directed against or centered on the sebaceous glands. Since its first description in the veterinary literature 20 years ago, sebaceous adenitis has been diagnosed with increasing frequency. Despite the fact that there is a strong breed predisposition for the development of the disease, the cause involves more than genetics. This article discusses the current information as to the cause, diagnosis, and treatment of sebaceous adenitis in companion animals.

Vesicular cutaneous lupus erythematosus (VCLE) is an uncommon to rare disease affecting adult Rough Collies and Shetland Sheepdogs. Although it has been recognized since the late 1960s, it has only recently been characterized as a form of lupus erythematosus. This article reviews the clinical diagnosis and management of VCLE and discusses the evidence supporting its reclassification.

GOAL STATEMENT

The goal of the *Veterinary Clinics of North America: Small Animal Practice* is to keep practicing veterinarians up to date with current clinical practice in small animal medicine by providing timely articles reviewing the state of the art in small animal care.

ACCREDITATION

The *Veterinary Clinics of North America: Small Animal Practice* offers continuing education credits, awarded by Cummings School of Veterinary Medicine at Tufts University, Office of Continuing Education.

Cummings School of Veterinary Medicine at Tufts University is a designated provider of continuing veterinary medical education. Veterinarians participating in this learning activity may earn up to 6 credits per issue up to a maximum of 36 credits per year. Credits awarded may not apply toward license renewal in all states. It is the responsibility of each participant to verify the requirements of their state licensing board.

Credit can be earned by reading the text material, taking the examination online at ***http://www.theclinics.com/home/cme***, and completing the program evaluation. Following your completion of the test and program evaluation, and review of any and all incorrect answers, you may print your certificate.

TO ENROLL

To enroll in the *Veterinary Clinics of North America: Small Animal Practice* Continuing Veterinary Medical Education Program, call customer service at 1-800-654-2452 or sign up online at ***http://www.theclinics.com/home/cme***. The CVME program is now available at a special introductory rate of $99.95 for a year's subscription.

FORTHCOMING ISSUES

RECENT ISSUES

PREFACE

Updates in Dermatology

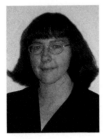

Karen L. Campbell, DVM, MS

Guest Editor

D ermatologic disorders are among the most common reasons clients seek professional help from veterinarians. The continued recognition of new dermatologic disorders and the development of new treatment modalities result in ongoing challenges for veterinarians desiring to provide accurate diagnoses and effective treatment plans for patients. The purpose of this issue is to provide veterinarians with state-of-the-art information regarding the recognition and management of important dermatologic diseases as well as with updates pertaining to new therapeutic modalities in dermatology.

The first article focuses on pain management strategies for patients who have dermatologic disorders and pain associated with diagnostic procedures. Pain management is a rapidly expanding area of veterinary medicine, and dermatology patients present numerous unique challenges; these challenges are reviewed in this article. The second article focuses on the use of CO_2 lasers, which have been proven to be highly useful in dermatology. This article includes multiple "before" and "after" photographs illustrating the use of CO_2 lasers in various skin disorders. Maintaining a current, practical database in veterinary therapeutics is an important challenge. The third article discusses several medications with new uses in veterinary dermatology.

There is growing interest in urban medicine, shelter medicine, and the placement of abandoned animals in new homes. Dermatology plays an important

0195-5616/06/$ – see front matter
doi:10.1016/j.cvsm.2005.10.002

role in shelter medicine for many reasons, including contagion, zoonoses, the importance of animal appearance in adoption decisions, and the amount of care certain skin disorders require for management. The fourth article discusses common skin diseases of shelter cats, and the fifth article focuses on updates regarding dermatophytosis—one of the most common problems encountered when large numbers of cats are housed in a shelter.

Cats now rank ahead of dogs as the most commonly owned household pet. Thus, it is highly important that veterinarians be familiar with feline dermatologic disorders. The sixth article reviews current knowledge regarding a variety of feline facial dermatoses, while the seventh article focuses on eosinophilic dermatoses, a heterogenous group of diseases commonly secondary to underlying hypersensitivity disorders. The diagnoses and management of these diseases in cats and dogs are reviewed.

Allergies have been the focus of increased attention and research in both humans and animals throughout the last decade. The eighth article discusses state-of-the-art information regarding the pathogenesis of atopy. The article emphasizes the importance of understanding the multifactorial nature of atopy and of using multiple therapeutic modalities individualized for each patient. The ninth article provides updates on the pathogenesis, diagnosis, and management of patients with food allergies.

Bacterial infections are one of the most common dermatologic disorders of dogs. Recent studies have identified several new species of *Staphylococcus* that cause disease in dogs. Some of these may be zoonotic. The tenth article reviews the various species of *Staphylococcus* that produce diseases in pets and discusses the importance of recognizing and treating emerging pathogens. One of the most frustrating forms of pyoderma is that which occurs in German shepherds. The eleventh article is devoted to reviewing the current state of knowledge of this disease and its treatment.

Cutaneous T cell lymphoma, the most common type of cutaneous lymphoma in dogs, has traditionally been reported to have a grave prognosis. However, through recent studies, several new treatment modalities have been identified that offer promising results. These are discussed in the twelfth article. Demodicosis continues to be an important common skin disease in dogs. Fortunately, many options are currently available for its treatment. These are reviewed in the thirteenth chapter. Sebaceous adenitis is being diagnosed with increasing frequency in dogs. It has also been described in cats and rabbits. The fourteenth article discusses current information pertaining to the cause, diagnosis, and treatment of this condition. Vesicular cutaneous lupus erythematosus is a disease affecting collies and Shetland sheepdogs. The diagnosis and treatment of this newly described disease are reviewed in the final article.

Hopefully, this issue of the *Veterinary Clinics of North America: Small Animal Practice* will achieve its goal of helping readers increase their understanding of recent advances in veterinary dermatology and, thereby, improve their ability to effectively diagnose and treat patients with skin disease. Special thanks are due to the authors for sharing their timely knowledge and professional expertise.

I am also appreciative of John Vassallo's editorial expertise and his willingness to include color illustrations within the articles.

Karen L. Campbell, DVM, MS
Department of Veterinary Clinical Medicine
College of Veterinary Medicine
University of Illinois
1008 West Hazelwood Drive
Urbana, IL 61802, USA

E-mail address: klcampbe@uiuc.edu

Pain Management and Anesthesia in Veterinary Dermatology

David D. Martin, DVM[a],*, Alondra L. Martin, DVM

[a]Companion Animal Division, Pfizer Animal Health, New York, NY, USA

Over the past 5 to 7 years, pain management has become a significant area of research and advancement in veterinary medicine. The International Association for the Study of Pain (IASP) has defined pain as "...the unpleasant sensory and emotional experience associated with actual or potential tissue damage, or described in terms of such damage." In the past few years, the IASP has added the following to that definition: "The inability to communicate in no way negates the possibility that an individual is experiencing pain and is in need of appropriate pain relieving treatment." This last statement is important in considering our veterinary patients.

Pruritus (itching) is an unpleasant sensation that seems to be physiologically associated with C-polymodal nociceptor activation. A-delta fibers carry signals for spontaneous, well-localized, pricking itch, whereas C fibers are slow conductors that produce unpleasant burning itch [1]. Many of the chemical mediators implicated in pruritus are the same as discussed in the instigation of many pain syndromes. Some examples are leukotrienes, prostaglandins, serotonin, trypsin, bradykinin, and substance P. Thus, most dermatologic conditions have a significant pain component (pruritus) that is the primary reason why owners seek veterinary care. There is a paucity of information on the treatment of pain in veterinary dermatologic patients, however.

CONCEPTS IN NOCICEPTION

It is important to have a basic understanding of the nociceptive pathway before developing an analgesic plan for a patient. The nociceptive process can be divided into four processes: transduction, transmission, modulation, and perception. Transduction is the translation of a chemical, mechanical, or thermal stimulus into electrical activity. Transmission is the propagation of this electrical signal (impulse) through the nervous system. Modulation is the modification of these transmissions via the endogenous opioid, serotonergic, and

*Corresponding author. 334 Old Sutton Road, Barrington, IL 60010. E-mail address: david.martin@pfizer.com (D.D. Martin).

0195-5616/06/$ – see front matter
doi:10.1016/j.cvsm.2005.09.010

noradrenergic pathways. Typically, this occurs within the spinal dorsal horn and is an inhibitory process, but it can have amplification effects as well. Finally, perception is the final conscious subjective response to the initial stimulus. If considered together, these sites along the nociceptive pathway present locations for affecting the final outcome of a painful stimulus and provide defined points for application of analgesia.

Some terminology is also important to understand. Preemptive analgesia is the concept of applying analgesia before the generation of a noxious stimulus. This decreases the intensity and duration of the pain associated with a procedure as well as minimizing the potential for the development of a chronic pain state. Although it is not always possible to apply analgesic therapy before a noxious stimulus, the earlier the intervention in the process, the more effective it is in preventing "wind-up." Wind-up is the result of cumulative increases in the number of electrical impulses that are produced in the dorsal horn, causing an increased excitability of the spinal cord neurons. Balanced or multimodal analgesia is the application of two or more analgesic therapies (eg, pharmacologic, acupuncture) in the effort to minimize pain better and reduce the dosage of any one drug. Multimodal analgesia arises from the application of therapies (drugs) that affect different portions of the nociceptive pathway via different mechanisms.

LOCAL ANESTHESIA

Local anesthesia has had a dramatic increase in use over the past 3 to 5 years in companion animal practice. Always a mainstay in large animal practice, it had been disregarded as unnecessary in small animal patients because of the advent of safer general anesthesia and sedative protocols. It is now realized that multimodal approaches to pain management have significant benefits over single-agent use.

It is not uncommon to use a local anesthetic as the sole agent for skin biopsies. Although this may be reasonable in a calm and manageable patient, sedation is also required many times. Sedation should not preclude the use of local analgesics as well, however, because these affect transmission along the pain pathway versus the spinal or central effects of most sedative and/or neuroleptanalgesic combinations. A similar multimodal approach is also beneficial in other painful diagnostic procedures.

Lidocaine is a typical local anesthetic that every veterinary practitioner has on the shelf. Lidocaine has a rapid onset (5–10 minutes) but short duration of action (60–120 minutes). For most simple biopsies, this would be the agent of choice. Lidocaine can be painful on injection because of the acidity (pH 6.5–6.8) of the solution. Addition of bicarbonate at a 1:9 ratio (1 mL bicarbonate to 9 mL lidocaine) can significantly decrease the burning sensation. It is important to remember that lidocaine, bicarbonate, and epinephrine can all inhibit growth of certain bacteria and fungi [1]. The smallest gauge needle (25–30 gauge) that is practical should be used, because the larger the diameter, the more painful is the injection [2]. Also, if a large area is to be blocked, a longer needle may decrease the number of sticks needed to desensitize the area. From a toxicity viewpoint, dosing should be less than 6 mg/kg (1.5 mL of 2% lidocaine per 10 lb) in the dog and 3 mg/kg (0.75 mL of 2% lidocaine per 10 lb) in the cat. Dilution of the lidocaine is sometimes necessary in smaller patients to achieve an adequate volume for multiple biopsy locations.

Bupivacaine is now being used for a longer duration of sensory blockade in many cases. Bupivacaine has a longer onset time of 15 to 20 minutes for peak effect compared with lidocaine, so it is not as useful for an immediate need in a case in which sedation is not used. It has a duration of effect of 6 to 8 hours, however, which may be beneficial in alleviating ongoing sensory input from a mass removal or area that has continuous stimulation and movement (eg, footpads). A typical dose for a regional technique is 1 to 2 mg/kg in the dog and 0.5 to 1 mg/kg in the cat. A much smaller volume than this is generally used for a simple local block (0.25–1.0 mL). From a toxicity viewpoint, using a total dose of less than 2 mL of 0.5% bupivacaine in a 5-kg (10-lb) dog or less than 1 mL in a 5-kg (10-lb) cat should keep the potential for overdose low. Always make sure that aspiration is performed before injection, because direct intravenous administration of bupivacaine can result in cardiac toxicity.

A combination of lidocaine and bupivacaine can be used to take advantage of the principles that each provides: the rapid onset of lidocaine and the longer duration of bupivacaine. A 50:50 mixture is used, and the volume is kept to less than 2 mL per 5-kg dog and to less than 1 mL per 5-kg cat as previously discussed.

Addition of a vasoconstrictor, most commonly epinephrine, may decrease the systemic absorption of local anesthetic and thus prolong the duration of action. Epinephrine is usually added at a concentration of 1:200,000 (5 µg/mL) or 0.1 mL per 20 mL of local anesthetic. Some precautions are in order when using epinephrine, however. First, intravenous injection must not occur so that systemic effects of the local anesthetic and the epinephrine do not both occur. Second, epinephrine should not be added to local anesthetics used in the distal extremities, where limited collateral circulation occurs (eg, paws, ear tips), because blood flow could be compromised. Also, in thin-skinned animals, epinephrine can delay wound healing or cause tissue necrosis of the wound edge. Third, the addition of epinephrine should probably be avoided in patients with preexisting cardiovascular disease, hypertension, or impaired circulation. In these authors' opinion, with the advent of longer acting local anesthetics, such as bupivacaine, and careful injection technique, the addition of a vasoconstrictor for most dermatologic applications is probably not warranted.

LOCAL AND REGIONAL ANALGESIC TECHNIQUES
There are several techniques that may be beneficial in alleviating discomfort after procedures in sedated pets using local anesthetics.

First is the standard field technique. Local anesthetic is injected in a circumferential pattern around the base of a mass to be removed and deeper into the subcutis. This can create increased skin tension and result in distortion of the biopsy site. Direct infiltration of a site can also create more pain and cause tissue distortion. Massaging the area after injection decreases this distortion. This same circumferential approach can be performed for a single-digit footpad biopsy, a tail mass biopsy, and other sites.

Specific nerve blocks may be used when more extensive biopsies are needed. These offer a more extensive area of desensitization and need to be performed in most cases on a sedated or anesthetized patient (diagrams illustrating these nerve blocks can be found elsewhere [3]).

The infraorbital nerve block may be beneficial when biopsying the nasal planum or areas of the muzzle and upper lip. Palpation of the infraorbital foramen can be performed using the caudal root of the third premolar as a landmark. Infiltration of local anesthetic under the buccal mucosa surrounding the foramen provides good desensitization of the muzzle rostral to the injection site. This can be useful for a nasal planum or lateral alar biopsy. If a more caudal nasal skin biopsy site is necessary, the needle can be inserted partially into the infraorbital foramen. The foramen is found dorsal to the third premolar and rostral to the zygomatic arch [4]. Aspiration before injection is important, because the artery and vein run with the nerve. Gentle pressure over the foramen during the injection forces the anesthetic to be pushed caudally, thus blocking the caudal branches of the nerve. The volume of injection is 0.25 to 1.0 mL depending on the size of the animal, with attention to the potential toxic doses previously discussed.

A distal radial, ulnar, or median nerve block can be used if more than one nail bed or footpad is to be biopsied on a foot. Subcutaneous infiltration of local anesthetic in a line at the point of flexion of the carpus on the dorsum of the paw and proximal to the carpal pad on the ventrum of the paw provides sensory blockade of all the digits [4]. The three-point technique may also be used. Here, local anesthetic (0.1–0.2 mL per site) is injected at points on the medial aspect of the carpal pad and proximal and lateral to the carpal pad to block the ulnar and median nerves. The superficial branches of the radial nerve are then blocked over the dorsal aspect of the proximal carpus [4]. Again, this needs to be performed in an anesthetized or heavily sedated patient.

A novel approach to a more painful systemic condition is to use lidocaine as a constant rate infusion in addition to opioids or ketamine, for example. At a dose of 50 µg/kg/min, lidocaine has been shown to reduce the minimum alveolar concentration by 18.7% [5]. Intravenous lidocaine has been shown to reduce the amount of morphine needed in the postoperative period, demonstrating how preemptive use is beneficial [6].

Topical anesthetics, such as a eutectic mixture of local anesthetics cream (EMLA cream; 2.5% lidocaine and 2.5% prilocaine) has had mixed results in these authors' hands. The key feature is that an occlusive dressing must be applied over the site of application of EMLA cream for 30 to 60 minutes for it to be effective. This, coupled with the differences in animal versus human skin and rate of systemic absorption, has limited its use and practicality in veterinary medicine.

PHARMACOTHERAPY

Glucocorticoid therapy may have a role in providing analgesia but is not discussed at length in this article. Suffice it to say that glucocorticoids are and should remain a mainstay in the treatment of many dermatologic conditions and that anti-inflammatory and analgesic properties are being applied through their use. The side effect profile of long-term steroid therapy is still of concern, however, and future studies on other agents may prove beneficial in reducing the use of glucocorticoids for the management of many conditions.

OPIOIDS

Opioid analgesics are too large an area to cover in detail, but a brief discussion is warranted. They produce their analgesia via the μ-, κ-, and δ-receptors by hyperpolarizing the cell (K+ channel) so that it becomes less responsive to stimuli.

Morphine is the "gold standard" for opioid comparison. It is a full-opioid agonist having spinal and supraspinal analgesic properties via the κ- and μ-receptors, respectively. Morphine produces profound analgesia for 4 to 6 hours in the dog but for a shorter period in the cat. Hydromorphone, oxymorphone, and fentanyl are other common choices of full agonists in veterinary medicine. These agents should be chosen as sedative and anesthetic adjuncts in cases in which moderate to severe pain is expected, such as in severe otitis externa. Morphine can also be used orally for chronic severe pain cases.

Butorphanol is an opioid agonist-antagonist that has primary analgesic properties at the κ-receptor. In a visceral model, the duration of analgesia was only 45 to 60 minutes, however [7]. This may be adequate for short-term mild pain settings, such as a simple skin biopsy (in conjunction with a local block), but not for severe otitis cases or large mass removals.

Buprenorphine is a partial agonist at the μ-receptor and has some unique properties that can be beneficial. The onset of the analgesia is 30 to 60 minutes, but the duration is 6 to 8 hours or potentially even longer. It is supplied only as an injectable but can be used transmucosally in cats at the same dosage as in other routes of administration [8]. Buprenorphine provides a potential dispensable analgesic agent for cats with more severe pain or those that cannot tolerate a nonsteroidal anti-inflammatory drug (NSAID). The dose is 0.005 to 0.03 mg/kg administered three to four times daily, but it may be reduced to twice daily for the oral route in those cats that exhibit mild inappetence and lethargy at higher doses.

Fentanyl patches have gained wide use in veterinary medicine and may be another useful "take-home" analgesic option for certain cases. Obviously, severe generalized skin disease would preclude the use of a patch because of the inability to apply it to unbroken skin. Severe otitis cases or large mass removals may warrant additional analgesic therapy for patients in their home environment, however. The usual dose is 2 to 5 μg/kg/h, and patch sizes are 25, 50, 75, and 100 μg/h.

Acetaminophen with codeine is another option for take-home medication that can be dispensed. For short-term administration, this can probably be added to steroid therapy, but be aware of possible gastrointestinal side effects of the combination. Acetaminophen is typically dosed as codeine, 1 to 2 mg/kg, two to three times per day, with the acetaminophen dose being correspondingly less than 10 to 15 mg/kg [9].

NONSTEROIDAL ANTI-INFLAMMATORY DRUGS

This class of drugs has experienced an explosion in options and availability over the past 3 years, such that an extensive discussion of each agent is beyond the scope of this article. This group of drugs can be quite useful in the dermatologic patient, however. Because inflammation is a common component of many skin diseases, NSAIDs can serve an important role in therapy. As an example from the field of human medicine, aspirin combined with antihistamines has been used for effective treatment of systemic mastocytosis [10]. Experimentally induced irritant dermatitis and the upregulated prostaglandin production that occur are inhibited by aspirin [11]. Finally, topical indomethacin was highly effective in relieving the redness, warmth, and tenderness of sunburn reactions [12].

NSAIDs produce their analgesic effects not only by the peripheral effects on inflammation (transduction) but via central mechanisms that are not fully understood at this time. Because of their effects on prostaglandin production via the cyclooxygenase (COX) enzymes (COX1 and COX2), these should not be used in conjunction with systemic steroids, because the potential for significant gastrointestinal side effects is increased. At this time, there are no published studies in the literature that have looked at the combination of topical steroids and systemic NSAIDs. There are also topical NSAIDs (eg, diclofenac) now available on the veterinary market, although currently only for use in equine osteoarthritis cases. These may prove to be useful in other areas of therapy.

Any of the current NSAIDs on the market should have efficacy in treating pain associated with an inflammatory process. Carprofen (injectable and oral) is the only NSAID that lists "control of postoperative pain associated with soft tissue AND orthopedic surgery" for dogs, and injectable meloxicam is the only NSAID that is approved for use in cats for postoperative pain. All the others have only osteoarthritis claims on the label. NSAIDs can cause cutaneous reactions as a side effect, but this seems to be rare in animals at this point.

One NSAID that deserves separate mention is tepoxalin. This product has COX and lipoxygenase (LOX) inhibitory mechanisms that could prove useful in certain dermatologic cases [13]. The LOX pathway is responsible for the conversion of arachidonic acid to leukotrienes. Leukotrienes (eg, LTB_4) cause leukocyte aggregation, chemotaxis, and release of lysosomal enzymes, all of which are components of inflammation. This LOX pathway has also been implicated in the pathogenesis of several inflammatory skin diseases, including atopic dermatitis [10]. The LOX pathway inhibition of tepoxalin lasts only a few hours, however; longer acting products may thus be more effective.

α_2 AGONISTS

The α_2 agonists are typically thought of only for sedation, but they carry the extra benefit of providing analgesia as well. The mechanism of this analgesia is similar to that of the opioids. Although the duration of the analgesia is short for these agents ($<$1 hour), they are useful for an intradermal test (IDT) or other minor procedures. Combination use with an opioid produces a much more profound and prolonged analgesia. Typically one quarter to one tenth of the label dose of the α_2 agonist is used when combined with an opioid. One study demonstrated that combining butorphanol at a dose of 0.2 mg/kg with medetomidine at a dose of 0.005 mg/kg provided up to 5.58 ± 2.28 hours of analgesia [14]. This combination use can provide profound analgesia alone for mild to moderate pain or when used as premedication for more painful procedures.

ADJUNCTIVE ANALGESICS

For those patients that are already on corticosteroids yet are still having significant discomfort, specifically chronic otitis externa cases, consideration should be given to the use of other options for the management of chronic pain. Adjunctive analgesics can be added to an NSAID to achieve more effective multimodal therapy. The interaction of these drugs with any antihistamines that may be used is unknown, so caution is warranted.

Tramadol

Tramadol is a synthetic opioid-like drug that is becoming more common in its use for pain management in companion animal medicine. Tramadol works by binding to the μ-opioid receptor but in a much weaker fashion than true opioids. It also inhibits reuptake of norepinephrine and serotonin, so it has actions much like the α_2 agonists as well. Tramadol can cause constipation with long-term administration. Tramadol is not a controlled substance. Typical dosing is 3 to 5 mg/kg administered two to three times daily [4]. It comes as a 50-mg tablet.

N-METHYL-D-ASPARTATE ANTAGONISTS

Unpublished studies have shown evidence that N-methyl-D-aspartate (NMDA) receptors play an important role in pruritus [15].

Dextromethorphan

Dextromethorphan has traditionally been thought of as an antitussive but was found to have NMDA receptor antagonistic properties that work as an analgesic adjunct similar to ketamine or amantadine. It has been found to be somewhat effective for the treatment (2 mg/kg administered twice daily) of self-directed scratching, biting, or chewing in dogs with allergic dermatitis [15]. Treated dogs had a slight but statistically significant decrease in their pruritus score. Based on the pharmacokinetics of this product, however, more frequent dosing would be needed in addition to the fact that there is wide variability in oral absorption [15,16]. Because of these factors, its usefulness as an analgesic may be limited.

Amantadine

Amantadine is a drug originally used as an antiviral agent that has also been shown to have efficacy for the treatment of Parkinson's disease [9]. More recently, it has been found to have NMDA receptor antagonist activity. This mechanism of action results in the prevention or improvement of the wind-up pain that occurs with chronic stimulation of the nociceptive pathway. It has been used in veterinary patients that are opioid tolerant and may have developed allodynia (the process by which a normal nonnoxious stimulus becomes painful). The typical dosage is 3 to 5 mg/kg administered once daily for a minimum of 21 days, with the potential for chronic administration [9]. Amantadine should be used in conjunction with an NSAID or steroid and potentially with an opioid for improved relief of pain. Mild gastrointestinal upset with diarrhea has been reported in dogs. There are only anecdotal reports of the use of this drug in veterinary patients.

Ketamine Infusions

For the acute pain case or for the case that has become nonresponsive to traditional NSAID therapy, adding ketamine in a constant rate infusion can help to minimize the development of wind-up or "unwind" the existing nociceptive pathway stimulation that develops in chronic pain cases. Ketamine as a drug was initially developed and used in pediatric burn patients because it provided sedation but also the profound short-term somatic analgesia needed for debridement of burns. Microdoses of 0.5 mg/kg administered intravenously before surgical stimulation, followed by 10 μg/kg/min during a procedure and 2 μg/kg during the recovery period and for the next 24 hours, have been shown to reduce pain scores significantly and improve activity in dogs with forelimb amputation [17]. Ketamine was not used as a sole agent but was added to systemic fentanyl. Ketamine should not be used as a sole analgesic agent.

A combination using morphine, lidocaine, and ketamine (MLK) in a constant rate infusion has been used as well for a multimodal approach in severe pain cases. This combination is primarily used during surgery but is also useful in the postprocedural period. The mixture for administration at a surgical rate of fluid therapy (10 mL/kg/h) is morphine (10 mg), lidocaine (150 mg), and ketamine (30 mg) in lactated Ringer's solution (LRS) at a volume of 500 mL [18]. This is not likely something that is used in a typical dermatologic practice, but certain severe cases, such as postoperative total ear canal ablation (TECA) or toxic epidermal necrolysis, may benefit from this combination.

GABAPENTIN

Gabapentin is an analogue of gamma-aminobutyric acid (GABA) that originally came on the market as an anticonvulsant. The mechanism of the analgesia is unclear. It has been used in human diabetic neuropathy and to relieve postherpetic (shingles) pain with good results. It has been used in numerous dermatologic conditions in human beings (eg, piloleiomyoma-related pain, glossodynia, allodynia, reflex sympathetic dystrophy) [19]. It has been shown to relieve cutaneous hyperalgesia in skin that has been hypersensitized to pain [20]. This type of neuropathic pain is undoubtedly present in dogs with chronic otitis; potentially, these cases could benefit from adjunctive analgesia. Gabapentin is most interesting in its use for chronic itch unresponsive to other treatment [19]. It has also been shown to be useful in the treatment of inflammatory pain. Typical dosing has been 1 to 10 mg/kg administered once daily for dogs and cats, starting at the lower end of the range and gradually increasing to effect [4]. Potential side effects are drowsiness and fatigue, at least initially. It seems to be a remarkably safe drug with few reported side effects across a wide dosage range. There are only anecdotal reports of the use of this drug in veterinary patients.

ALTERNATIVE THERAPY
Acupuncture
We cannot forget about the potential benefit of acupuncture as an adjunctive therapy in some cases. Acupuncture is most commonly performed in combination with standard pharmacologic therapy. One technique that has been described and reported to be effective is the "surrounding the dragon" technique. This has been used for the treatment of acral lick granulomas. Four to 12 needles are inserted around the lesion a few millimeters from the edge with the needle tips pointing toward the lesion. This is done for 15 to 20 minutes once weekly for 4 weeks [21].

SAMPLE CASE
To illustrate use of the options that have been presented, a sample case for multimodal analgesia is presented.

Otitis Externa
Many of these cases are extremely painful, some to the point of the animals not wanting to be touched anywhere on the body because of the chronic pain that has developed, resulting in potential allodynia (pain produced by nonnoxious stimuli). Many of these patients are already being given a steroid for the inflammation, which precludes the use of an NSAID; however, NSAIDs should be considered if steroids have not been administered recently. For otic examination, culture, and biopsy as well as for an ear flush, general anesthesia is usually required. Even then, these animals can react vigorously during the procedure as well as at recovery. Here, a significant multimodal approach is warranted. Obviously, the general health of the patient has to be the first concern. Preemptive use of a full-agonist opioid, such as morphine, in combination with an α_2 agonist can be quite effective. If general anesthesia is needed, this can be added to effect. After an ear culture and flush, these dogs are quite painful. Sending home tramadol or acetaminophen with codeine for short-term therapy can be effective adjuncts to the steroids or NSAIDs. If more chronic pain management is needed, the addition of amantadine or even gabapentin may be

Table 1
Common drug doses

Drug	Dog (mg/kg)	Cat (mg/kg)	Duration (hours)
Local anesthetics			
Lidocaine	<6.0 perineural	<3.0 perineural	1–2
Bupivacaine	<2.0 perineural	<1.0 perineural	6–8
Opioids			
Morphine	0.2–2.0 IM, SC; 0.05–0.5 IV	0.05–0.2 IM, SC	3–6 dog 2–4 cat
Hydromorphone	0.05–0.2 IM, SC, IV	0.05–0.1 IM, SC 0.01–0.025 IV	3–4 dog 3–4 cat
Oxymorphone	0.05–0.2 IM, SC, IV	0.05–0.1 IM, SC	3–4 dog 3–4 cat
Butorphanol	0.2–0.8 IM, SC, IV	0.1–0.4 IM, SC, IV	1–2 dog 1–4 cat
Buprenorphine	0.005–0.3 IM, SC, IV	0.005–0.02 IM, SC, IV, buccal/ sublingual	6–8 dog 6–12 cat
Acetaminophen with codeine	10–15 acetaminophen + 1–2 codeine (dose based on codeine)	Not for use in cats	8–12 dog
α 2 agonists (when used in combination)			
Xylazine	0.1–0.5 IM, IV	0.1–0.5 IM, IV	0.5–1.0
Medetomidine	0.005–0.02 IM, IV	0.005–0.04 IM, IV	0.5–1.5
Adjunctive agents			
Tramadol	2–5 PO	1–4 PO (limited information)	8–12 in both
Amantadine	3 PO	3 PO	24
Gabapentin	1–10 PO	1–10 (limited information)	24

Abbreviations: IM, intramuscular; IV, Intravenous; PO, per so; SC, subcutaneous.

Agents that are contraindicated for use in IDT are acepromazine, oxymorphone, and morphine. Other opioids could also probably be included in this list, because most have some level of histamine-releasing properties. Acepromazine has vasodilatory effects as well as antihistamine effects that have been shown to decrease the skin reactions in IDT significantly.

SUMMARY
Available analgesic therapies have expanded dramatically in the past few years. Although some represent anecdotal reports of success, there is growing information about many agents that could be effective in alleviating our patients' pain. Local analgesics, NSAIDs, opioids, and other adjunctive therapies can prove quite helpful in the treatment of the pruritus and inflammation associated with many dermatologic conditions. Doses and duration of activity of commonly used analgesics are summarized in Table 1.

References
[1] Scott DW, Miller WH, Griffin CE. Structure and function of skin. In: Muller and Kirk's small animal dermatology. 6th edition. Philadelphia: WB Saunders; 2001. p. 1–70.
[2] Koay J, Orengo I. Application of local anesthetics in dermatologic surgery. Dermatol Surg 2002;28(2):143–8.
[3] Lemke KA, Dawson SD. Local and regional anesthesia. Vet Clin North Am Small Anim Pract 2000;30(4):839–57.
[4] Tranquilli WJ, Grimm KA, Lamont LA. Pain management for the small animal practitioner. 2nd edition. Jackson (WY): Teton New Media; 2004.
[5] Valverde A, Doherty TJ, Hernandez J, et al. Effect of lidocaine on the minimum alveolar concentration of isoflurane in dogs. Vet Anaesth Analg 2004;31(4):264–71.
[6] Koppert W, Weigand M, Neumann F, et al. Perioperative intravenous lidocaine has preventive effects on postoperative pain and morphine consumption after major abdominal surgery. Anesth Analg 2004;98(4):267–73.
[7] Sawyer DC, Rech RH, Durham RA, et al. Dose response to butorphanol administered subcutaneously to increase visceral nociceptive threshold in dogs. Am J Vet Res 1991;52(11): 1826–30.
[8] Robertson SA, Taylor PM, Bloomfield M, et al. Systemic uptake of buprenorphine after buccal administration in cats. In: Proceedings of the Annual Meeting of the American College of Veterinary Anesthesiologists. New Orleans, LA, 2001.
[9] Gaynor JS, Muir WW, editors. Handbook of veterinary pain management. St. Louis (MO): Mosby; 2002.
[10] Friedman ES, LaNatra N, Stiller MJ. NSAIDs in dermatologic therapy: review and preview. J Cutan Med Surg 2002;6(5):449–59.
[11] Plummer NA, Hensby CN, Kobza Black A, et al. Prostaglandin activity in sustained inflammation of human skin before and after aspirin. Clin Sci Mol Med 1977;52:615–20.
[12] Snyder DS, Eaglestein WH. Topical indomethacin and sunburn. Br J Dermatol 1974;90: 91–3.
[13] Agnello KA, Reynolds LR, Budsberg SC. In vivo effects of tepoxalin, an inhibitor of cyclooxygenase and lipoxygenase, a prostanoid and leukotriene production in dogs with chronic osteoarthritis. Am J Vet Res 2005;66(6):966–72.
[14] Grimm KA, Tranquilli WJ, Thurmon JC, et al. Duration of nonresponse to noxious stimulation after intramuscular administration of butorphanol, medetomidine, or a butorphanol-medetomidine combination during isoflurane administration in dogs. Am J Vet Res 2000;61(1): 42–7.
[15] Dodman NH, Shuster L, Nesbitt G, et al. The use of dextromethorphan to treat repetitive self-directed scratching, biting, or chewing in dogs with allergic dermatitis. J Vet Pharmacol Ther 2004;27:99–104.
[16] Kukanich B, Papich MG. Plasma profile and pharmacokinetics of dextromethorphan after intravenous and oral administration in healthy dogs. J Vet Pharmacol Ther 2004;27: 337–41.
[17] Wagner AE, Walton JA, Hellyer PW, et al. Use of low doses of ketamine administered by constant rate infusion as an adjunct for postoperative analgesia in dogs. J Am Vet Med Assoc 2002;221(1):72–5.
[18] Muir WW, Wiese AJ, March PA. Effects of morphine, lidocaine, ketamine, and morphine-lidocaine-ketamine drug combination on minimum alveolar concentration in dogs anesthetized with isoflurane. Am J Vet Res 2003;64(9):1155–60.
[19] Scheinfeld N. The role of gabapentin in treating diseases with cutaneous manifestations and pain. Int J Dermatol 2003;42:491–5.
[20] Dirks J, Petersen KL, Rowbotham MC, et al. Gabapentin suppresses cutaneous hyperalgesia following heat-capsaicin sensitization. Anesthesiology 2002;97:102–7.
[21] Schoen AM. Veterinary acupuncture: ancient art to modern medicine. St. Louis (MO): Mosby; 2001.

[22] Frank LA, Kunkle GA, Beale KM. Comparison of serum cortisol concentration before and after intradermal testing in sedated and nonsedated dogs. J Am Vet Med Assoc 1992;200(4):507–10.

[23] Beale KM, Kunkle GA, Chalker L, et al. Effects of sedation on intradermal skin testing in flea-allergic dogs. J Am Vet Med Assoc 1990;197(7):861–4.

[24] Vogelnest LJ, Mueller RS, Dart CM. The suitability of medetomidine sedation for intradermal skin testing in dogs. Vet Dermatol 2000;11:285–90.

[25] Moriello KA, Eicker SW. Influence of sedative and anesthetic agents on intradermal skin test reactions in dogs. Am J Vet Res 1991;52(9):1484–8.

[26] Codner EC, Lessard P, McGrath CJ. Effect of tiletamine/zolazepam sedation on intradermal allergy testing in atopic dogs. J Am Vet Med Assoc 1992;201(12):1857–60.

[27] Kennis RA, Robertson SA, Rosser EJ, et al. Effects of propofol anesthesia on intradermally injected histamine phosphate in clinically normal dogs. Am J Vet Res 1998;59(1):7–9.

[28] Graham LF, Torres SM, Jessen CR, et al. Effects of propofol-induced sedation on intradermal test reactions in dogs with atopic dermatitis. Vet Dermatol 2003;14:167–76.

Lasers in Veterinary Dermatology

David Duclos, DVM

Animal Skin and Allergy Clinic, 16418 7th Place West, Suite B, Lynnwood, WA 98037, USA

HISTORY OF LASERS

Laser is an acronym that means light amplification by stimulated emission of radiation [1]. The stimulated emission of light and its properties was first described in the early 1900s by Einstein. Forty years later (in 1960), the first laser was developed at Bell Laboratories, and during the 1970s, lasers were introduced for use in medicine. Over the next decade, smaller and less expensive lasers were introduced and their use in medicine expanded. By late 1980s, many different types of lasers had been developed and were being used by many medical specialties, including veterinary medicine [2–8].

HOW LASERS WORK

Lasers are devices that generate electromagnetic radiation that is essentially monochromatic, a single wavelength, and can be compressed into a small beam that is able to travel wide distances with little divergence. Lasers produce a high-intensity beam so intense that their light is 10 times brighter than the sun [9].

The lasers in use for medical purposes are referred to as light lasers. Light, by definition, is that portion of the electromagnetic spectrum that is visible to the human eye; however, lasers in use in medicine emit beams of radiation that are in the visible range as well as in the near-infrared or ultraviolet regions. These beams behave in the same way as the visible spectrum in that they can be focused with lenses and reflected with mirrors; thus, for simplicity, they are called light lasers [7]. Lasers are named for the medium that is used to produce the laser light beam. Each laser's properties depend on the medium used to produce the laser beam and the ways in which that beam is delivered. The laser beam's interaction with tissue depends on the wavelength, power, and time that the beam is exposed to the tissue [4]. Some lasers, for example, the Q-switched ruby laser, do not interact with the surface tissue but penetrate deeper to interact with pigmented or vascular targets, such as pigmented nevi, tattoos, or vascular lesions. In human dermatology alone, there are currently at least nine different lasers available to the dermatologist for use in the removal of

E-mail address: animalskinallergy@msn.com

0195-5616/06/$ – see front matter
doi:10.1016/j.cvsm.2005.10.001

pigmented nevi, vascular lesions, or tattoos. All these lasers have slightly different behaviors, and learning to use one does not transfer to knowing how to use
another. Most of the lasers used to interact with vascular or pigmented lesions
emit beams in the visible spectrum [10]. Conversely, the carbon dioxide (CO_2)
laser, which is the primary laser used in veterinary dermatology, emits a beam
in the infrared region with a wavelength of 10,600 nm. Because this laser beam
is in the invisible range, it is not affected by the color of the tissue. The CO_2
laser beam is absorbed by water. Because water is the main component of all
living cells, the CO_2 laser beam is absorbed efficiently with minimal thermal
scattering and limited thermal damage [11]. CO_2 lasers are the most efficient
of all the lasers, and powers of several hundred watts can be generated from
reasonably sized devices [7]. This efficiency, together with the ability for the
operator to control the effect of the laser beam essentially to the area that
you can see with no collateral damage, has led to wide use of this laser in
many areas of medicine, including veterinary dermatology.

LASERS IN VETERINARY MEDICINE

The early lasers in veterinary medicine were neodymium:yttrium-aluminum-
garnet (Nd:YAG) and argon lasers, which were used primarily in endoscopic
procedures to coagulate tumors and treat ulcers in the respiratory and intestinal
tracts. These lasers produce wide zones of collateral tissue damage and were
found to be poor choices for incisions or for ablations of surface lesions. The
CO_2 laser proved to be an excellent choice for laser surgery because of the ability to limit the zones of damage to microsurgery with little to no collateral damage. This laser is the primary laser in use today in veterinary dermatology. The
operator can easily control the device for use in three ways: skin incision, lesion
excision, and ablation. It can be readily controlled for precise microsurgery or
can be used for ablating larger lesions. Because of its high absorption by water,
there is little to no collateral tissue damage with this laser when used properly.

CONSIDERATIONS

The effective and safe use of lasers in surgery is dependent on the training of
the user and attention to important safety measures. There are numerous publications dealing with the use of lasers as well as educational seminars in laser
use [2,7–9,11–15]. The CO_2 laser does not penetrate into deep tissue; the penetration depth of the beam is approximately 0.3 mm. Cells in tissue exposed to
the high-intensity beam of the CO_2 laser are disintegrated by vaporization,
steam production, and ejection of solids. The solids that are ejected with the
steam are heated to the point of combustion. The combustion of solids results
in a smoke plume of carbonized material. Some of the carbonized debris is deposited along the path of the laser beam, giving the false impression that the
tissue is burnt. The poor heat conduction of water-filled cells limits tissue destruction to a thin layer of cells. With the CO_2 laser, the collateral zone of necrosis is less than 0.3 mm; however, the carbonized debris deposited along the
beam's path can act as a heat sink. After each pass, this carbonized material

must be removed with a saline-soaked gauze pad. If this carbon is not removed, it can conduct heat into the adjacent tissue and thereby increase the collateral damage. The depth of the incision depends on the power used, the spot size, and the speed with which the beam is swept across the area. These three variables (spot size, power, and time of exposure) are used by the operator to control how much tissue is removed [4,7,16].

ADVANTAGES AND DISADVANTAGES OF CARBON DIOXIDE LASERS

Hemostasis

The CO_2 laser is well known to have excellent hemostasis; in fact, in most of the procedures amenable to laser surgery, this is the main advantage for the use of this laser over conventional scalpel surgery. The CO_2 laser is only effective in sealing blood vessels less than the beam diameter (0.5 mm or less). The hemostatic effect of the CO_2 laser can be improved by temporarily clamping the main blood supply to the tissue.

Healing

Although hemostasis is good, the healing time for the CO_2 laser is extended when compared with conventional scalpel surgery, especially if the exposure time is extended. Also, biopsy samples taken with this laser have small zones of char (0.31 mm) on the edges. The operator must take this zone into consideration if interested in removing a lesion for histopathologic margins. It is recommended to keep 0.4 to 0.5 mm away from the edge of lesions for which you want histopathologic evaluation of the margins [16–18]. Finally, operators must be aware that many lesions being removed by laser ablation are small and can easily be entirely ablated with the laser. If you want histopathologic evaluation, a biopsy must be taken before laser ablation. As a general rule, if you are ablating lesions for which you have a previous histopathologic diagnosis, there is no problem in proceeding with ablation; however, if the lesions have changed, look different, or have an ulcerated nonhealing appearance, a repeat biopsy should be obtained for additional histopathologic evaluation.

Selected Cases for Use of the Carbon Dioxide Laser in Veterinary Dermatology

The following conditions have been treated by this author effectively with CO_2 laser surgery. In many cases, laser surgery is easier, more effective, and less harmful to the animal. In some cases, laser treatment is the only method to achieve adequate results.

Viral papillomas

There are several types of viral papillomas [19], and the exophytic types can be treated with laser ablation. Exophytic viral papillomas consist of two types: the oral type and the cutaneous form. Many papillomas spontaneously resolve in weeks to months; however, clients usually want something done sooner, especially when their pet is being exposed to other dogs in boarding or day care facilities. Treatment with interferon-α-2a recombinant often results in complete resolution, especially when used in conjunction with CO_2 laser ablation in human beings [20–23]. In this author's experience, use of CO_2 laser ablation alone is successful in the treatment of single viral papillomas, but it is unpredictable in cases of multiple papillomas. Some of these cases recur, and because of the contagious nature of papillomas, recurrence is a problem. The combination of laser ablation and interferon therapy seems to offer better resolution. Interferon therapy is usually given at a rate of 1 million U/m^2 subcutaneously three times per week. Interferon therapy is typically initiated 4 weeks before laser surgery, and some papillomas resolve without the need for surgery. In the cases with lesions still present after 4 weeks of interferon therapy, laser ablation is performed, removing every lesion and continuing interferon therapy for another 6 to 8 weeks (Fig. 1).

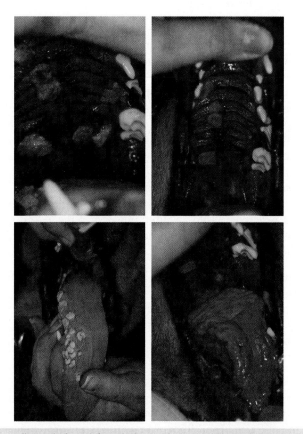

Fig. 1. Oral papillomas before (*left*) and after (*right*) laser ablation. Systemic interferon therapy was used for 6 weeks before and 4 weeks after laser ablation.

The laser ablation is performed with the continuous-wave (CW) mode at a power of 10 W using a 0.8-mm tip to excise the tumors; the remaining tumor beds are then ablated with the superpulse (SP) mode at 3 to 5 W.

Papilloma-like lesions that do not respond to laser ablation are the paw pad keratomas of Greyhound dogs and the cutaneous horns on the paw pads of cats. In the cat, some, although not all, of these paw pad keratomas are associated with the feline leukemia virus (FeLV). In Greyhound dogs, the cause is unknown; it has been proposed that these lesions may be caused by papillomavirus, but this has not been proven [19]. The current understanding is that canine viral-induced papillomas of the feet do not involve the footpads [19]. Other papilloma-like lesions are associated with some infundibular keratinizing acanthomas, which may have keratin horn-like projections. These may clinically appear to be papillomas; however, histopathologic evaluation of these lesions is diagnostic for acanthomas. Infundibular keratinizing acanthomas can be removed using laser excision; however, there is really no advantage to using a laser over conventional surgery for these or any of the other follicular tumors. These lesions are deep in the subcutaneous tissue and require deep incisions and sutures. Because laser incisions have delayed healing, it is this author's opinion that laser excision is actually less desirable than excision with a conventional scalpel. The CO_2 laser is most advantageous for surface lesions where suturing is not required or for deeper lesions where the superior hemostasis provided by CO_2 laser surgery allows the operator to identify the lesion, excise it, and spare the normal tissue. It is important to biopsy lesions whenever possible before laser ablation so that you have a definitive diagnosis. This enables the surgeon to make an informed judgment regarding the prognosis, decide what kind of surgical treatment is most appropriate, and know what kind of surgical margins are needed.

Canine pigmented viral plaques, bowenoid in situ carcinoma, and feline viral plaques

These three diseases have several features in common; they all are associated with papillomavirus cytopathologic changes, they have melanin pigmentation, and there is a tendency to progress in the number of lesions and in severity toward squamous cell carcinoma. All these diseases may represent a continuum of a single disease caused by a single papillomavirus. In veterinary medicine, we currently are not able to identify the subtype of papillomavirus present in each of these different conditions. Knowing the subtype of these viruses could help us to understand the relation between these conditions.

Feline viral plaques have been described as a single entity [19]. Because pigmented plaques and macules are also seen in cats with bowenoid lesions, however, viral plaques could be a mild form of a disease that later progresses to bowenoid lesions.

In Figs. 2 and 3, note the similarities between canine pigmented viral plaques and feline bowenoid in situ carcinomas; note the pigmented nodules, macules, and plaques that are similar in both diseases.

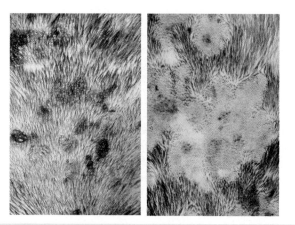

Fig. 2. Feline bowenoid lesions on the trunk before (*left*) and after (*right*) laser treatment; note the plaques and pigmented macules.

Canine pigmented viral plaques have only recently been found to contain papillomavirus. It seems that these are less likely to progress to carcinoma; however, this impression could change as dermatologists become more familiar with these lesions and begin to recognize and follow their progression in more dogs. Clinically, all three of these lesions have similarities, which we need to learn to recognize. In the dog, the lesions are often asymptomatic, beginning as darkly pigmented papules and progressing to plaques that increase in number, prompting the owner to seek veterinary advice. On closer observation, what appears to be pigmented macules can be seen to be slightly raised and slightly roughened on the surface. They vary in size from 2 mm to 1 to

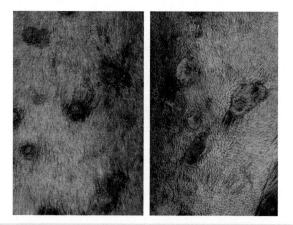

Fig. 3. Canine pigmented viral plaques before (*left*) and after (*right*) laser ablation; note the similarity to feline bowenoid lesions.

2 cm. They are reportedly most common in Miniature Schnauzers and Pugs but are also seen in other breeds. The lesions are located most often on the dorsal or ventral trunk or on the pinnae and base of the ears. Because they increase in number, the owners want something done about them. Histopathologic evaluation of the canine lesions show mild to moderate papulations of the surface, heavy hypergranulosis of the granular cell layer, and papillomavirus-induced koilocytosis [19]. Often, these histologic lesions are subtle and can be easily missed by an untrained eye, especially if the pathologist is not given any clinical or historical information. Clinically, many of these lesions seem to be cosmetic diseases, but because they are associated with a virus and could potentially progress to carcinoma, removal seems reasonable. With the option of CO_2 laser ablation, removal is simple and, in the dog, is often curative, because the lesions rarely recur (Fig. 4).

In the cat, it is clearer that removal is important to prevent progression to squamous cell carcinoma. Of importance is that in cats there tends to be a mixture of progressive lesions on the same cat. Lesions typical of feline viral plaques, bowenoid in situ carcinoma, and invasive squamous cell carcinoma can all be seen on the same cat. In fact, this may be more common than currently reported. It is important in this condition, more so than in almost any other, that multiple biopsy samples be taken of each separate lesion type. In addition to this, as always, a complete history and physical description of the lesions must be sent to the pathologist, and, if possible, the different lesions should be identified for the histopathologist. In my practice, digital photographs of these separate lesions are also sent to the pathologist. Sending in samples labeled something like "cat skin, itching" is sure to render an incomplete and possibly totally incorrect diagnosis. As veterinarians become more familiar with these cases, perhaps a different clinical picture will develop.

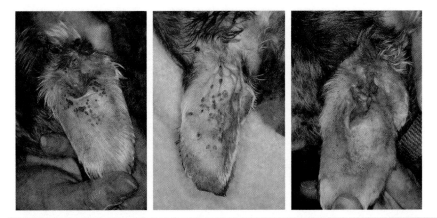

Fig. 4. Canine pigmented viral plaques on the pinnae before (*left*) and after (*middle, right*) laser ablation.

Treatment of these conditions with laser ablation is successful, even in cases in which the entire trunk has crusted lesions (Fig. 5). It may take several laser procedures, but you can make the animal comfortable and prevent progression of precancerous lesions into invasive cancer at the same time. One should not be misled by the diagnosis "in situ carcinoma" into thinking that these lesions are a minor problem. Often, these are older animals, and the tendency is to think that they will outlive progression of the lesions into cancer. This thinking perhaps dates from the time when the only mode of therapy was conventional surgical excision, which was not possible in most of these cases because of the large body areas affected. With the availability of laser surgical ablation, we now have a surgical option that is well tolerated by the patient. Topical antiviral therapy, such as imiquimod, is also currently used, especially for small localized lesions; both of these therapies can be part of our therapeutic considerations. In this author's experience, laser surgery is a much easier treatment because it offers immediate and long-term relief. Ablation of lesions with the laser in this disease is not curative, but it gives the cat immediate relief from discomfort, which lasts for long periods, often a year or more, before new lesions recur and need treatment. Generally, the subsequent laser ablation procedures are not as extensive; because the client is aware of the diagnosis and the nature if the disease, he or she brings the animal in for repeat procedures sooner.

To remove the lesions in cats with bowenoid in situ carcinoma or with pigmented plaques, you have to shave the hair from the lesions to expose all the lesions. In these animals, the lesions extend far beyond what is visible before clipping. This is commonly a condition that is much more extensive than it appears on physical examination. When the hair is clipped, you can remove all the affected lesions. The laser is set in the CW mode with the power at

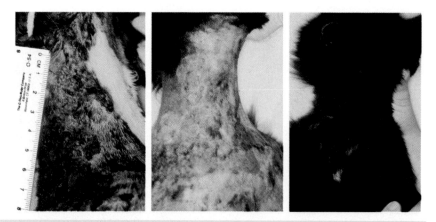

Fig. 5. Feline bowenoid in situ carcinoma on the trunk before laser ablation (*left*), during laser ablation (*middle*), and after healing (*right*).

10 W, and the scanner tip is used for ablation of these lesions. It takes a lot of energy to remove these lesions. Only the epidermis and the upper layer of the dermis are removed, so suturing is not necessary. Any lesions that are deep or ulcerated or appear to be invasive should be biopsied for histologic evaluation. Cats tolerate the ablation procedure well, even when large areas of the body are treated. They heal within 3 to 4 weeks, and hair regrowth covers any small nonhaired areas where lesions were deeper and leave scars. Scars with CO_2 laser ablation are smooth and often barely noticeable. Fig. 6 shows a cat with bowenoid lesions on the foot, which were painful to the cat. After laser ablation, the cat was no longer in pain, and the foot healed and was normal.

Sequential surgical sessions are common with laser procedures. The cases shown here (see Figs. 5 and 6) had repeat ablation procedures every 12 to 18 months. This is similar to the situation in human beings with conditions like oral papillomatosis, bowenoid in situ carcinomas, and other lesions, where repeat laser ablation sessions are common [10,20,24]. With laser surgery, the surgeon needs to be prepared for the possibility that repeat ablation sessions are required and also needs to convey this possibility to the client. In some cases, laser treatment is not meant to remove the disease completely; rather, it is palliative, debulking and removing the lesions causing the animal the most discomfort. This is true in many of the cats with extensive bowenoid disease. In this author's experience, clients come seeking a different answer than just "wait and see." The owners are worried about cancer or they just do not like the crusts and bumps or both on their pet. With laser ablation as a therapeutic option, veterinary medicine is beginning to develop different recommendations for diseases such as these. Conditions that could not be ameliorated with conventional surgery are now often treated because of the ease of laser

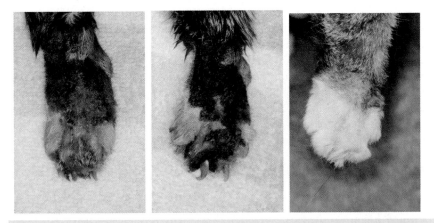

Fig. 6. Feline bowenoid in situ carcinoma on the foot before laser ablation (*left*), during laser ablation (*middle*), and after healing (*right*).

ablation. (Additionally, in treating conditions previously not recognized as a problem, such as follicular cysts in canine pododermatitis, laser ablation is helping to identify and resolve a previously unrecognized problem.)

Squamous cell carcinoma
Not all squamous cell carcinomas can be treated effectively with CO_2 laser excision or ablation. This tumor has different presentations; some are extremely invasive, and surgical excision and ablation with the CO_2 laser are ineffective. The dermatologist must learn to select the patients with early squamous cell carcinoma that is treatable with laser ablation. The lesions need to be on the surface rather than deep and without visible evidence of invasion into adjacent structures that could not be surgically excised. Squamous cell carcinomas most commonly occur in sun-exposed areas and may be preceded by or occur with actinic in situ carcinoma lesions. In the early stages, most squamous cell tumors have not metastasized and are only locally invasive. In the cat, they present most commonly on the nose, pinnae, or face, whereas they are most commonly located on the ventrum in dogs [19]. Other non–sun-exposed squamous cell carcinomas can occur anywhere; in dogs, the oral cavity and nail beds are locations that this author has seen frequently. In cats with squamous cell carcinomas on the nasal planum, when the entire tumor is removed, the lesions heal quickly, within 3 to 4 weeks. If the lesions do not heal with simple surface ablation of the nasal lesions, a radical nasal planectomy can be performed to prevent the tumor from invading deep into the adjacent facial structures (Fig. 7).

The more aggressive tumors can be highly invasive. If the tumor has progressed past the nasal planum, surgical removal alone is not indicated. Careful examination of the planum and adjacent structures is important before choosing to perform a radical planectomy with the laser. Biopsy of the lesion and of any suspicious adjacent potentially invaded structures is important. Fig. 8 shows a cat with squamous cell carcinoma on the planum nasale that has been present too long and has invaded beyond the nasal planum. This tumor has progressed from the planum up along the left side of the nasal bridge toward the left eye. The first panel (see Fig. 8) shows the cat on first presentation, at the time of the biopsy. The second panel (see Fig. 8) shows the cat at follow-up 3 weeks later, after the biopsy had confirmed that this tumor was far beyond the planum and was extremely invasive. It was deep in the facial musculature and was in the tissue all the way up to the eye. Clinically, one can see that this tumor is way beyond just simple ablation or even a nasal planectomy. A nasal planectomy can prevent this from occurring if performed early in the disease. Cases amenable to a nasal planectomy need to be chosen carefully, and the procedure must be done before the tumor has time to invade beyond the superficial tissues.

Fig. 9 shows a cat that was presented to its veterinarian with a small pigmented lesion on the nasal planum. The client was told to just "watch it." Four months later, the cat was presented to this author's clinic with a 2.5-cm, crusted, ulcerated nodule on the planum. A combination of a biopsy

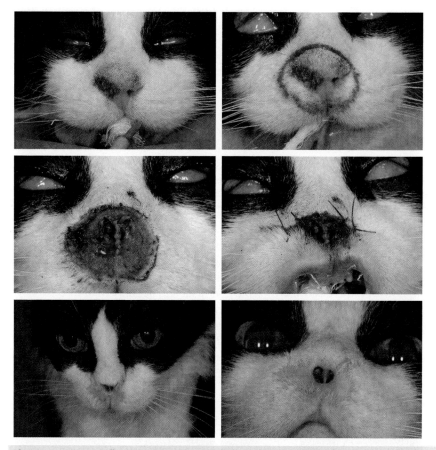

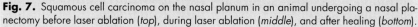

Fig. 7. Squamous cell carcinoma on the nasal planum in an animal undergoing a nasal planectomy before laser ablation (*top*), during laser ablation (*middle*), and after healing (*bottom*).

and nasal planectomy was performed. The entire planum with the tumor was submitted for histopathologic evaluation. It was found to be a spindle-cell form of squamous cell carcinoma that, fortunately, had not progressed beyond the borders of the excision. This cat was 19 years old and lived another 4 years with no recurrence of this tumor. This is a good example of the changing nature of veterinary medicine now that laser surgery is an option. The previous pigmented and crusted spot on the planum was not biopsied but was most likely actinic in situ carcinoma, an early stage of squamous cell carcinoma. At that time, simple laser ablation of the surface of the planum could have prevented the later need for a radical planectomy.

Actinic in situ carcinoma (actinic keratosis)
These lesions are one of the conditions for which the CO_2 laser is the only means of treatment. Without laser ablation, treatment would consist of

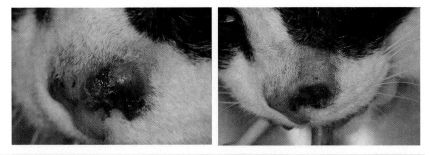

Fig. 8. Squamous cell carcinoma on the nasal planum; note that the tumor has progressed under the skin along the bridge of the nose toward the eye. The tumor has progressed too far, and the animal is not a candidate for a nasal planectomy.

"watching the lesion for change." Actinic keratoses are sun-induced skin lesions and are seen as roughened to crusted lesions. Often, the crusting has a dark color and could be confused with dirt. If this dark material is scraped off, however, there is usually visible erythema and possibly mild ulceration beneath the lesions. These lesions are seen in dogs and cats and occur in lightly haired nonpigmented skin that is exposed to the sun. In cats, they are most common on the planum nasale, the adjacent haired skin of the bridge of the nose, and the tips of the pinnae. In dogs, they are usually found on the

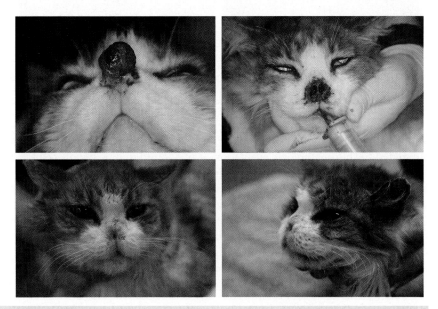

Fig. 9. Spindle-cell form of squamous cell carcinoma in an animal undergoing a nasal planectomy before laser ablation, during laser ablation, and after healing.

ventrum. Studies have demonstrated that the cells from these lesions have similar mutations in their DNA to that found in cells from squamous cell carcinoma. It is suspected that these cells, if allowed to grow, eventually develop into squamous cell carcinoma. Because of this potential to develop into an invasive carcinoma, it has been suggested that the histopathologic diagnosis for these lesions be termed *actinic carcinoma in situ* because they are likely just an early form of this carcinoma [19,25]. Because these lesions are small and do not extend deep into the epidermis, they are easily removed with laser ablation. Repeat laser ablation may be required if new lesions develop over time. The frequency of recurrence varies with the patient; in this author's practice, the average time is 6 to 18 months between treatments. This recurrence rate is in the northwestern United States; in the more southern sunny regions of the world, recurrence rates may be different. The laser procedure can be performed with light sedation using medetomidine or with short general anesthetic gas anesthesia. These procedures are brief, usually taking 5 to 10 minutes for the entire procedure. It is well tolerated by the patient and can be done on an outpatient basis. A biopsy of these lesions on repeat procedures is more invasive than simple laser ablation and is not necessary most of the time; on the initial presentation, histopathologic examination is usually obtained to confirm the diagnosis. With subsequent recurrences, a biopsy is not necessary unless lesions change or do not respond to the laser ablation. One of the disadvantages of laser ablation for lesions that are small and confined to the surface is that laser excision completely evaporates the lesion, making histopathologic examination of the lesion impossible. In Fig. 10, you can see a typical nasal planum on a cat that has had recurrent laser ablations of actinic in situ carcinoma lesions.

Pinnal tumors (histiocytomas, papillomas, fibrous tumors, and nodular sebaceous gland hyperplasia)
Tumors on the pinnae are often difficult to remove with conventional scalpel surgical excision without causing some disfiguration of the pinnae. Additionally, with conventional surgery, bleeding occurs and the lesions require sutures to control this bleeding. Furthermore, it is difficult to remove just the lesion; thus, adjacent normal skin and cartilage are often excised, resulting in further deformities of the pinnae. With the CO_2 laser, hemostasis allows tumor removal without the need for sutures, and the operator is able to limit removal to just the lesion, thereby avoiding damage to adjacent normal structures. Laser ablation results in much less scar formation, and thus no to minimal deformity of the pinnae (Fig. 11).

Feline ceruminous cystomatosis
This disorder is a nonneoplastic disorder that may be associated with previous otitis or a senile change, or it may be an inherited disorder in cats. Clinically, it is seen as bluish papular discoloration at the external orifice to the ear. Frequently, the lesions are asymptomatic, but the client is concerned about them, particularly when there are numerous lesions on the ears. In some cases, large blue- to black-colored irregularly shaped apocrine cystadenomas [26] are

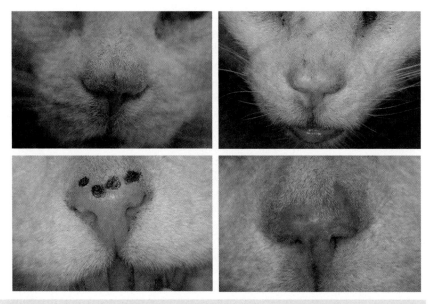

Fig. 10. Actinic in situ carcinoma (actinic keratosis) in a cat that has had recurrent laser ablations. Actinic lesions typically respond well to laser ablation, but new lesions usually develop in 6 to 12 months.

present along with the smaller benign lesions of ceruminous cystomatosis. They are usually confined to the external ear, rarely extending beyond the vertical ear canal. As is the case with other lesions on the ears, laser ablation is the best mode of therapy because of the ability to fine-tune the laser ablation by variation of the spot size, the power setting, and the duration of exposure.

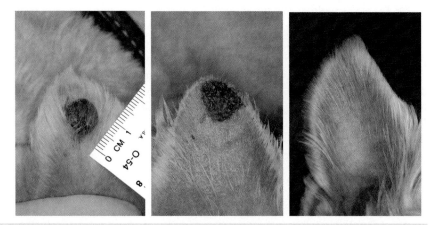

Fig. 11. Pinnal tumor before laser ablation (*left*), during laser ablation (*middle*), and after healing (*right*). Typically, there is no scarring and no bleeding, with good cosmetic results.

The trained laser operator can confine removal to the affected tissue, sparing the normal structures. Laser excision and ablation are well tolerated and curative. In some cats, the lesions are so numerous that it could take two or three sequential procedures to remove all of them. On the pinnae, the power settings for all these procedures are much lower than on haired skin. Usually, the SP mode is used, with power settings of 2 to 4 W. The lesions of feline ceruminous cystomatosis are readily identifiable because of their distinctive bluish color. Most of these lesions are inherited or represent senile changes; once removed, it is rare for them to recur. Fig. 12 shows a cat with feline ceruminous cystomatosis; you can see some of the smaller typical lesions around the larger tumor. Removal was completely curative in this cat.

Calcinosis circumscripta

This condition most often occurs as single nodules that are easily removed surgically; in some animals, metastatic lesions can develop with renal failure [27]. In most cases, a single lesion occurs and simple excision is curative. This author had one case of severe multiple lesions of calcinosis cutis in the tongue of a young kitten. The tongue was so severely affected that the kitten could not eat. The tongue protruded from the mouth and, on palpation, was quite firm, like a "wooden tongue." Laser excision was chosen over conventional surgery because of the hemostatic properties that the CO_2 laser gives to surgical procedures. All the palpable, firm, calcium-filled nodules were opened with the laser, and removal of the calcium was then done by conventional curettage. By the following day, the cat was starting to eat some food on its own, and within 3 days, it was able to eat entirely on its own. Although this is an example of an unusual case, it demonstrates how an otherwise impossible operation using conventional means was able to be performed using the laser. Fig. 13 shows the cat before surgery, during surgery, and 6 weeks after surgery.

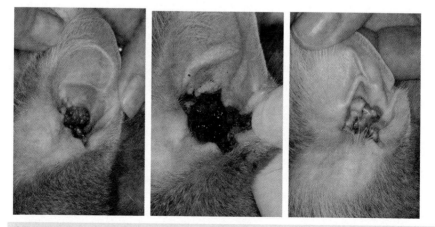

Fig. 12. Feline ceruminous cystomatosis on the external ear and pinna before laser ablation (*left*), during laser ablation (*middle*), and after healing (*right*).

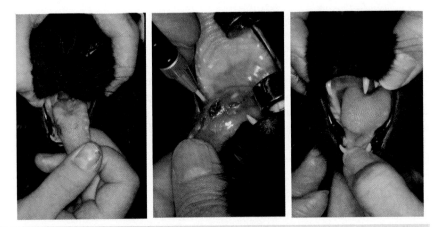

Fig. 13. Calcinosis circumscripta in the tongue of a young kitten before laser ablation (*left*), during laser ablation (*middle*), and after healing (*right*).

Follicular cysts and tumors

A cyst is a nonneoplastic sac-like structure that is defined by identification of the tissue that lines the structure [28]. Most cysts in the dog or cat are of follicular origin. Follicular cysts that are curable by laser therapy occur in dogs on the elbows and the feet. Follicular cysts as a cause of deep furunculosis on the elbow and feet have been largely unrecognized. In fact, most cases of recurrent sterile pododermatitis in dogs have been thought to represent an inflammatory disease of unknown cause; few have recognized that some cases are the result of cysts [29]. In this author's experience, some cases of recurrent sterile nodular pododermatitis are the result of cysts, and removal of these cysts leads to complete permanent cure of this problem (author's personal case material, publication in progress). These lesions present as draining tracts on the dorsal surface in the interdigital toe webs, and on the ventral portion of the foot, one can see a visible comedo. Using the scanner tip on the CO_2 laser, surgical ablation of these lesions allows the removal of numerous follicular cysts (Figs. 14 and 15). A similar problem develops on the elbows of some dogs, although less commonly than on the feet.

It should be stressed that not all cases of pedal folliculitis are caused by follicular cysts; the clinician must be thorough in following all the dermatologic protocols for evaluation of this disease [29] and learn to recognize which cases may be caused by the presence of follicular cysts. Most cases of pedal folliculitis are caused by complications of allergy as bacterial or yeast infections, or deep pyoderma, either idiopathic deep pyoderma or deep pyoderma caused by parasites (demodicosis). Less commonly pedal folliculitis is the result of one of the many other differentials listed in dermatologic texts. There are just a few cases with these follicular cysts that are curable using laser ablation.

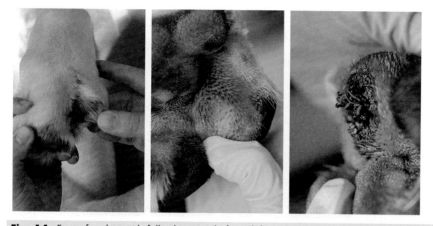

Fig. 14. Foot of a dog with follicular cysts before (*left*) and during laser ablation (*middle, right*).

Gingival hyperplasia and epulis

Gingival hyperplasia and epulis can be removed using the CO_2 laser. One must be careful to obtain a histologic diagnosis of these conditions, because some can be neoplastic and some are recurrent (Fig. 16) [30–34]. Gingival hyperplasia is a condition caused primarily by cyclosporine, although other drugs, such as phenytoin, are known to cause it in human beings. Good dental hygiene can help to minimize the development of these drug-associated lesions, and in the case of cyclosporin, lowering the dose, if possible, can also help. In the more severe cases, CO_2 laser removal is helpful. Fig. 17 shows a severe case of gingival hyperplasia caused by cyclosporin [35,36].

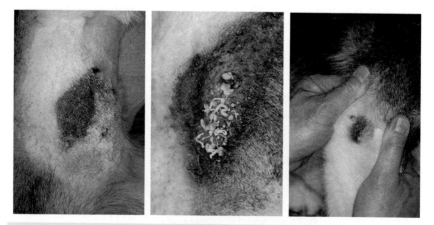

Fig. 15. Dog with follicular cysts on the elbow callus before laser ablation (*left*), during laser ablation (*middle*), and after healing (*right*).

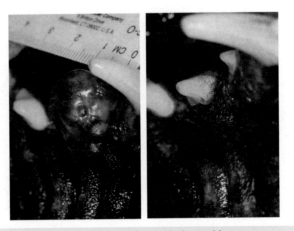

Fig. 16. Dog with epulis before (*left*) and after (*right*) laser ablation.

Nodular sebaceous hyperplasia

These tumors are the most common lesions removed with the CO_2 laser. Nodular sebaceous hyperplasia is a common nonneoplastic tumor of dogs (Fig. 18). Lesions can be focal or multifocal and are commonly referred to as warts by clients but can be distinguished from true papillomas (warts) by their shiny oily to waxy surface. They are often of concern to the pet owner, can be a nuisance to groomers, and sometimes bother the pet to the point where it licks or chews at them. Because of the ease in removal by laser ablation, many more of these tumors are removed today than in the past, when the only means of removal was with conventional surgical excision. As in other laser procedures, repeat surgery is common, because new lesions do continue to develop. Most dogs return for follow-up tumor removal every 6 to 12 months. In some dogs, the number of nodular sebaceous gland tumors can be extreme, but their removal, even at one setting, is not difficult (Fig. 19).

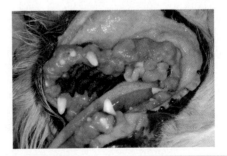

Fig. 17. Dog with cyclosporin-induced gingival hyperplasia.

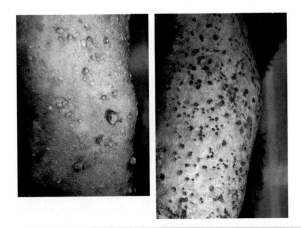

Fig. 18. Dog with numerous nodular sebaceous tumors before (*left*) and after (*right*) laser ablation.

Plasma cell pododermatitis

Plasma cell pododermatitis affects only the footpads of cats and usually only the large central paw pads (Fig. 20). The cause is unknown; the presenting signs are large, soft, spongy footpads, and the surface of the affected pads has a white, scaly, silvery appearance. Occasionally, one or more pads ulcerate, resulting in hemorrhage and lameness; otherwise, these lesions are asymptomatic [37]. In asymptomatic cats, no treatment may be necessary. Treatment with corticosteroids may help some cats. Surgical excision is reported to be successful, and in the author's experience, the easiest mode of surgery is with CO_2 laser. It is well tolerated, with no recurrence [38,39].

Examples of Other Conditions or Lesions That Can Be Treated with the Carbon Dioxide Laser

Some other conditions amenable to treatment with the CO_2 laser include but are not limited to the following: fibropruritic nodules, actinic comedones,

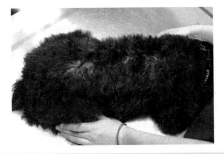

Fig. 19. Same dog as in Fig. 18 after healing.

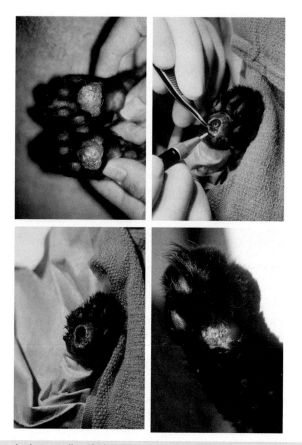

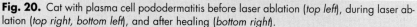

Fig. 20. Cat with plasma cell pododermatitis before laser ablation (*top left*), during laser ablation (*top right, bottom left*), and after healing (*bottom right*).

canine leproid granuloma, foreign body reactions, melanocytomas, nodular perianal gland tumors, histiocytomas, and meibomian gland tumors.

Acral lick dermatitis (ALD) is listed by some veterinarians as a condition that is treatable with laser ablation. These suggestions should be taken cautiously, because ALD often has a long history of treatments that are often only partially helpful [40–46]. One must keep in mind that there are numerous underlying problems involved with ALD, the most common of which are allergic diseases and infection. When these two conditions are dealt with, most of these lesions are adequately controlled. Laser ablation of an acral lick lesion should only be considered after all the underlying causes are addressed and the underlying infections are thoroughly treated. Only then, if there is a significant remaining lesion, would laser ablation potentially offer some additional help. Laser ablation should never be considered as the first treatment for ALD. Laser ablation is only potentially useful for the removal of deep pyogranulomatous tracts that are trapped deep in the overlying collagen and fail to resolve with appropriate antibiotic therapy. ALD is a complicated condition, and laser surgery does not offer some new magical cure; we still need to work on trying to identify the underlying cause of the licking, which can be a complicated problem. Laser surgical ablation is not likely to be a permanent cure; it can help by removing deep draining tracts but is not the single cure for this complicated disease.

SUMMARY

Laser use is becoming more common in veterinary medicine. Technologic advances have resulted in the development of smaller devices, and the cost has also decreased, making their use more feasible for private as well as university veterinary hospitals. In the early years of laser development, many of their potential uses were not known. Presently, with the increased number of veterinarians using these devices, the potential indications for their use are expanding. This article has summarized some of the more important dermatologic uses of the CO_2 laser in veterinary medicine. The diseases mentioned here are the ones for which the laser is better than conventional scalpel surgery; in many of these conditions, conventional surgery would not even be possible. There is no single laser that can do everything, and most lasers have limited and specific applications. The CO_2 laser is a laser that has numerous applications, and because of this, it is currently the most used laser in veterinary medicine.

References
  [1] Glover JL, Bendick PJ, Link WJ. The use of thermal knives in surgery: electrosurgery, lasers, plasma scalpel. Curr Probl Surg 1978;15:1–78.
  [2] Bartels KE. Lasers in medicine and surgery [preface]. Vet Clin North Am Small Anim Pract 2002;32:xiii–xv.
  [3] Crane SW. State of the art message: lasers in veterinary surgery. Lasers Surg Med 1986;6: 427–8.
  [4] Fuller TA. The characteristics in operation of surgical lasers. Surg Clin North Am 1984;64: 843–9.
  [5] Goldman L, Blaney DJ, Kindel DJ Jr, et al. Effect of the laser beam on the skin. Preliminary report. J Invest Dermatol 1963;40:121–2.
  [6] Petrick SW. [Laser treatment for a dog.] J S Afr Vet Assoc 1988;59:176–7 [in Afrikaans].
  [7] Polanyi TG. Physics of surgery with lasers. Clin Chest Med 1985;6:179–202.
  [8] Schick RO, Schick MP. CO2 laser surgery in veterinary dermatology. Clin Dermatol 1994;12:587–9.
  [9] Parrish JA, Wilson BC. Current and future trends in laser medicine. Photochem Photobiol 1991;53:731–8.
  [10] Alster TS, Bettencourt MS. Review of cutaneous lasers and their applications. South Med J 1998;91:806–14.
  [11] Durante EJ. The carbon dioxide laser scalpel. J S Afr Vet Assoc 1991;62:191–4.
  [12] Fry TR. Laser safety. Vet Clin North Am Small Anim Pract 2002;32:535–47.
  [13] Holt TL, Mann FA. Soft tissue application of lasers. Vet Clin North Am Small Anim Pract 2002;32:569–99.
  [14] Kurkomelis J. Introduction to lasers and laser safety. Contemp Top Lab Anim Sci 2004;43: 100–2.
  [15] Peavy GM. Lasers and laser-tissue interaction. Vet Clin North Am Small Anim Pract 2002;32. 517–34.

[16] Durante EJ, Kriek NP. Clinical and histological comparison of tissue damage and healing following incisions with the CO2-laser and stainless steel surgical blade in dogs. J S Afr Vet Assoc 1993;64:116–20.

[17] Durante EJ. Breaking strength of CO2-laser and scalpel blade incisions in the dog. J S Afr Vet Assoc 1992;63:141–3.

[18] Rizzo LB, Ritchey JW, Higbee RG, et al. Histologic comparison of skin biopsy specimens collected by use of carbon dioxide or 810-nm diode lasers from dogs. J Am Vet Med Assoc 2004;225:1562–6.

[19] Gross T, Ihrke P, Walder E, et al. Epidermal tumors. In: Skin diseases of the dog and cat: clinical and histopathologic diagnosis. 2nd edition. Oxford, United Kingdom: Blackwell Science; 2005. p. 561–603.

[20] Akyol A, Anadolu R, Anadolu Y, et al. Multifocal papillomavirus epithelial hyperplasia: successful treatment with CO2 laser therapy combined with interferon alpha-2b. Int J Dermatol 2003;42:733–5.

[21] Bonnem EM. Alpha interferon: the potential drug of adjuvant therapy: past achievements and future challenges. Eur J Cancer 1991;27(Suppl 4):S2–6.

[22] Mattot M, Ninane J, Hamoir M, et al. Combined CO2-laser and alfa recombinant interferon treatment in five children with juvenile laryngeal papillomatosis. Acta Clin Belg 1990;45:158–63.

[23] Strander HA. Interferon in the treatment of human papilloma virus. Med Clin North Am 1986;(Suppl):19–23.

[24] Canning S, Kurban AK. Laser treatment of cutaneous malignancies. Dermatol Nurs 1993;5:447–51.

[25] Gross T, Ihrke P, Walder E, et al. Hyperplastic diseases of the epidermis. In: Skin diseases of the dog and cat: clinical and histopathologic diagnosis. 2nd edition. Oxford, United Kingdom: Blackwell Science; 2005. p. 136–60.

[26] Gross T, Ihrke P, Walder E, et al. Sweat gland tumors. In: Skin diseases of the dog and cat: clinical and histopathologic diagnosis. 2nd edition. Oxford, United Kingdom: Blackwell Science; 2005. p. 665–94.

[27] Gross T, Ihrke P, Walder E, et al. Degenerative, dysplastic and depositional diseases of the dermal connective tissue. In: Skin diseases of the dog and cat: clinical and histopathologic diagnosis. 2nd edition. Oxford, United Kingdom: Blackwell Science; 2005. p. 373–99.

[28] Gross T, Ihrke P, Walder E, et al. Follicular tumors. In: Skin diseases of the dog and cat: clinical and histopathologic diagnosis. 2nd ed. Oxford, United Kingdom: Blackwell Science; 2005. p. 604–40.

[29] Scott D, Miller W, Griffin C. Bacterial skin diseases. In: Muller and Kirk's small animal dermatology. 6th edition. Philadelphia: WB Saunders; 2001. p. 274–335.

[30] Bjorling DE, Chambers JN, Mahaffey EA. Surgical treatment of epulides in dogs: 25 cases (1974–1984). J Am Vet Med Assoc 1987;190:1315–8.

[31] Bostock DE, White RA. Classification and behaviour after surgery of canine 'epulides.' J Comp Pathol 1987;97:197–206.

[32] Dubielzig RR, Goldschmidt MH, Brodey RS. The nomenclature of periodontal epulides in dogs. Vet Pathol 1979;16:209–14.

[33] Pollock S, Turk MH. Gingival hyperplasia: a case study of an inflammatory response. Vet Med Small Anim Clin 1979;74:691–4.

[34] Reichart PA, Philipsen HP, Durr UM. Epulides in dogs. J Oral Pathol Med 1989;18:92–6.

[35] Greenwood AM, O'Brien FV. The fibrous epulis in the dog. J Oral Pathol 1975;4:67–72.

[36] Luomanen M. Oral focal epithelial hyperplasia removed with CO2 laser. Int J Oral Maxillofac Surg 1990;19:205–7.

[37] Gross T, Ihrke P, Walder E, et al. Nodular and diffuse disease of the dermis with prominent eosinophils, neutrophils, or plasma cells. In: Skin diseases of the dog and cat: clinical and histopathologic diagnosis. 2nd edition. Oxford, United Kingdom: Blackwell Science; 2005. p. 342–72.

[38] Dias PP, Faustino AM. Feline plasma cell pododermatitis: a study of 8 cases. Vet Dermatol 2003;14:333–7.

[39] Scott D, Miller W, Griffin C. Miscellaneous skin diseases. In: Muller and Kirk's small animal dermatology. 6th edition. Philadelphia: WB Saunders; 2001. p. 1125–83.

[40] Dodman NH, Shuster L, White SD, et al. Use of narcotic antagonists to modify stereotypic self-licking, self-chewing, and scratching behavior in dogs. J Am Vet Med Assoc 1988;193:815–9.

[41] Hewson CJ, Luescher UA, Parent JM, et al. Efficacy of clomipramine in the treatment of canine compulsive disorder. J Am Vet Med Assoc 1998;213:1760–6.

[42] Rapoport JL, Ryland DH, Kriete M. Drug treatment of canine acral lick. An animal model of obsessive-compulsive disorder. Arch Gen Psychiatry 1992;49:517–21.

[43] Sischo WM, Ihrke PJ, Franti CE. Regional distribution of ten common skin diseases in dogs. J Am Vet Med Assoc 1989;195:752–6.

[44] Virga V. Behavioral dermatology. Vet Clin North Am Small Anim Pract 2003;33. 231–51.

[45] White SD. Naltrexone for treatment of acral lick dermatitis in dogs. J Am Vet Med Assoc 1990;196:1073–6.

[46] Wynchank D, Berk M. Fluoxetine treatment of acral lick dermatitis in dogs: a placebo-controlled randomized double blind trial. Depress Anxiety 1998;8:21–3.

Updates in Therapeutics for Veterinary Dermatology

Stephanie R. Bruner, DVM

Greater Cincinnati Veterinary Specialists, 11 Beacon Drive, Wilder, KY 41076, USA

Perhaps some of the most important developments in veterinary dermatology over the past 5 years have not been the introduction of new drugs but rather our expanded knowledge and use of established medications. Whether previously used in human medicine or other facets of veterinary medicine, these "oldies but goodies" have contributed substantially to our updated and improved treatment formulary. This article introduces some new therapeutics as well as presenting some newly revised uses for more well-known medications.

ANTIVIRAL AND ANTIPROLIFERATIVE THERAPY

Imiquimod is a heterocyclic imidazoquinolone amide that demonstrates antiviral and antitumor properties [1,2]. Originally developed and approved by the US Food and Drug Administration (FDA) for the treatment of external genital and perianal warts caused by papillomaviruses in human beings, imiquimod was also approved in 2004 for the treatment of actinic keratoses.

The exact mechanism of action of imiquimod is unknown. The drug has no direct antiviral or antiproliferative activity in vitro. Imiquimod affects the innate and acquired and/or adaptive immune systems, primarily through the Toll-like receptors (TLRs) [3]. The innate immune system is activated by increasing the natural killer (NK) cell activity, inducing proliferation and differentiation of B lymphocytes, and activating macrophages to secrete various cytokines and nitric oxide. Imiquimod stimulates the adaptive immune system by activating antigen-presenting cells, including dendritic cells, Langerhans cells, macrophages, and B lymphocytes [3]. Langerhans cells, for example, develop increased mobility after topical application of imiquimod and migrate more readily to the lymph nodes for antigen presentation to T lymphocytes [4]. Additionally, imiquimod may have direct proapoptotic capabilities against tumor cells by setting off a cascade of events ultimately resulting in caspase enzyme activation and fragmentation of cellular DNA [5].

E-mail address: brunerderm@bigfoot.com

0195-5616/06/$ – see front matter
doi:10.1016/j.cvsm.2005.09.011

The human medical literature relates numerous off-label applications of imiquimod in various stages of clinical development, ranging from anecdotal reports to clinical trials in progress. Among the dermatoses reporting some success with imiquimod are extragenital warts, molluscum contagiosum, herpes simplex, superficial or nodular basal cell carcinoma, sclerodermiform basal cell carcinoma, Bowen's disease (squamous cell carcinoma in situ), invasive squamous cell carcinoma, lentigo maligna (melanoma in situ), mycosis fungoides, keratoacanthoma, metastatic melanoma, and extramammary Paget's disease [6,7]. Imiquimod has been reported as a useful adjunct medication in the treatment of cutaneous leishmaniasis [8].

Anecdotal reports in veterinary medicine suggest that imiquimod may prove useful in the treatment of Bowen's disease in cats as well as in the treatment of cutaneous papillomatosis. Although imiquimod treatment protocols have not been definitively established for veterinary medicine, extrapolations from the human protocols are likely to occur. The patient prescribing information for one brand of imiquimod recommends twice-weekly applications for a 16-week period for actinic keratoses. Superficial basal cell carcinoma is treated with five topical applications of imiquimod weekly for 6 weeks. External genital warts respond to imiquimod when it is applied three times weekly for a maximum of 16 weeks.

Imiquimod is well tolerated in human beings. Side effects include erosions, excoriations, flaking, edema, and erythema at the site of application. Of these, erythema is the most common [3]. The severity of the local reaction is dose related. Less than 1% of the topically applied medication is absorbed systemically [9]. Imiquimod is contraindicated in individuals with known sensitivity to this product.

HORMONE MODULATION THERAPY

Trilostane interferes with adrenal steroidogenesis by competitive inhibition of the 3β-hydroxysteroid dehydrogenase enzyme (3β-HSD) [10]. This enzyme converts pregnenolone to progesterone and 17-hydroxypregnenolone to 17-hydroxyprogesterone in the adrenal cortex. Trilostane has been in use since the 1970s in human patients for the treatment of Cushing's syndrome [11] and breast cancer [12] and for the termination of pregnancy in women [13,14]. Although not currently available in the United States, trilostane can be obtained from England with a written prescription and a new drug waiver permit from the FDA.

Currently available for veterinary use in Europe, trilostane represents a treatment alternative for hyperadrenocorticism in small animals. Induction doses of trilostane vary widely (range: 5.3–50 mg/kg, median of 16.7 mg/kg administered per os once daily) [15]. Control of hyperadrenocorticism is achieved at doses that do not disrupt peripheral steroidogenesis. The administration of trilostane at 30 mg/d for dogs weighing less than 5 kg, 60 mg/d for dogs weighing 5 to 20 kg, and 120 mg/d for dogs weighing more than 20 kg has been suggested. Larger dogs typically require lower doses per kilogram of body weight to control their disease. Many dogs are sensitive to trilostane during the initial 10 to 30 days of administration but may subsequently require dosage increases to maintain good disease control until a long-term maintenance or plateau level is achieved. Monitoring the efficacy of trilostane involves corticotropin stimulation testing with the target serum or plasma cortisol concentrations between 1 and 2 μg/dL 2 to 6 hours after drug administration. Urinary cortisol/creatinine ratio measurement and abatement of clinical signs can also be useful in monitoring these patients. Re-evaluations are recommended at 7 to 10 days, 30 days, and 90 days after initiating therapy and every 6 months thereafter.

Trilostane has recently demonstrated efficacy for Alopecia X in Pomeranians and Miniature Poodles. In one study, trilostane administered at a mean dose of 10.85 mg/kg/d resulted in complete hair regrowth in 85% of Pomeranians (16 total) and all Miniature Poodles (8 total) treated for Alopecia X [14]. A response was usually noted within 4 to 8 weeks after initiating therapy. Trilostane administration could be tapered in some dogs after hair coat regrowth was complete. The authors hypothesized that trilostane's mechanism of action for Alopecia X may be related to downregulation of adrenal steroid production or competitive inhibition of estrogen receptors at the hair follicles.

Trilostane is generally well-tolerated in veterinary patients, with vomiting and lethargy observed infrequently [15]. This perceived advantage over traditional therapies for adrenocortical disease encourages practitioner interest in trilostane in spite of its often substantial expense. Life-threatening adrenal necrosis has been reported in the dog, however. Likewise, careful cardiac monitoring is recommended for patients with preexisting heart disease. Two Pomeranians died suddenly in the initial report of trilostane therapy for Alopecia X, and anecdotal reports of similar incidents seem to be increasing as trilostane use gains popularity [14]. Pet owners should be educated about these potential complications before the onset of treatment.

IMMUNOMODULATION THERAPY

Tetracycline and niacinamide administered in combination have an increasingly long list of dermatologic uses in veterinary medicine. Although the exact anti-inflammatory and immunomodulatory mechanism(s) of action for tetracycline and niacinamide is(are) not known, tetracycline is capable of suppressing lymphocyte blastogenesis in vitro and leukocyte chemotactic responses in vivo [16]. Tetracycline also inhibits C3 activation, prostaglandin synthesis, and various lipases and collagenases. Niacinamide blocks antigen–immunoglobulin E–induced histamine release in vivo and in vitro as well as preventing degranulation of mast cells. Niacinamide also inhibits phosphodiesterases and protease release [17].

Tetracycline and niacinamide are routinely administered at an empiric dose rate of 500 mg of each medication per os three times daily for dogs weighing greater than 10 kg and at 250 mg of each medication per os three times daily for dogs weighing less than 10 kg [17]. Doxycycline may be substituted for tetracycline at a dose of 5 mg/kg administered orally one to two times daily [18].

Clinical improvement may not be observed for 4 to 6 weeks after initiation of therapy. In many cases, this regimen can be tapered as the dermatosis is controlled.

Tetracycline and niacinamide have been successful at controlling discoid lupus erythematosus (subacute cutaneous lupus) and pemphigus erythematosus in 25% to 65% of affected dogs [19,20]. This combination also serves as adjunct therapy for pemphigus foliaceus in association with prednisone and azathioprine. Other dermatoses in which tetracycline and niacinamide may be efficacious include vesicular cutaneous lupus erythematosus [21], lupoid onychodystrophy [22], dermatomyositis [18], German Shepherd Dog metatarsal fistulae [23,24], sterile granulomatous and/or pyogranulomatous dermatitis and/or panniculitis [25,26], vasculitis, cutaneous histiocytosis [22], sebaceous adenitis, and arteritis of the nasal philtrum [27].

Adverse drug events are relatively uncommon but can include vomiting, diarrhea, anorexia, and lethargy [22]. Although either medication may be implicated in these reactions, niacinamide is usually not tolerated as well as tetracycline. Niacinamide has also been anecdotally reported to increase the frequency of seizures in dogs. Dose reduction or discontinuation of niacinamide alone may permit continued treatment in some patients [17].

Pentoxifylline is a trisubstitute xanthine derivative of methylxanthine. It has rheologic as well as numerous immunomodulatory effects. The rheologic, or blood flow modulation, properties are achieved by increasing erythrocyte and leukocyte deformability, decreasing platelet aggregation, decreasing leukocyte adhesion and aggregation, and increasing neutrophil motility and chemotaxis [28]. The end result is improved peripheral tissue circulation and subsequent oxygenation.

Immunomodulation is accomplished by decreasing leukocyte responsiveness to interleukin (IL)-1 and tumor necrosis factor-α (TNFα); decreasing production of TNFα from macrophages; decreasing production of IL-1, IL-4, and IL-12; inhibition of T- and B-lymphocyte activation; decreasing NK cell activity; and inhibition of phosphodiesterases and T-cell adherence to keratinocytes [28,29]. Pentoxifylline also affects wound healing and connective tissue disorders through the increased production of collagenases and fibrinolytic activity and decreased production of collagen, fibronectin, and plasma fibrinogen [30].

Pentoxifylline is metabolized by the red blood cells and liver, with extensive enterohepatic recycling of the metabolites [28]. Urinary excretion of the metabolites eliminates more than 90% of the drug from the body. The bioavailability of pentoxifylline after oral administration is 15% to 32% [31]. The medication reaches its peak plasma levels in dogs within an hour after oral administration and has a short elimination half-life of an hour or less [32]. This rapid elimination, with no drug detectable in dogs 4 hours after administration, has led to the consideration of a thrice-daily dosing schedule for some disorders. This philosophy may be countered, however, with pharmacokinetic data suggesting that repetitive dosing in dogs results in decreased concentrations.

Numerous uses for pentoxifylline have been proposed in veterinary medicine. Dermatoses for which pentoxifylline may be helpful, as single-agent or adjunctive therapy, include canine familial dermatomyositis [31], allergic contact dermatitis [33], pinnal thrombovascular disease, ear margin dermatosis [31], vasculitis of various causes [34], vaccine-induced ischemic dermatopathies, erythema multiforme [35], discoid lupus erythematosus, idiopathic mucinosis of the Chinese Shar Pei, lupoid onychodystrophy and/or onychitis, German Shepherd Dog deep pyoderma [36], vesicular cutaneous lupus erythematosus, acral lick dermatosis, Greyhound vasculopathy, metatarsal fistulae of the German Shepherd Dog, sterile nodular pyogranulomatous and/or granulomatous panniculitis, deep pyoderma, interdigital furunculosis, and, possibly, atopy [30]. Recommended doses vary as widely because of the diseases this drug treats, ranging from 10 to 40 mg/kg administered once daily to three times daily. Treatment suggestions for dermatomyositis alone range from recommendations of 400 mg per dog per day to up to 30 mg/kg administered twice daily or 15 mg/kg administered three times daily [37]. Dogs with allergic contact reactions to plants demonstrated improvement at a dose of 10 mg/kg administered orally twice daily, with a response in as little as 2 days [33]. Even this report, however, noted that the effect may be dose related. In general, a response to therapy is anticipated in 1 to 3 months.

Various generic formulations of pentoxifylline are available, although some authors report decreased efficacy or increased side effects with these products [37]. Because pentoxifylline is only manufactured as 400-mg sustained-release tablets, accurate dosing in veterinary patients often necessitates crushing, breaking, or compounding the tablets. Consequently, the patient may not receive the bioavailability benefits of the sustained-release formulation [31]. Storage in a light-protective container is recommended.

Pentoxifylline is generally well tolerated and considered quite safe in veterinary patients. The most common adverse drug effects are vomiting and diarrhea, which may largely be avoided by giving it with food. Central nervous system or cardiovascular stimulation has been observed in people [28]. Pentoxifylline should be used in caution with patients with known sensitivity to other methylxanthine derivatives, patients at risk for hemorrhage, or patients with recent cerebral or retinal hemorrhage [31]. This drug may increase the risk of hemorrhage in patients on warfarin and may result in drug interactions in human patients receiving cisplatin, alkylating agents, and amphotericin B [28,31]. Pentoxifylline may synergize with ciprofloxacin in inhibiting TNFα production [38]. Pentoxifylline is excreted in human milk, and its safety in pregnancy has not been established [31].

Cyclosporine A (CsA) is a fat-soluble cyclic polypeptide metabolite derived from the telluric fungus *Tolypocladium inflatum gams* [39,40]. CsA has been used to aid in the prevention of organ transplant rejection in human beings since 1977 and is employed as an immunomodulator for inflammatory dermatoses, such as atopic dermatitis and psoriasis [41–43].

CsA binds to the intracellular protein cyclophilin-1, forming a complex that inhibits calcineurin [44]. Hence, CsA is classified as a calcineurin inhibitor. Calcineurin is a calcium- and calcimodulin-dependent protein phosphatase that is responsible for transmission of signal information from the cell membrane to the nucleus. Calcineurin transmits information by dephosphorylating nuclear factor of activated T cells (NF-AT), a transcription factor that penetrates the nucleus and induces cell activation. One of the essential processes in cellular activation is the transcription of genes controlling the synthesis of IL-2. Inhibition of IL-2 transcription and T-cell responsiveness to IL-2 results in impaired T helper and T-cytotoxic lymphocytes. Inhibition or impaired production of other cytokines, such as interferon-α (IFNα), IL-3, IL-4, IL-5, and TNFα, has an impact on mononuclear cell function, mast cell and eosinophil production and survival, cytoplasmic granule release, cytokine secretion, prostaglandin production, neutrophil adherence, NK cell activity, and growth and differentiation of B cells. In addition, CsA decreases the number of Langerhans cells in the epidermis, inhibits the lymphocyte-activating function of Langerhans cells, and diminishes cytokine secretion by keratinocytes [44]. CsA does not alter humoral immunity and has not been demonstrated to have a significant effect on serum allergen-specific IgE levels and immediate-phase intradermal test results [45]. Likewise, vaccinations that stimulate a humoral protective response are not negatively affected [39].

Because of its lipophilic properties, CsA is widely distributed in most tissues, with the exception of low passage across the blood-brain barrier [39]. CsA is metabolized by the cytochrome P450 enzyme system, specifically CYP3A4, in the liver and intestines [46]. Drugs that inhibit CYP3A4 or compete with P-glycoprotein may alter CsA metabolism substantially [39]. Although numerous medications have been documented to affect CsA metabolism in human beings, few clinically relevant drug interactions have been reported in veterinary medicine. Ketoconazole represents one of these important and useful drug interactions. Ketoconazole suppresses the cytochrome P450 enzymes, thereby decreasing CsA clearance and increasing CsA blood concentrations [47]. Concurrent administration of CsA and ketoconazole at 5 to 10 mg/kg/d orally for the treatment of perianal fistulae has been estimated to result in a 50% to 75% CsA dose reduction at a potentially substantial cost savings [48].

CsA is currently marketed in veterinary medicine in a microemulsion formula to enhance bioavailability and produce more consistent blood levels. Absorption is also enhanced by administering the drug 2 hours before or after feeding, but fasting may be less important with the microemulsified product [39]. Measurement of CsA blood levels is not widely used or recommended for veterinary dermatologic disorders, largely because of the drug's wide margin of safety and lack of definitive relations between efficacy and blood levels [49]. Drug monitoring may be desirable if a patient is not improving, if toxicosis is suspected, or if a CsA-sparing medication is being used concurrently [39,50]. If blood levels are measured, high-pressure liquid chromatography (HPLC) is the preferred assay technique, because it avoids cross-reactivity with CsA; metabolites [39,44]. Unfortunately, HPLC is not widely available commercially, and this further limits the utility of drug level monitoring. CsA is primarily eliminated through the biliary system. with a minor fraction being excreted by the kidneys [39].

Atopy and perianal fistulae and/or furunculosis are the dermatologic conditions for which CsA has been evaluated most often in dogs. CsA has been recommended as a single agent at an initial dose of 5 mg/kg/d administered orally. Recent studies of CsA for the control and treatment of atopic dermatitis in dogs have reported 71% to 75% client satisfaction rates [51,52]. In one of these studies, 55% of dogs required ongoing therapy, although not necessarily on a daily basis, whereas 45% discontinued therapy because of limited response or drug cost (22%) or after achieving and maintaining remission of clinical signs. The mean time of remission after cessation of therapy was 12 months [52]. Perianal fistulae and/or anal furunculosis studies have reported 72% to 100% remission rates with CsA with or without ketoconazole [50]. Long-term remission rates greater than 50% make CsA the most effective medical treatment for anal furunculosis in the dog at this time [50,53]. Many other applications have been reported or suggested and include cutaneous lupus erythematosus [54], eosinophilic granuloma complex in the cat [55–57], feline pseudopelade, feline atopy [49], pemphigus erythematosus [54], pemphigus foliaceus [17,54], sebaceous adenitis [55], sterile nodular panniculitis [39], chronic pedal furunculosis [49], dirty face syndrome of Persian cats [49], erythema multiforme [49], follicular hyperkeratosis of the Cocker Spaniel [49], primary seborrhea and/or epidermal dysplasia [55,58], end-stage proliferative otitis externa [59], German Shepherd Dog deep pyoderma [49,55], metatarsal fistulae [49,60], ulcerative dermatosis of the philtrum of St. Bernard and Newfoundland dogs [55], and feline plasma cell pododermatitis. Some of these reports used CsA as an adjunct medication to other immunomodulators, including glucocorticoids. Because CsA does not act on the glucocorticoid receptor, it may suitable for dogs using glucocorticoids or experiencing glucocorticoid tachyphylaxis [61].

Nephrotoxicity, hypertension, and hepatotoxicity occur with a relatively high incidence in human patients receiving CsA [62]. Major adverse drug reactions occur uncommonly in veterinary medicine at dose levels of 5 to 10 mg/kg/d [63]. Gastrointestinal upset (vomiting, diarrhea, and anorexia) may be seen at these levels but can usually be resolved by drug withdrawal and reintroduction, administration with a small amount of food, division of the dose into a twice-daily schedule, or coadministration with an antiemetic [44,49]. Other adverse drug reactions in dogs, usually associated with high-dose drug administration up to 45 mg/kg/d, include gingival hyperplasia; papillomatosis; bacteriuria; hirsutism; involuntary shaking; psoriasiform- or lichenoid-like dermatosis [64]; spurious serum chemistry panel elevations; and, possibly, nephropathy, bacterial skin infections, and bone marrow suppression [49,51,53,63,65]. Drug withdrawal and dose reduction may result in resolution of some of these reactions [49]. In comparison to methylprednisone administration, however, CsA has been associated with a decreased frequency of bacterial skin infections [51]. CsA is contraindicated in dogs with a prior history of malignancy [44]. In addition, cost may be a limiting factor for the use of this product in veterinary dermatology.

Side effects in cats are currently considered rare [44]. Concerns have arisen about increased susceptibility to viral and other latent infections. Fatal acute systemic toxoplasmosis has recently been diagnosed in a cat after 8 months of CsA therapy for feline atopy [66]. No other immunosuppressive medications or viral infections were detected. The authors suspected acute systemic illness attributable to a recently acquired infection. It is reasonable to expect that more adverse drug reactions may be reported in cats as CsA is evaluated more thoroughly in this species.

Tacrolimus was launched on the human medical market in the United States in 2001. It is indicated for topical use in human patients with moderate to severe atopic dermatitis. The 0.03% ointment is labeled for children older than 2 years of age. A macrolide lactone, tacrolimus is derived from the *Streptomyces tsukubaensis* [67]. It is chemically distinct from CsA but has similar properties. Tacrolimus is estimated to be 10 to 100 times more potent than CsA [68]. Tacrolimus is considered better suited than CsA for topical use because of its lower molecular weight, which enhances its ability to penetrate skin [69,70]. The drug penetrates inflamed skin readily but penetrates normal epidermis poorly, leading to the hypothesis that penetration may decrease as inflammation diminishes [69,71]. Tacrolimus is not atrophogenic, which represents a major advantage over glucocorticoids for the treatment of atopic eczema in human beings [72].

After binding a cyclophilin-like protein (FK506-binding protein [FKBP]) intracellularly, the tacrolimus complex inhibits calcineurin, resulting in immunomodulation that is pharmacologically similar to that obtained with CsA. Topical administration to dogs is generally well tolerated, with only mild skin irritation at the site of application reported. In studies measuring blood levels of tacrolimus in dogs for atopic dermatitis, pemphigus erythematosus, and discoid lupus erythematosus, blood levels of the active medication were detected but did not correlate with any clinical or laboratory signs of toxicity [68,69], In fact, no adverse changes in complete blood cell counts or serum biochemistry profiles were observed in these patients. Immediate skin test reactivity in dogs is not affected by the topical use of tacrolimus [73]. Late-phase reactions may be suppressed, however. A 4-week withdrawal is recommended if late-phase reactions are to be evaluated as a component of the intradermal skin test.

Topical tacrolimus therapy has been evaluated for the treatment of canine atopic dermatitis, pemphigus erythematosus, discoid lupus erythematosus, and anal furunculosis [68,69,74–76]. An early pilot study of topical tacrolimus for the treatment of atopy used a compounded 0.3% lotion that decreased clinical signs, primarily erythema, but improvement was not perceived to be significant by the pet owners [69]. More recently published works have used commercially available 0.1% tacrolimus ointment and demonstrated a statistically significant improvement in lesions associated with atopic dermatitis

[75,76]. Results of each study indicated that tacrolimus is particularly effective for the treatment of localized lesions, with improvement noted as early as 2 weeks after initiating therapy. In a limited study of topical tacrolimus for the treatment of pemphigus erythematosus and discoid lupus erythematosus, 10 of 12 dogs exhibited improvement over an 8-week trial period [68]. In some cases, clinical improvement was accompanied by discontinuation of systemic immunosuppressant therapy. Evaluation of tacrolimus as a single agent applied topically once to twice daily for mild to moderate perianal fistulae resulted in complete lesion resolution in 50% of dogs [74]. Noticeable improvement was observed in 90% of dogs participating in the study. Tacrolimus has been anecdotally suggested for the treatment of focal lesions of vesicular cutaneous lupus erythematosus [21], metatarsal fistulae of the German Shepherd Dog [60], eosinophilic granuloma complex lesions in cats (Joseph M. Bruner, DVM, personal communication, 2005), and localized lesions of pemphigus foliaceus [77].

In a recent public health advisory, the FDA issued a notice of intent to require a label warning for tacrolimus ointment regarding the drug's potential carcinogenicity [78]. The data on which this advisory is based used extremely high doses of orally administered tacrolimus in rodent models. Regardless, owners should be apprised of this information before purchasing the tacrolimus ointment and should be advised to wear gloves when handling this product. Although the cost of tacrolimus per tube may be considerable, the lack of requirement for drug monitoring, potential displacement of other medication requirements, and length of time that each tube lasts if carefully applied may make this a viable treatment alternative for some veterinary patients.

ANTIFUNGAL THERAPY

Lufenuron is a benzyl-phenoluria compound marketed in the United States for the control of fleas. It is effective by inhibition of chitin synthesis, polymerization, and deposition [79]. Because chitin is a critical component of the outer cell wall of many fungi, a retrospective study published in 2000 evaluated the use of this product for the treatment of dermatophytosis in dogs and cats [80]. This study reported rapid mean durations from time to initiation of treatment to time of negative fungal culture (14.5 days in dogs and 8.3 days in cats) and to time of resolution of gross lesions (20.75 days in dogs and 12 days in cats) with no adverse treatment effects. The doses administered to dogs ranged from 54.2 to 68.3 mg/kg by mouth. Revised dose recommendations, published by the same authors in 2001, advocated the use of lufenuron for cats housed in catteries at a dose of 100 mg/kg administered orally and at a dose of 80 mg/kg administered orally for house cats [81]. Each group of animals was to be retreated in 2 weeks, followed by monthly maintenance dosing at the manufacturer's recommended dose for flea control. A 5% reinfection rate was anticipated in dogs and cats.

Unfortunately, more recently published prospective work indicates that lufenuron has not fulfilled its initial promise in the prevention or treatment of dermatophytosis. In a placebo-controlled study using oral lufenuron at dosages ranging from 30 to 133 mg/kg administered every 28 days for two treatments, cats were subsequently challenged with 10^5 *Microsporum canis* spores applied to the skin under occlusion [82]. All cats, treated and control alike, developed infections that progressed and regressed in a similar manner. In another study, cats received four monthly doses of lufenuron at 100 to 133 mg/kg administered orally or 40 mg/kg administered subcutaneously before exposure to a subclinically infected cat [83]. Five monthly doses were administered subsequent to exposure. Although dermatophyte infections were established more slowly, the infection rates and speed of resolution were not affected by the use of lufenuron. In either case, the authors concluded that oral lufenuron, at these dosages and under these conditions, neither prevented nor changed the course of dermatophytosis in cats. Treatment may have failed because of the high spore exposure or a flawed dosing scheme; however, lufenuron is not currently recommended for the prevention or treatment of dermatophytosis in dogs and cats [82,84].

Terbinafine is an allylamine antifungal agent used for the treatment of superficial dermatomycoses, including sporotrichosis, and onychomycoses in human beings. Terbinafine is fungicidal for dermatophytes [85].

Terbinafine inhibits squalene epoxidase, an enzyme that converts squalene to lanosterol [86]. This action results in depletion of ergosterol within the cell membrane as well as accumulation of squalene intracellularly, leading to cell death. The outer and inner layers of the dermatophyte arthroconidia cell wall are the initial targets for terbinafine, followed by changes in the cytosol and intracellular organelles, suggesting possible applications for terbinafine with dermatophyte prophylaxis in the future [87].

Terbinafine is highly keratophilic and lipophilic, with high concentrations detected in the stratum corneum, hair, sebum, and subcutaneous fat [22,88]. Delivery to the stratum corneum is via sebum and basal keratinocytes and, to a lesser extent, diffusion through the dermis and epidermis [88–90]. High drug levels are noted in the stratum corneum within the first 2 days of treatment. In human patients, therapeutic levels are maintained for 2 to 3 weeks in the skin and 2 to 3 months in the nails after cessation of therapy. Terbinafine is well absorbed in human beings, with greater than 70% bioavailability, and is not significantly affected by food [86,91]. Extensive biotransformation occurs in the liver, primarily through *N*-demethylation and oxidation of the tertiary butyl group [92]. Of at least 15 metabolites that are produced through this process, none is known to be active. Excretion is primarily renal, with only approximately 20% being excreted in the feces [86].

Terbinafine is currently recommended at a dose of 30 to 40 mg/kg administered orally once daily for the treatment of dermatophytosis [84]. At least one report used terbinafine for the successful treatment of dermatophytosis in cats and dogs at a lower dose of 10 to 30 mg/kg once daily. Another study, however, found that cats receiving 10 to 20 mg/kg had no difference in outcome than untreated control cats [93,94]. In comparison, cats on a high-dose protocol of 30 to 40 mg/kg were cured after approximately 4 months of therapy.

Terbinafine may represent a treatment alternative for other superficial mycoses in veterinary medicine. Daily administration of 30 mg/kg orally had comparable efficacy to ketoconazole in reducing baseline levels of *Malassezia* organisms in healthy Basset Hounds [95]. Expense is likely to limit the routine use of terbinafine for *Malassezia* dermatitis. This drug may be useful in cases in which concurrent disease or potential drug interactions contraindicate the azoles.

This drug may also prove helpful in management of the often-frustrating oomycoses. Combination therapy with terbinafine and itraconazole has successfully treated pythiosis in human patients [96]. Early work with this combination in veterinary medicine suggests that combination therapy may likewise be preferred to itraconazole or amphotericin B alone, although clinical outcomes still require a guarded prognosis in dogs and cats [97].

The highly keratophilic and lipophilic nature of this medication makes it a good candidate for a pulse therapy regimen (intermittent dosing after an initial period of daily loading doses) or cycle therapy (continuous administration followed by a rest and fungal culture) [84]. In an early report of terbinafine use in veterinary dermatology, 92% of cats receiving only 14 to 21 days of terbinafine at 30 mg/kg/d orally achieved mycologic cure [98]. The time to cure ranged from 44 days to 134 days after treatment, however. To the author's knowledge, neither a pulse nor cycle therapy protocol has been developed for terbinafine at this time.

Terbinafine is typically quite well tolerated in cats and dogs [99]. Vomiting is an infrequently reported adverse effect. No embryonic or fetal toxicity is observed in human beings, and teratogenicity has not been documented. Although some medications (rifampin, cimetidine, and cyclosporine) may alter drug clearance when used concurrently with terbinafine, drug reactions are considered rare.

ANTIBACTERIAL THERAPY

Cefpodoxime proxetil is an extended-spectrum cephalosporin marketed in the United States for the treatment of bacterial infections in dogs. Classified as a group 5 cephalosporin, this drug demonstrates resistance to many β-lactamases and is suitable for oral administration. It is intended for the treatment of infections caused by *Staphylococcus intermedius, Staphylococcus aureus, Streptococcus canis* (group G and β-hemolytic), *Escherichia coli, Pasteurella multocida,* and *Proteus mirabilis.* This drug is not active against most obligate anaerobes, *Pseudomonas* species, or enterococci [100].

Administered as the prodrug cefpodoxime proxetil, this medication is de-esterified in the intestinal wall to yield its active metabolite, cefpodoxime. The mechanism of cefpodoxime's bactericidal activity against susceptible organisms involves inactivation of the transpeptidase enzymes in the bacterial cell walls [101]. These enzymes are responsible for catalyzing the cross-linking reactions of the peptidoglycans that are integral to the rigidity of the cell wall. Inactivation of the transpeptidase enzymes results in cell lysis. Cefpodoxime is widely distributed and not significantly metabolized in dogs [102]. Elimination is primarily via renal excretion, with an elimination half-life of 5 to 6 hours after oral administration. Approximately 33% of cefpodoxime may be recovered in the feces.

Cefpodoxime proxetil is administered at a dosage of 5 to 10 mg/kg orally every 24 hours for a maximum of 28 days. This once-daily schedule makes it an attractive option to many veterinarians as a first-line treatment for pyoderma. It may be administered with or without food [100]. Unfortunately, independent clinical studies evaluating the use and efficacy of this drug in dogs are currently lacking.

Cefpodoxime is generally well tolerated in the dog. Vomiting, diarrhea, and decreased appetite are the most commonly reported adverse drug events. The manufacturer's studies demonstrate an excellent margin of safety and low level of toxicity. The author is aware of no studies regarding the clinical use of this drug in gestating or lactating bitches, breeding male dogs, or cats. Cefpodoxime is excreted in human milk (data on file, Pfizer Animal Health Services). It is contraindicated in patients with known hypersensitivities to cephalosporins and may occasionally cause a positive direct Coombs' test.

Marbofloxacin is a synthetic fluoroquinolone developed exclusively for use in animals. It is indicated for the treatment of skin, soft tissue, and urinary tract infections associated with susceptible bacteria. *Staphylococcus* species, *Pseudomonas* species, *Proteus* species, and *E coli* are examples of common skin pathogens that frequently demonstrate drug susceptibility [103–105].

Marbofloxacin is approved for use in dogs and cats at 2.5 to 5.5 mg/kg/d administered orally. A DNA-gyrase inhibitor, it is bactericidal in a concentration-dependent manner [106]. Like other fluoroquinolones, marbofloxacin accumulates in inflammatory cells, especially macrophages [107]. This drug has high bioavailability after oral administration, approaching 100% in dogs [108]. It is widely distributed and has a significantly longer plasma half-life than enrofloxacin, ciprofloxacin, enrofloxacin combined with ciprofloxacin, or difloxacin [109]. Whether this latter observation offers any clinical advantage remains unknown at this time. Excretion is primarily by the kidneys and in the feces, with a small amount of hepatic metabolism occurring in dogs [108]. Marbofloxacin is used frequently in veterinary medicine for the treatment of cutaneous infections, superficial and deep pyoderma, and otitis externa or media, especially if the infection is caused by *Pseudomonas aeruginosa*. Evaluation of marbofloxacin, administered at 2.75 mg/kg/d orally for 21 or 28 days, resulted in resolution of superficial or deep pyoderma in 86.1% of treated dogs [110]. The authors speculated that extending treatment duration beyond 28 days might have resulted in a 94.4% success rate, producing outcomes comparable to those of enrofloxacin and other antibiotics commonly prescribed for pyoderma. Selection of marbofloxacin should be based on bacterial culture and antimicrobial sensitivity test results. Consequently, marbofloxacin is not recommended as a first-line antibiotic for canine pyoderma or otitis [110].

Marbofloxacin is generally well-tolerated, with a low occurrence of adverse drug events reported. Inappetence, decreased activity, and vomiting are most commonly reported at doses up to 5.5 mg/kg/d [111–113]. This drug is contra-indicated in immature dogs during their rapid growth phase because of potential toxicity to chondrocytes. Central nervous system signs may occur after high doses or rapid intravenous infusions [107]. This is believed to be caused by inhibition of the inhibitory neurotransmitter gamma-aminobutyric acid (GABA). Marbofloxacin can precipitate seizures and should be avoided in patients with a history of seizure activity. This medication should not be administered with other drugs containing di- and trivalent cations, such as antacids or sucralfate, because this may decrease absorption from the gastrointestinal tract [114]. Cost may be a factor limiting the use of this medication.

ANTIPARASITIC THERAPY

Selamectin is a novel semisynthetic avermectin derived from a new strain of *Streptomyces avermitilis* [115]. It is labeled in the United States for the prevention and control of flea (*Ctenocephalides felis*) infestations, prevention of heartworm (*Dirofilaria immitis*) disease, treatment and control of ear mite (*Otodectes cynotis*) infestations, treatment and control of sarcoptic mange (*Sarcoptes scabiei*), and control of tick infestations caused by *Dermacentor variabililis* in dogs. In cats, this product is labeled for the prevention and control of flea infestations (*C felis*), prevention of heartworm disease, treatment and control of ear mite (*O cynotis*) infestations, and treatment and control of roundworm (*Toxocara cati*) and intestinal hookworm (*Ancylostoma tubaeforme*) infestations.

The mechanism of action of selamectin has not been completely defined but probably involves increased permeability to chloride ions through interaction with GABA binding sites [116]. The rapid influx of chloride ions inhibits electrical activity of nerve cells in nematodes and muscle cells of arthropods, resulting in rapid flaccid paralysis and death or elimination by the host. After topical administration, selamectin is rapidly absorbed from the skin into the bloodstream and selectively redistributed back into the sebaceous glands (data on file, Pfizer Animal Health). The drug can be identified in the sebaceous glands, hair follicles, and basal layers of the epithelium. Selamectin is further eliminated from the body by excretion into the intestinal tract.

In addition to its label indications, selamectin has been successfully reported to control cheyletiellosis in cats when administered monthly for three doses [117]. In addition, many veterinary dermatologists advocate readministering selamectin for canine scabies every 2 to 3 weeks for a minimum of three treatments because of perceived delayed responses to therapy when applied monthly [118].

Selamectin is typically well tolerated in dogs and cats. Although cutaneous reactions, such as alopecia at or near the site of application, pruritus, erythema, and urticaria, are reported (infrequently), other systemic adverse reactions are considered to be quite rare [119].

Doramectin is another macrocyclic lactone of the avermectin family. It is derived from the fermentation of selected strains of *S avermitilis* [120]. To the author's knowledge, there is currently not a product labeled for small animal use in the United States.

Sharing the same proposed mechanism(s) of action as selamectin and the other avermectins, doramectin has a half-life in plasma that is approximately twice that of ivermectin [121]. Doramectin also provides a longer duration of residual protection that varies depending on the species of parasite in question [122]. The long plasma half-life is attributed to its oily formulation and its non-polar cyclohexil group located at carbon 25 of the ivermectin ring [123].

Doramectin has been evaluated for the treatment and control of scabies in the dog and notoedric mange in the cat at subcutaneously administered doses of 0.2 to 0.3 mg/kg and 0.2 mg/kg, respectively [120,124]. Doramectin has also been investigated for use in the treatment of canine demodicosis when dosed at 0.6 mg/kg subcutaneously weekly for 5 to 23 weeks [125]. This study requires further follow-up, however, because only 10 of 23 dogs were considered cured on a long-term basis. Doramectin has been reported successful for the treatment of *Demodex cati* in three cats at a dosage of 0.6 mg/kg administered subcutaneously weekly for two to three treatments [125].

Moxidectin is an avermectin derived from fermentation products of *Streptomyces cyanogriseus* subspecies *noncyanogenus* [120]. A moxidectin formulation is not currently approved in the United States for small animals. A recently marketed injectable product intended for the prevention of heartworm disease in dogs was withdrawn after the FDA issued a recall because of adverse drug reactions, including death.

In the future, further consideration may be given to moxidectin as an ectoparasiticide. Moxidectin has been reported for the successful treatment of scabies in the dog when administered at 0.2 to 0.25 mg/kg orally or subcutaneously every 7 days for 3 to 6 weeks [126]. Adverse effects were reported in 7 of 41 dogs, however, and included urticaria, angioedema, and ataxia. Moxidectin has been used to treat otoacariasis in dogs at a dosage of 0.2 mg/kg orally or subcutaneously every 10 days for two treatments and in cats at a dosage of 0.2 mg/kg subcutaneously for one treatment [127,128]. Reinfestation was problematic in cats, suggesting that repeated treatments are probably necessary. The response of canine demodicosis to moxidectin has also been preliminarily investigated. Doses ranged from 0.2 mg/kg administered subcutaneously every week or every other week to 0.2 to 0.4 mg/kg/d administered orally [126,129–132]. Although overall remission and cure rates seemed to be comparable with those of other avermectins, further study is warranted, particularly in light of the adverse drug effects recently associated with some formulations of this product.

SUMMARY

This article discusses current and future treatment options for some common small animal dermatoses. Some of these medications may already be familiar to veterinarians but should now have a broader spectrum of use. Other drugs may be entirely new or represent growing opportunities for research.

[49] Robson D, Burton G. Cyclosporin: applications in small animal dermatology. Vet Dermatol 2003;14(1):1–9.

[50] Patterson A, Campbell K. Managing anal furunculosis in dogs. Compend Contin Educ Pract Vet 2005;27(5):339–60.

[51] Steffan J, Alexander D, Brovedani F, et al. Comparison of cyclosporine A with methylprednisolone for treatment of canine atopic dermatitis: a parallel, blinded, randomized controlled trial. Vet Dermatol 2003;14(1):11–22.

[52] Radowicz S, Power H. Long-term use of cyclosporine in the treatment of canine atopic dermatitis. Vet Dermatol 2005;16(2):81–6.

[53] Marks SL. Perianal fistula disease. In: Campbell K, editor. Small animal dermatology secrets. Philadelphia: Hanley & Belfus; 2004. p. 341–4.

[54] Rosenkrantz WS, Griffin CE, Barr RJ. Clinical evaluation of cyclosporine in animal models with cutaneous immune-mediated disease and epitheliotropic lymphoma. J Am Vet Med Assoc 1989;25:377–84.

[55] Rosenbaum M. Cyclosporine. Topeka (KS): Hill's Pet Nutrition; 1999.

[56] Rosenbaum MR. Feline eosinophilic granuloma complex. Topeka (KS): Hill's Pet Nutrition; 2005.

[57] Guaguere E, Prelaud P. Efficacy of cyclosporin in the treatment of 12 cases of eosinophilic granuloma complex [abstract]. Vet Dermatol 2000;11(Suppl 1):31.

[58] Kwochka KW. Therapy of cornification and keratinization disorders. Presented at the 18th Annual Meeting of the American Academy of Veterinary Dermatology and American College of Veterinary Dermatology. Monterey, CA, April 9–12, 2003.

[59] Hall J, Waisglass S, Yager J, et al. Oral cyclosporin in the treatment of cystic/polyploid proliferative otitis externa in a cocker spaniel: a case report [abstract]. Vet Dermatol 2003;14(4):223.

[60] Crow D. Treatment of canine interdigital and metatarsal fistulas. Topeka (KS): Hill's Pet Nutrition; 2003.

[61] Marsella R. Calcineurin inhibitors: a novel approach to canine atopic dermatitis. J Am Anim Hosp Assoc 2005;41(2):92–7.

[62] Koo J. Cyclosporine in dermatology. Fears and opportunities. Arch Dermatol 1995; 131(7):842–5.

[63] Steffan J, Parks C, Seewald W. Clinical trial evaluating the efficacy and safety of cyclosporine in dogs with atopic dermatitis. J Am Vet Med Assoc 2005;226(11): 1855–63.

[64] Werner A. Psoriasiform-lichenoid-like dermatosis in three dogs treated with microemulsified cyclosporine A. J Am Vet Med Assoc 2003;223(7):1013–6.

[65] Ryffel B, Donatsch P, Madorin M, et al. Toxicological evaluation of cyclosporin A. Arch Toxicol 1983;53(2):107–41.

[66] Last R, Suzuki Y, Manning T, et al. A case of fatal systemic toxoplasmosis in a cat being treated with cyclosporin A for feline atopy. Vet Dermatol 2004;15(3):194–8.

[67] Kino T, Hatanaka H, Hashimoto M, et al. FK-506, a novel immunosuppressant isolated from a Streptomyces. I. Fermentation, isolation, and physico-chemical and biological characteristics. J Antibiot (Tokyo) 1987;40(9):1249–55.

[68] Griffies JD, Mendelsohn CL, Rosenkrantz WS, et al. Topical 0.1% tacrolimus for the treatment of discoid lupus erythematosus and pemphigus erythematosus in dogs. J Am Anim Hosp Assoc 2004;40(1):29–41.

[69] Marsella R, Nicklin C. Investigation on the use of 0.3% tacrolimus lotion for canine atopic dermatitis: a pilot study. Vet Dermatol 2002;13(4):203–10.

[70] Lauerma AI, Surber C, Maibach HI. Absorption of topical tacrolimus (FK506) in vitro through human skin: comparison with cyclosporin A. Skin Pharmacol 1997;10(5–6): 230–4.

[71] Bieber T. Topical tacrolimus (FK 506): a new milestone in the management of atopic dermatitis. J Allergy Clin Immunol 1998;102(4 Pt 1):555–7.

[72] Rico MJ, Lawrence I. Tacrolimus ointment for the treatment of atopic dermatitis: clinical and pharmacologic effects. Allergy Asthma Proc 2002;23(3):191–7.

[73] Marsella R, Nicklin C, Saglio S, et al. Investigation on the effects of topical therapy with 0.1% tacrolimus ointment (Protopic) on intradermal skin test reactivity in atopic dogs. Vet Dermatol 2004;15(4):218–24.

[74] Misseghers B, Binnington A, Mathews K. Clinical observations of the treatment of canine perianal fistulas with topical tacrolimus in 10 dogs. Can Vet J 2000;41(8):623–7.

[75] Marsella R, Nicklin C, Saglio S, et al. Investigation on the clinical efficacy and safety of 0.1% tacrolimus ointment (Protopic) in canine atopic dermatitis: a randomized, double-blinded, placebo-controlled, cross-over study. Vet Dermatol 2004;15(5):294–303.

[76] Bensignor E, Olivry T. Treatment of localized lesions of canine atopic dermatitis with tacrolimus ointment: a blinded randomized controlled trial. Vet Dermatol 2005;16(1):52–60.

[77] Olivry T, Bloom P. Treatment of canine pemphigus foliaceus. Topeka (KS): Hill's Pet Nutrition; 2005.

[78] US Food and Drug Administration. FDA Public health advisory; March 10, 2005. Available at: www.fda.gov.

[79] Dean SR, Meola RW, Meola SM, et al. Mode of action of lufenuron in adult Ctenocephalides felis (Siphonaptera: Pulicidae). J Med Entomol 1999;36(4):486–92.

[80] Ben-Ziony Y, Arzi B. Use of lufenuron for treating fungal infections of dogs and cats: 297 cases (1997–1999). J Am Vet Med Assoc 2000;217(10):1510–3.

[81] Ben-Ziony Y, Arzi B. Updated information for treatment of fungal infections in cats and dogs [letter to the editor]. J Am Vet Med Assoc 2001;218(11):1718.

[82] Moriello K, Deboer D, Schenker R, et al. Efficacy of pre-treatment with lufenuron for the prevention of Microsporum canis infection in a feline direct topical challenge model. Vet Dermatol 2004;15(6):357–62.

[83] DeBoer DJ, Moriello KA, Blum JL, et al. Effects of lufenuron treatment in cats on the establishment and course of Microsporum canis infection following exposure to infected cats. J Am Vet Med Assoc 2003;222(9):1216–20.

[84] Moriello K. Treatment of dermatophytosis in dogs and cats: review of published studies. Vet Dermatol 2004;15(2):99–107.

[85] Hazen K. Fungicidal versus fungistatic activity of terbinafine and itraconazole: an in vitro comparison. J Am Acad Dermatol 1998;38(5 Pt 3):S37–41.

[86] Leyden J. Pharmacokinetics and pharmacology of terbinafine and itraconazole. J Am Acad Dermatol 1998;38(5 Pt 3):S42–7.

[87] Rashid A. New mechanisms of action with fungicidal antifungals. Br J Dermatol 1996;134(Suppl 46):1–6.

[88] Faergemann J, Zehender H, Denouel J, et al. Levels of terbinafine in plasma, stratum corneum, dermis-epidermis (without stratum corneum), sebum, hair and nails during and after 250 mg terbinafine orally once per day for four weeks. Acta Derm Venereol 1993;73(4):305–9.

[89] Colombo S, Hill P, Shaw D, et al. Effectiveness of low dose immunotherapy in the treatment of canine atopic dermatitis: a prospective, double-blinded, clinical study. Vet Dermatol 2005;16(3):162–70.

[90] Scott DW. Fungal skin disease. In: Scott D, Miller W, Griffin C, editors. Small animal dermatology. 6th edition. Philadelphia: WB Saunders; 2001. p. 336–422.

[91] Gupta A, Shear N. Terbinafine: an update. J Am Acad Dermatol 1997;37(6):979–88.

[92] Kovarik JM, Kirkesseli S, Humbert H, et al. Dose-proportional pharmacokinetics of terbinafine and its N-demethylated metabolite in healthy volunteers. Br J Dermatol 1992;126(Suppl 39):8–13.

[93] Chen C. The use of terbinafine for the treatment of dermatophytosis [abstract]. Vet Dermatol 2000;11(Suppl 1):41.

[94] Kotnik T. Drug efficacy of terbinafine hydrochloride (Lamisil) during oral treatment of cats experimentally infected with Microsporum canis. J Vet Med B Infect Dis Vet Public Health 2002;49(3):120–2.

[95] Guillot J, Bensignor E, Jankowski F, et al. Comparative efficacies of oral ketoconazole and terbinafine for reducing Malassezia population sizes on the skin of Basset Hounds. Vet Dermatol 2003;14(3):153–7.

[96] Shenep JL, English BK, Kaufman L, et al. Successful medical therapy for deeply invasive facial infection due to Pythium insidiosum in a child. Clin Infect Dis 1998;27(6):1388–93.

[97] Grooters A. New developments in oomycosis and zygomycosis. Presented at the 17th Annual Meeting of the American Academy of Veterinary Dermatology and American College of Veterinary Dermatology. New Orleans, LA, April 10–14, 2002.

[98] Mancianti F, Pedonese F, Millanta F, et al. Efficacy of oral terbinafine in feline dermatophytosis due to Microsporum canis. J Feline Med Surg 1999;1(1):37–41.

[99] de Jaham C, Paradis M, Papich MG. Antifungal dermatologic agents: azoles and allylamines. Compend Contin Educ Pract Vet 2000;22(6):548–59.

[100] Pfizer Animal Health Services. Technical monograph on cefpodoxime. New York: Pfizer Animal Health Services.

[101] Mason I, Kietzmann M. Cephalosporins—pharmacological basis of clinical use in veterinary dermatology. Vet Dermatol 1999;10:187–92.

[102] Caprile KA. The cephalosporin antimicrobial agents: a comprehensive review. J Vet Pharmacol Ther 1988;11(1):1–32.

[103] Spreng M, Deleforge J, Thomas V, et al. Antibacterial activity of marbofloxacin. A new fluoroquinolone for veterinary use against canine and feline isolates. J Vet Pharmacol Ther 1995;18(4):284–9.

[104] Thomas VM, Guillardeau LD, Thomas ER, et al. Update on the sensitivity of recent European canine and feline pathogens to marbofloxacin. Vet Q 1997;19(Suppl 1):S52–3.

[105] Lloyd D. Fluoroquinolone sensitivity among Pseudomonas aeruginosa isolate from canine skin and ears. In: Proceedings of the WSAVA, BSAVA, and the FECAVA World Congress. Birmingham, United Kingdom; 1997. p. 282.

[106] Ihrke P, Papich M, Demanuelle T. The use of fluoroquinolones in veterinary dermatology. Vet Dermatol 1999;10:193–204.

[107] Pfizer Animal Health Services. Technical monograph on marbofloxacin. Exton (PA): Pfizer Animal Health Services; 2004.

[108] Schneider M, Thomas V, Boisrame B, et al. Pharmacokinetics of marbofloxacin in dogs after oral and parenteral administration. J Vet Pharmacol Ther 1996;19(1):56–61.

[109] Frazier DL, Thompson L, Trettien A, et al. Comparison of fluoroquinolone pharmacokinetic parameters after treatment with marbofloxacin, enrofloxacin, and difloxacin in dogs. J Vet Pharmacol Ther 2000;23(5):293–302.

[110] Paradis M, Abbey L, Baker B, et al. Evaluation of the clinical efficacy of marbofloxacin (Zeniquin) tablets for the treatment of canine pyoderma: an open clinical trial. Vet Dermatol 2001;12(3):163–9.

[111] Carlotti DN, Guaguere E, Pin D, et al. Therapy of difficult cases of canine pyoderma with marbofloxacin: a report of 39 dogs. J Small Anim Pract 1999;40(6):265–70.

[112] Cotard JP, Gruet P, Pechereau D, et al. Comparative study of marbofloxacin and amoxicillin-clavulanic acid in the treatment of urinary tract infections in dogs. J Small Anim Pract 1995;36(8):349–53.

[113] Gough AW, Kasali OB, Sigler RE, et al. Quinolone arthropathy—acute toxicity to immature articular cartilage. Toxicol Pathol 1992;20(3 Pt 1):436–49. [discussion: 449–50].

[114] Nix DE, Watson WA, Lener ME, et al. Effects of aluminum and magnesium antacids and ranitidine on the absorption of ciprofloxacin. Clin Pharmacol Ther 1989;46(6):700–5.

[115] Pfizer Animal Health Services. Technical monograph on selamectin. Exton (PA): Pfizer Animal Health Services.

[116] Arena JP, Liu KK, Paress PS, et al. The mechanism of action of avermectins in Caenorhabditis elegans: correlation between activation of glutamate-sensitive chloride current, membrane binding, and biological activity. J Parasitol 1995;81(2):286–94.

[117] Chailleux N, Paradis M. Efficacy of selamectin in the treatment of naturally acquired chey-letiellosis in cats. Can Vet J 2002;43(10):767–70.

[118] Curtis C. Current trends in the treatment of Sarcoptes, Cheyletiella and Otodectes mite in-festations in dogs and cats. Vet Dermatol 2004;15(2):108–14.

[119] Pfizer Animal Health Services. Selamectin package insert. Exton (PA): Pfizer Animal Health Services; 2003.

[120] Scott DW. Parasitic skin diseases. In: Scott D, Miller W, Griffin C, editors. Small animal dermatology. 6th edition. Philadelphia: WB Saunders; 2001. p. 423–516.

[121] Goudie AC, Evans NA, Gration KA, et al. Doramectin—a potent novel endectocide. Vet Parasitol 1993;49(1):5–15.

[122] Clymer BC, Janes TH, McKenzie ME. Evaluation of the therapeutic and protective efficacy of doramectin against psoroptic scabies in cattle. Vet Parasitol 1997;72(1):79–89.

[123] Wicks SR, Kaye B, Weatherley AJ, et al. Effect of formulation on the pharmacokinetics and efficacy of doramectin. Vet Parasitol 1993;49(1):17–26.

[124] Delucchi L, Castro E. Use of doramectin for treatment of notoedric mange in five cats. J Am Vet Med Assoc 2000;216(2):193–216.

[125] Johnstone I. Doramectin as a treatment for canine and feline demodicosis. Aust Vet Pract 2002;32(3):98–103.

[126] Wagner R, Wendlberger U. Field efficacy of moxidectin in dogs and rabbits naturally in-fested with Sarcoptes spp., Demodex spp. and Psoroptes spp. mites. Vet Parasitol 2000;93(2):149–58.

[127] Bourdeau P. The probable role of environmental conditions in the efficacy of treatment of Otodectes cynotis infestation in dogs. An example with moxidectin (Cydectin®) in 60 dogs. Presented at the 15th Annual Congress of the European Society of Veterinary Der-matology/European College of Veterinary Dermatology. Maastricht, September 2–5, 1998.

[128] Bourdeau P, Chohen P. Evaluation of a 10% pyriproxyfen spot-on for the control of Oto-dectes cynotis in cats [abstract]. Vet Dermatol 2000;11(Suppl 1):58.

[129] Mueller R. Treatment protocols for demodicosis: an evidence-based review. Vet Dermatol 2004;15(2):75–89.

[130] Sushma C, Khahra S, Nauriyal D. Efficacy of ivermectin and moxidectin in treatment of ec-toparasitic infestation in dogs. Indian J Vet Med 2001;21:91–2.

[131] Bensignor E, Carlotti D. Moxidectin in the treatment of generalized demodicosis in the dog. A pilot study: 8 cases. In: Kwochka KW, Willemse T, Von Tscharner C, editors. Ad-vances in veterinary dermatology. Oxford, United Kingdom: Butterworth-Heinemann; 1998. p. 554–5.

[132] Burrows A. Evaluation of the clinical efficacy of two different doses of moxidectin in the treatment of generalized demodicosis in the dog. Presented at the Annual Meeting of the American Academy of Veterinary Dermatology and American College of Veterinary Dermatology. Nashville, TN, April 17–20, 1997.

Skin Diseases of Animals in Shelters: Triage Strategy and Treatment Recommendations for Common Diseases

Sandra Newbury, DVM[a],*, Karen A. Moriello, DVM[b]

[a]Director of Animal Medical Services, Dane County Humane Society, 5132 Voges Road, Madison, WI 53718–6941, USA
[b]Department of Medical Sciences, School of Veterinary Medicine, University of Wisconsin–Madison, 2015 Linden Drive, West Madison, WI 53706, USA

D ermatology is an important medical specialty in animal shelters for many reasons. First, many skin diseases are infectious or contagious, and core knowledge of these diseases is needed by veterinarians caring for shelter animals so as to prevent outbreaks and spread of zoonotic diseases. Second, the general appearance of the animal influences adoption decisions by potential new owners. Finally, many skin diseases of dogs and cats are manageable but not curable. The care needed to manage some of these diseases often exceeds many well-intentioned owners' capabilities, resulting in the surrender of many animals because of chronic skin diseases. Also, many "severe" skin cases may be nothing more than a manageable chronic skin disease that has relapsed. Lack of simple dermatologic treatments often gives the mistaken impression that the animal is not a suitable pet. A basic knowledge of the common skin diseases seen in animal shelters and how to triage and sort out these animals can greatly enhance their opportunities for rehoming.

The culture and environment of shelters differ greatly from those of private practice. Also, animals presented to shelters often come with little or no historical information. This article is divided into three sections. Part 1 is a "primer" on dermatology in shelter medicine. Part 2 outlines a triage approach to identifying common diseases. Finally, in part 3, treatment options for the most common diseases or diseases unique to shelters are discussed. These recommendations are based on collaborative work conducted by the authors at the Dane County Humane Society in Wisconsin.

*Corresponding author.

0195-5616/06/$ – see front matter
doi:10.1016/j.cvsm.2005.09.007

DERMATOLOGIC SHELTER MEDICINE PRIMER
Contagion, Zoonoses, and Herd Health
Implementation of an effective infectious disease control plan

Several contagious and zoonotic dermatologic disorders seen less frequently in private practice may be quite common in animal shelters. Shelters have a public responsibility to protect the community from potential zoonoses spread by animals in foster care or animals adopted from the shelter. From a public health standpoint, zoonoses should be the highest priority for disease prevention. Shelters must also limit spread of disease from animal to animal so that animals coming into the shelter can stay healthy enough to be adopted and limited resources can be conserved rather than spent on outbreak management.

Although these treatable dermatologic conditions rarely cause mortality in house pets, in shelters that must euthanize responsibly to maintain a healthy population, animals with infectious, although treatable, conditions are often those selected for euthanasia. The beauty of an infectious disease control plan is that by controlling infectious disease, shelter managers or veterinarians rather than infectious agents are able to select which animals to place up for adoption.

Because infectious dermatologic diseases as well as other infectious systemic diseases cause such a high rate of morbidity and mortality in animal shelters, there is a pressing need to introduce and evaluate infectious disease control plans. Implementing an infectious disease control plan requires an understanding of the factors affecting immunity, exposure, infection, and cure. The importance of each of these causative factors may vary from shelter to shelter.

Management of infectious disease within an animal shelter is small animal population medicine and follows a production medicine model. The product is healthy animals adopted into loving homes [1]. Production can be measured by the save rate. The save rate reflects the number of animals admitted to the shelter that were returned to their owners or adopted into homes. The save rate is the positive counterpart of the euthanasia rate [2]. An animal cannot be included in the save rate until an outcome is finalized, however. In other words, if an animal is still in the shelter contributing to the population, it should not yet be considered saved. An effective plan should positively affect the save rate through increased successful adoptions, more efficient use of resources, improved staff and volunteer morale, and better public relations.

In a typical production model, individual animal value is tied to production. In many shelters, the value of individual animals is determined, in large part, by temperament or emotional attachment of staff and volunteers. In the production model, investment of resources is based on the likelihood of future production, whereas in a shelter, financial decisions may be based on public relations or staff morale. In some cases, it is a sick or injured animal that may bring in the most resources to the organization. Although, ultimately, it is the admission and adoption rates that mathematically determine the save rate, public relations, staff morale, and volunteer participation dramatically affect the resources available [3]. Staff and volunteer compliance can often make or break implementation of an infectious disease control plan.

Management decisions in animal shelters may be fraught with conflict. Changes are often made based on anecdotal information and evaluated based on unsupported impressions. Evidence-based medicine is the ideal means of decision making; however, there is little literature specific to naturally occurring disease in animal shelters. Many shelters cannot find the time to track and evaluate changes that are implemented. Because of population dynamics, animal shelters present unique and difficult challenges in the area of infectious disease. An infectious disease plan, careful monitoring, and assessment of results can conserve resources and optimize the save rate. A plan to control infectious disease may be the most beneficial act a veterinarian can contribute to homeless animals.

Admission as the control point for infectious disease
Admission is the control point for infectious disease. Many of the primary infectious or contagious disorders that should be monitored for and treated at admission to an animal shelter affect the skin. Dermatophytosis and external parasites are the most common zoonotic skin diseases of small animals in animal shelters [4]. Identifying resources to screen for and control infectious dermatologic disease at the point of entry to the shelter can conserve resources by preventing outbreaks. In most cases, the cost of preventative treatment is minimal in comparison to the resources expended when a contagious disease spreads throughout a shelter. When implementing an infectious disease control plan for an animal shelter, it is crucial to evaluate the available resources and budget and to prioritize what is needed for admitting animals safely to the animal shelter. The budget must be based on a protocol that lay staff or admitting technicians can understand and follow (Table 1).

In this example, testing for feline leukemia virus (FeLV) and feline immunodeficiency virus (FIV) is included in the costs. FeLV and FIV testing almost doubles the cost of admission. An argument could be made that when resources are limited, because of the relative risk of contagion in caged housing,

Table 1
Admitting cost breakdown example

Feline	Cost
Eclipse 3	$1.19
Heska Feline Ultra Intranasal	$2.00
Revolution >5 lb cats	$6.37
Revolution <5 lb cats	
Fungal culture	$3.00
Toothbrush	$0.20
FeLV/FIV test	$8.99
Strongid, pyrantel pamoate qt ($0.024/mL)	$0.02
Total	$21.77

Abbreviations: FeLV, feline leukemia virus; FIV, feline immunodeficiency virus.

testing for FeLV and FIV at admission, which may be common shelter practice, is less of a priority than testing for dermatophytosis. Although testing for FeLV and FIV is a key component of adoption decision making, unrecognized dermatophytosis, which is spread more readily by fomite transmission, may be a far greater risk to the individuals making up the population as a whole.

In many cases, admission is the closest thing to a fixed cost that a shelter may have, because each animal is given the same treatments according to a set protocol. Many shelters have a fairly constant admission rate. It is wise to plan for a slight increase in admissions each year. Even though there has been an overall national downward trend in shelter admissions in the last 10 years, shelters in many regions may continue to experience increases [5]. Having a set protocol allows protection with a margin for error, because many dermatologic diseases are difficult to diagnose. Although technicians or admitting staff may recognize disease effectively, a preventative protocol can protect against unseen disorders. Protocols may vary depending on the availability of isolation and quarantine facilities within the shelter or trained foster homes. Open-admission shelters (ie, shelters that do not turn animals away) with a higher turnover are likely to expend more resources at admission than limited-admission shelters, but screening is equally important.

Considerations for Monitoring and Treating Skin Disease in a Shelter Setting

As mentioned previously, infectious disease is often the primary consideration for treating and monitoring skin disease in the shelter setting. Although "recognize and euthanize" policies (RE) are commonly and responsibly implemented as a means of controlling infectious diseases, in some cases, because of issues with staff and volunteer compliance and public relations, treatment protocols may actually be a more effective tool. One example of this is dermatophytosis. This disease targets the most adoptable and gregarious population of cats. In our shelter, generalized reluctance to comply with an RE policy led to failure to control this disease when compared with the success of a screening and treatment protocol [6].

Shelters are staffed primarily with lay people. Medical training and experience vary widely from shelter to shelter. Although some shelters may have veterinary staff regularly at the shelter, others may have a part-time veterinarian, a consulting veterinarian from private practice, fee for service, or no veterinary care [7]. In every case, veterinary care is at a premium.

Training and advice on protocols may be the most important assistance a veterinarian can give an animal shelter. Treatment protocols should be set in writing with clear case definitions and clinical signs that help staff to identify the target disease and use the appropriate treatment. Clear written protocols are essential to any admitting or medical plan and must include any special information, including weight, health, or age restrictions, for treatments that may be indicated. A complete plan should include where to house animals, alternative treatments, follow-up treatment schedules, and what to do if an animal cannot be treated. Because dermatologic conditions are so visible, a color atlas or set of "classic pictures" can be an invaluable aid to lay staff. Specific staff members should be identified and trained to use each protocol before it is implemented. Because veterinary care is often a scarce resource at shelters, effective protocols allow staff to monitor or treat many more readily identifiable conditions (eg, ear mite infestations, flea infestations), saving veterinary time for herd health management or animals with less well-defined dermatologic disorders.

Resources: Choose Your Battles

Shelter resources are rarely unlimited. Adoptive homes as well as money for medical treatments are commonly in short supply. Implementing guidelines to determine which dermatologic conditions are to be treated is a helpful way of organizing expenditures. It is often the case that because of the mathematic difference between the numbers of animals coming into a shelter and the numbers of animals being adopted that euthanasia is an inevitable and responsible choice for some animals. By limiting the population density within a shelter, the health of the individuals making up the group may be protected. When making such difficult decisions, it may be best to prioritize treatment efforts for skin diseases that (1) affect otherwise adoptable animals, (2) have a generally good prognosis for complete resolution, and (3) have limited impediments to adoption after treatment. Risk of contagion as well as cost and duration of treatment must also be considered.

Examples of conditions that are generally less practical to treat in a shelter setting are definitively diagnosed immune-mediated diseases, deep pyoderma, and demodicosis in dogs older than 1 year of age. Because generalized demodicosis is known to have a heritable component in its pathogenesis, it is especially important to spay or neuter dogs with a known history of demodicosis before adoption. In addition, it is important to spay or neuter breeds in which this disease is common. Breed predilections may vary by region; in our area, demodicosis is most common in Pit Bull Terriers. Animals with complicated or multiple problems or with endocrine diseases, such as hyperadrenocorticism, that are difficult to treat or work up may also be chosen for euthanasia. External parasites and uncomplicated dermatophytosis are examples of conditions with a good prognosis if they can be treated appropriately in the shelter setting.

Compliance

Guidelines instituted with no flexibility for individual animals may be met with great resistance. Leaving room for a few special cases improves staff and volunteer morale and compliance as well as improving public relations. Without "buy in" from staff and volunteers, protocols are unlikely to succeed.

Animal Care Days and Housing as It Relates to Skin Diseases

Animal care days may be one the greatest expenses encountered when treating skin disease in a shelter setting. (An animal care day is the calculated cost of keeping an individual animal in the shelter.) Many times, an ongoing diet trial or diagnostic response to treatment causes an impediment to adoption for an animal. Many potential owners are willing to take on dermatologic problems but not when they are uncertain of the diagnosis. If treatment is going to be long term and an animal is not likely to be adopted or would not be made available for adoption until treatment is completed, it becomes important to consider the stress of long-term shelter housing. Unlike the case in owned animals in private practice, where animal care days are less of an issue, more frequent rechecks (eg, days versus weeks) for shelter animals with skin disease are often more cost-effective than prolonged treatment. In some cases, the shelter environment may exacerbate an existing skin condition through increased humidity, irritant contact, kennel flooring, difficulties with compliance, or stress. Developing a network of foster parents who are trained and willing to provide medical treatments and care for animals can be a viable alternative to treating animals in the shelter. Trained foster parents can function as reliable advocates for the animal and provide feedback and progress reports on treatments and clinical signs. Because of the emotional bond that develops between the animal and the foster parent, foster homes are best used for animals in need of care with a favorable prognosis for adoption. The best way to develop a successful network of foster homes is to move animals effectively through the system. An animal in foster care that cannot be made available for adoption is a disheartening experience for the foster family.

Rescue Opportunities

There are often several rescue groups in the community that are willing to take on animals with special circumstances making them difficult to place or difficult to treat in a shelter. Rescue groups can be a great alternative for animals that do not quite fit into treatment guidelines. There are different types of rescue groups. Many established rescue groups are breed specific. More recently, newer rescue groups have sprung up with the primary goal of supporting their local shelters by taking difficult-to-treat or difficult-to-place animals and finding homes through their own networks. Good communication and relationships with rescue groups can help to conserve resources and may improve the save rate for the shelter.

Many veterinarians in private practice are asked to work with rescue groups. All the dermatologic conditions described as commonly seen in shelter animals are also seen in the rescue population. When consulting or working with rescue groups or individuals, it is important to remember that they need to consider themselves like shelters with respect to infectious disease control. Veterinarians who work with rescue groups should keep in mind the diseases of shelter animals. Although in some cases, the shelter the animals are rescued from may have taken first steps to help control contagion, in other cases, unfortunately, the animal's first stop at the shelter may have caused exposure and increased risk. Families associated with rescue groups should not assume that the shelter has treated or screened an animal for contagious or infectious diseases. Considerations for treating skin disease in a rescue setting are similar to those within the shelter, but drug licensing likely varies. Because many rescue groups are breed-related caregivers, they are often well informed, or opinionated, about breed-related disorders.

Surrender Reasons

Because the skin is so visible, owners often notice skin diseases long before they become aware of other illnesses. In our experience, skin disease is a common reason for relinquishment to our shelter. Although often treatable or curable, dermatoses may lead to euthanasia if an owner becomes frustrated with chronic care, disappointed in an animal's appearance, or overwhelmed by medical expenses. "Not enough time" and "cost" are among the most frequently cited reasons for surrender [2].

Neglected Patients

Dermatologic neglect is commonly seen in surrendered animals as well as in stray animals. Neglect may include but is not limited to pododermatitis caused by improper housing or hard kennel flooring; injuries caused by spike collars or tight collars or friction injuries from collars or halters; fight or bite wound injuries; rubber band, string, or collar injuries; "burdock granuloma tongue" with associated lip granulomas and dental disease; abscesses or pyoderma caused by severe hair coat matting (Fig. 1); myiasis; and chronic urinary or fecal scalding. Diseases of neglect are easily overlooked in the ears and mouth.

Cruelty and neglect often seem to be unintentional. Many owners call in to report their lost animal and happily describe neglected conditions as part of the pet's general appearance. Some seemingly neglected pets are surrendered to the shelter with a long medical history. Often, animals have been improperly treated or poorly diagnosed as a result of financial decisions made by the owners. Other times, diagnostic or treatment choices seem to have been made inappropriately. Some owners surrender the animal after they believe they have exhausted every possible treatment option.

Cruelty and neglect cases should be carefully documented with medical records and photographs to serve as a legal record. Education is a crucial component when neglected animals are returned to their owners. Documentation

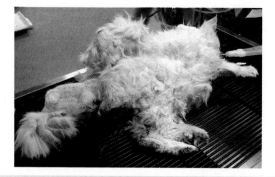

Fig. 1. Severe hair coat matting in a cat because of neglect.

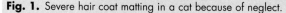

may serve to sway the owner to be more dutiful in his or her care if the animal is redeemed, or it may be crucial evidence if the situation warrants legal action against the owner. In some cases, animals reunited with their owners may be accompanied by abatement orders and requirements to seek appropriate veterinary care. Veterinarians and humane officers must work closely with local authorities to institute and enforce these protections for owned animals.

Private practitioners function as the first defense animals have against neglect. Veterinarians who are willing to tell owners that they are not appropriately caring for their pet can help to educate owners and protect pets from harm, which, once chronic, may be irreversible. Veterinarians should understand what constitutes neglect under local law and what resources are available for follow-up in such cases.

Medical History

Addressing and reporting the dermatologic medical history from previous veterinarians and medical staff at the animal shelter are other crucial components of a successful adoption. Health waivers are documents given to potential adopters as a means of describing particular medical conditions. Signing a health waiver indicates that the adopter has been informed of the special needs of his or her new pet. Addressing the previous medical history of surrendered animals may be more complicated. Although it is important to provide previous medical records to new adopters when available, it is also possible for veterinarians working with the shelter to provide a second opinion if clinical signs presented while at the shelter point to alternative diagnoses.

When reporting medical history, it may be tempting to minimize the consequences of clinical conditions. Everyone wants to see animals adopted into loving homes. Accurate and realistic reporting is the most effective means of successfully rehoming animals. Information given to potential adopters before adoption allows them to make informed choices that make relinquishment and disappointment less likely. New adopters take their new pet and its medical records to a veterinarian in practice. Winning the respect of local veterinarians influences them to encourage shelter adoption and assist their local shelter.

Adopter's View: Why Treat Skin Disease?

Shelter animals must sell themselves to potential adopters. Although most of us are taught to never judge a book by its cover, skin and hair coat are one of the first things new adopters may notice about a shelter animal. Although there is an occasional adopter coming to the shelter hoping to rescue the most pathetic looking creature he or she can find, in most cases, adopters are interested in finding a cute healthy animal they can take home to be their pet. The shelter's job is to help animals put their best face forward while, at the same time, informing potential adopters what issues or problems they may face with their new pet so that they can make informed choices about which animal may be the best match for their experience, time, family, and budget. Careful matchmaking improves the likelihood of a successful placement. Each successful placement is positive public relations for the shelter. Positive public relations within the community help to increase the available resources and adoption rate, and thus the save rate for the other animals in the shelter.

Chronic Dermatoses and Matchmaking: Finding the Right Owner for That Skin

Animals with chronic or hereditary skin diseases may not seem adoptable; however, there is a segment of the pet-owning population that is willing to adopt these animals for many reasons. For example, one of the authors had a client actively search shelters and rescue groups for a dog with ichthyosis because the client had that disease. Shelters may consider posting animals with special needs on a web site to help find that "special owner."

WORKING WITH DERMATOLOGY PATIENTS WHEN ALL YOU HAVE IS THE SKIN

Unlike private practice, shelter dermatology must be practiced more with one's eyes and clinical acumen than with benefit of the animal's history. Obviously, this is not the optimum situation, but it is possible to use the skin and common diagnostic tests as a "questionnaire." The following summarizes our approach to working with shelter animals with skin disease.

Figure 2 is a visual flow chart of "if you see this…think." Box 1 is a list of common differential diagnoses for skin conditions presented at admission. Table 2 is a list of basic in-house diagnostic tests that can be used to help make a diagnosis. This latter section is brief, and more detailed explanations of how to perform and interpret these diagnostic tests can be found in other sources [8].

Quick Unbiased Assessment of Chemical Kickback

Obviously, it is always best to treat according to a clear diagnosis. Sometimes, even with the aid of many tables and a long list of differential diagnoses, a diagnosis cannot be made. Clinical trials for response to therapy may be a reasonable way to proceed, taking into consideration that average treatment days are likely to be longer, and risk of contagion may be higher, when treating without a definitive diagnosis. Treatment trials should be targeted toward likely diagnoses as determined by potential rule outs. For example, if a dog has crusty ear tips and multifocal erythema as well as crusting, scaling, and pruritic alopecia, it is reasonable to treat for scabies even if no mites can be found. It is well known that for scabies, the absence of mites on a scraping does not rule out their presence. In shelters, secondary skin infections are common and underdiagnosed. Serious consideration should be given in this type of patient to treat concurrently for secondary infections. The bottom line is that respond-to-treatment trials, or quick unbiased assessments of chemical kickback (QUACKs), are not all bad, especially when treatment decisions may literally be a life or death decision. If the QUACK approach seems appropriate for a case, be sure to record what question you are trying to answer with your treatment trial. In other words, if it works, what was the most likely diagnosis, and if it does not work, what was ruled out and what is the next step?

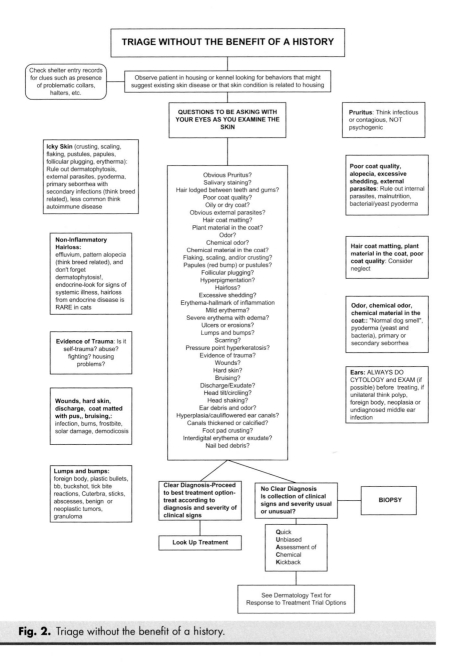

Fig. 2. Triage without the benefit of a history.

TREATMENT PROTOCOLS FOR COMMON SKIN DISEASES AND DISEASES WORTH SPECIAL MENTION

The scope of this article does not allow for a detailed discussion of the treatment of all of the diseases a shelter veterinarian may encounter. The reader is referred to *Mueller and Kirk's Small Animal Dermatology* [9] for the most complete review of specific diseases and treatment options. The books that are most useful on a day-to-day basis are problem-oriented textbooks or texts with concise formats and color pictures, however. Two excellent and affordable resources are the *BSAVA Manual of Small Animal Dermatology* [10] and *Small Animal Dermatology: A Color Atlas and Therapeutics Guide* [11].

The recommendations here are those in use at the Dane Country Humane Society and those that the authors find clinically most effective. In selecting treatment protocols, we focus on therapies that are aggressive and decrease "animal medical care days" so that the patient can return to the adoptable population as soon as possible. We respect the fact that others may disagree with our treatment suggestions; use what works best in your particular situation. More detailed discussions of treatment options can be found in the texts mentioned previously. This discussion focuses on diseases that represent a contagious risk to the general population or a zoonotic risk to employees or potential adopters, diseases for which the outcome is positive, and diseases for which immediate and aggressive intervention is needed to save the animal or stabilize it during the stray holding period (see the article in this issue by Moriello and Newbury on recommendations for the management and treatment of dermatophytosis in animal shelters).

Safely Using Glucocorticoids in the Treatment of Skin Disease in a Shelter

The most difficult transition for one of the authors (KM) from a specialty private practice to shelter medicine dermatology was the inability to use glucocorticoids as part of routine therapy for many diseases. The use of systemic glucocorticoids in a shelter patient is always a difficult decision. In general, both authors avoid using systemic glucocorticoids if an alternative can be found. In some cases (eg, severe otitis externa/media), there may be no better option given that relief of discomfort and resolution of the infection as quickly as possible is the goal. Most ear cases resolve well with deep ear cleaning or middle ear irrigation, appropriate topical and systemic steroids, and systemic antibiotics. Animals needing prolonged anti-inflammatory or immunosuppressive doses of glucocorticoids are best treated in foster care, where they are less stressed and not constantly bombarded by infectious and contagious agents. With that said, we have had few if any problems associated with the use of topical glucocorticoids (otic treatments, lotions, or sprays) for treatments or when humane relief is needed. One of the most beneficial but easily overlooked treatments for pruritus is bathing and, if necessary, topical lime sulfur (LymDyp; DVM Pharmaceuticals, Inc., St. Joseph, Missouri) for its antipruritic benefit. Other topical leave-on rinses (eg, Resicort Leave on Conditioner; Virbac Animal Health, Peakhurst, NSW, Australia) with antipruritic benefits are often helpful but tend to be cost-prohibitive in a shelter unless donated.

Box 1: Problem-oriented differential diagnosis of skin diseases seen in animal shelters[a]

Odor
- Normal pet odor
- Oral: rule out uremia, foreign body, dental disease, lip fold pyoderma, oral injuries, and calicivirus
- Ear disease
- Feces or urine
- Fold infections (axillary, inguinal, or perineal)
- Whole body: secondary bacterial and yeast infections with or without the rancid smell of seborrhea
- Neglect (eg, matted hair coat, urine or fecal scalding)
- Undetected injuries
- Abscesses with or without maggots

Crusting and scaling throughout the hair coat but spares the footpads and nose
- Bacterial and yeast pyoderma
- Primary disorders of keratinization
- *Cheyletiella* or *Sarcoptes* infestation
- Poor nutrition
- Poor coat quality: almost always associated with secondary infections

Crusting or scaling involving the face, ears, nose, or footpads
- Breed-related nasodigital crusting caused by a primary disorder of keratinization
- Digital hyperkeratosis caused by lameness and abnormal pad wear
- Dermatophytosis
- Demodicosis
- Zinc deficiency, especially in sled dogs or puppies
- Hepatocutaneous syndrome
- Norwegian scabies (large numbers of mites causing severe scaling and crusting)
- Pemphigus complex

Oily skin with or without odor
- Bacterial and yeast pyoderma in dogs or cats
- Poor grooming in cats
- Primary disorders of keratinization with or without secondary infections

- Underlying endocrine disorders with or without secondary infections
- Older cat: consider feline hyperthyroidism

Malodorous ears
- Seborrheic otitis externa with or without secondary bacterial and yeast infections: dog is usually grossly seborrheic
- Severe otitis externa/media caused by mixed infections with yeast, cocci, and rods
- Undiagnosed middle ear infections
- Foreign body and secondary infections
- Ear polyps and secondary infections
- Neoplasia (rarely)

Whole-body pruritus
- Mild: bacterial pyoderma, dermatophytosis, demodicosis, lice, or flea infestation
- Moderate: cheyletiellosis, bacterial and yeast infections, lice, fur mites, flea infestation, allergy (atopy or food allergy), insect bite hypersensitivity, or contact allergy (especially after shampoo therapy)
- Severe: feline demodicosis, *Sarcoptes* infestations in dogs, *Notoedres* concurrent yeast and bacterial infections of dogs, flea allergy dermatitis, "mad itch of cats," pyotraumatic dermatitis, "eosinophilic plaques" of cats, or atopy or food allergy in some animals

Pruritic ears or face
- Ear mites: pruritus can be mild to severe from overt infestation or hypersensitivity reaction
- Flea infestation in cats
- Yeast otitis: yeast is a significant finding in a symptomatic animal and needs to be treated
- Feline demodicosis: young cats, found on cytology
- Sarcoptes: pruritic ear margins or positive "pruritic ear flap test" result
- Insect bite hypersensitivity
- Allergic otitis in dogs or cats
- Chin acne in cats

Inflammatory hair loss (eg, scales, crust, erythema, broken hairs, salivary staining)
- Focal: dermatophytosis, demodicosis, or bacterial pyoderma

(continued on next page)

Box 1 (continued)

- Multifocal or diffuse patchy hair loss: demodicosis, bacterial and yeast pyoderma, dermatophytosis, or primary seborrheic disorders with secondary infections
- Generalized: demodicosis, dermatophytosis, bacterial or yeast pyoderma, primary seborrheic disorders with secondary infections, feline symmetric alopecia, atopic dermatitis or food allergy, or epitheliotropic lymphoma

Noninflammatory hair loss

- Focal area: dermatophytosis, adverse reaction to topical spot-on parasiticidal agents, feline or canine demodicosis, scar, steroid injection or vaccine vasculitis, postclipping alopecia, or traction alopecia (alopecia in areas in which ribbons or rubber bands have been placed)
- Multifocal or diffuse patchy hair loss: follicular dysplasia, keratinization defects, color dilution alopecia, or dermatomyositis
- Generalized or symmetric: endocrine disorders (hypothyroidism or hyperadrenocorticism), pattern baldness and/or follicular dysplasia, congential alopecia, effluviums, color dilution alopecia, or feline symmetric alopecia syndrome

"Hard skin or fur"

- Matting of the hair coat because of neglect or poor grooming
- Matting of the hair coat because of accumulations of skin exudate from a focal or generalized deep pyoderma
- Burn eschar: there is often a lag time between exposure to a heat source and development of clinical signs
- Chin, lip, or lineal lesions on caudal thighs or hard plaque-like area in a cat: "true eosinophilic granuloma"
- Calcinosis cutis (this can be focal or generalized) in an adult dog
- Calcinosis cutis in a puppy: found coincidentally in young dogs with acute onset of severe illness
- Dystrophic mineralization caused by trauma
- Focal calcification in pad or on flexor surface: calcinosis circumscripta
- Calcified ear canal: "end-stage ear disease" caused by chronic otitis

Ulcers and erosions

- Mucocutaneous ulceration on lips or nose-lip fold pyoderma, yeast pyoderma and secondary trauma, eosinophilic feline lip ulcers, intranasal vaccine reaction (cats), respiratory disease complex, or viral infections
- Nasal or facial ulceration: nasal pyoderma, eosinophilic furunculosis, insect bite hypersensitivity, trauma, vaccine reaction, thermal injury (cats), neoplasia (squamous cell carcinoma, lymphoma), or immune-mediated disease (rare)
- Multiple sites of mucocutaneous ulcerations (rare): drug reactions or immune-mediated diseases

- Focal ulceration: pyotraumatic dermatitis, "eosinophilic plaque" in cats, fungal kerion, thermal burn or clipper burn, or sporotrichosis (cat)
- Large areas of ulceration or erosion: generalized deep pyoderma, generalized demodicosis, systemic fungal infections (eg, sporotrichosis), thermal injuries, physical trauma (eg, automobile, collar), chemical burn, or immune-mediated diseases
- Ulceration in axillary, inguinal, or genital fold area: bacterial or yeast infections (fold pyoderma), urine or fecal scald, trauma from halter harness, or clipper burns
- Thermal injuries from clipping are underrecognized and may take weeks to become evident

Nail or paw abnormalities
- Individual nail injury: trauma
- Corkscrew nails or brittle nails with or without inflammation around nailbed: dermatophytosis
- Sloughing or soft nails, with dog usually being painful or lame: lupoid nail dystrophy (dogs)
- Worn bloody nails in a cat: trauma, especially if cat was captured in live trap
- "Claw like horn on foot pad": cutaneous horn or callous, especially in cats

Pad or interdigital lesions
- Swollen purple pads in a cat: insect bite hypersensitivity reaction or plasma cell pododermatitis
- Bleeding interdigital areas in a dog: interdigital abscesses
- Chronic recurrent interdigital abscesses or infection
- Focal hard interdigital nodule: previous site of foreign body reaction or interdigital abscess
- Pruritic foot chewing: *Malassezia, Pelodera,* or hookworm dermatitis
- Erythematous ventral pads: irritant reactions or contact allergies, atopic dermatitis, or yeast or bacterial infections

Lumps and bumps
- Three major causes of lumps or bumps: infection, granuloma, or tumor (malignant or benign)
- Fluctuant lumps in kittens: after vaccination, *Cuterebra*
- Hard lumps on chin, lip, ears, or backs of legs in young cats: eosinophilic granulomas
- Pea-sized lumps: tick bite reactions in dogs or cats, inclusion cysts, lead or steel shot, or tumor
- Plastic bullets, reactions to microchip

(continued on next page)

Box 1 (*continued*)

- Large masses that exude blackish gray material: inclusion cyst
- Large mass that is cool to the touch or seems to be developing slowly: fungal or bacterial granuloma, scar tissue site, tumor, or lick granuloma
- Large mass that is painful or warm to touch: infection, fungal kerion, foreign body, or tumor

Pigment change

- Depigmented lesions are rarely a concern in shelter animals, with a few exceptions.
- Any dog presented with depigmented mucocutaneous areas should be examined immediately for signs of uveitis. These are key findings in uveodermatologic syndrome that can lead to blindness if the uveitis is left untreated. This disease is most common in sled dog breeds.
- Depigmented focal sites are usually the result of trauma or idiopathic vaccine reactions. Seasonal depigmentation on the nose of dogs is common. A congenital or hereditary disease usually causes widespread depigmentation. These do not present a risk to other shelter animals.
- Hyperpigmentation is a common finding, is a sign of chronicity, and is caused by inflammation (or possibly normal skin color).
- Flat patches with well-demarcated borders: normal pigmentation, especially in orange cats
- Raised or thickened areas: nevus or tumor for which fine needle aspirate or biopsy is indicated
- Hyperpigmentation associated with inflammation or crusting demodicosis, dermatophytosis (especially in cats), or bacterial pyoderma lesions
- Lacy hyperpigmentation in axilla or groin or on ears: most commonly caused by inflammation secondary to atopic dermatitis

Fragile or easily bruised skin

- Feline hyperadrenocorticism: rare disease of older cats
- Cutaneous asthenia: animal is usually young and skin is stretchy
- Idiopathic feline fragility skin syndrome
- Canine hyperadrenocorticism
- Excessive exogenous glucocorticoid use

Skin diseases associated with signs of systemic illness (fever, depression, pain, and anorexia)

- Canine demodicosis with secondary deep bacterial infection
- Severe otitis externa or media
- Panniculitis
- Immune-mediated diseases (eg, pemphigus, bullous pemphigoid, lupus, toxic epidermal necrolysis)

- Hepatocutaneous syndrome
- Juvenile cellulitis
- Feline herpes or calicivirus infections with skin involvement

[a]Unless otherwise noted, the list applies to dogs and cats. The list is not intended to be all-inclusive but, instead, focuses on those diseases commonly encountered in shelters.

Clinical Infestations with Fleas, Ticks, Lice, or *Cheyletiella* Mites

Fleas and ticks are best prevented at admission via the use of spot-on therapies (fipronil, selamectin, or imidacloprid). Animals with clinical infestations are best treated via whole-body application of a topical flea spray and an oral dose of nitenpyram, because there is a lag time of approximately 24 hours before spot-on therapies are maximally effective. There are pros and cons to the use of all spot-on therapies. The spot-on treatment of choice is shelter specific, and factors like cost, regional flea and tick burden, and heartworm risk factor into what is best to use. Lice, fleas, ticks, and *Cheyletiella* mites are highly contagious and, with the exception of lice, zoonotic. Treatment for lice and *Cheyletiella* mites in a shelter must be focused on the most rapid kill of adults and removal of eggs, with the latter being attached to hairs. It is important to remember that any therapy that does not coat the hair coat cannot kill migrating parasites or parasites in egg sacs. These hatchlings are only killed after they emerge and come into contact with the skin. Given that most problematic parasites generally have a 3- to 4-week lifespan, at least two treatments of topical spot-on therapies are needed. During this time, lack of whole-body treatment puts other animals at risk for contagion. Animals with contagious parasites should be isolated.

The most effective and rapid resolution of these infestations occurs with aggressive topical parasiticidal therapy for at least 4 weeks, or 1 week longer than the parasite's life cycle. In private practice, the rule of thumb is to treat for at least two life cycles, or 6 weeks, but this is not practical or possible in many shelters. In a shelter, it is ideal if animals can be bathed to facilitate mechanical removal of gross ectoparasites. Clipping of the hair coat is helpful in the treatment of *Cheyletiella* mites and lice because these parasites deposit their eggs on the hair shafts. In all cases, the initial treatment of choice is whole-body application of a parasiticidal agent, such as fipronil spray (Frontline; Merial, Duluth, Georgia), lime sulfur (8 oz/gal), or a flea spray labeled as safe to use on kittens and puppies. The key to eradication is a follow-up therapy, such as weekly lime sulfur for 4 to 6 weeks, biweekly fipronil sprays, or biweekly treatments of a spot-on flea control product. Permethrins are toxic to cats, and serious consideration should be given to not stocking products containing this insecticide in a shelter so as to minimize the potential for accidental poisoning of cats. All in-contact animals should be treated. With regard to environmental decontamination, routine cleaning of the environment should be adequate. If there is

Table 2
In-house diagnostic tests for shelter animals with skin disease

Test	Key points	Comments
Key in-house diagnostic tests at admission		
Fungal culture	Prompt sampling for fungal culture at admission provides a solid rule-out for a pathologic condition that may look like or exacerbate many others Early identification Most positive fungal cultures are identifiable in 7–10 days, some as early as 5–7 days In a study by the authors of more than 4000 fungal cultures from cats, all untreated fungal infections were identified within 10 days of inoculation	Hair loss in dogs is more commonly related to pyoderma or *Demodex* than to dermatophytosis Fungal kerion reactions are seen more commonly in dogs
Flea dirt test, flea combing	Black pepper–like material from the hair coat that turns red on wet gauze or white paper towel Flea combings are helpful to find lice, *Cheyletiella* mites, ticks, and other macroparasites If you find a flea infestation, consider PCV/total protein (see below)	Flea-allergic dogs and cats often do not have large numbers of fleas on their coat, treat anyway
PCV/total protein	Rule out blood loss anemia secondary to external parasites	Especially important in young puppies, kittens, and debilitated animals
Ear swab with mineral oil for mites	Ear swabs can identify ear mites, ear mite eggs, and *Demodex* mites	For ear mites, one egg or ear mite is compatible with an infestation, treat
5-minute itch watch	A 3–5-minute observation of a cat in its cage may help to differentiate those cats that are truly pruritic and uncomfortable Watching quietly for a few minutes while the cat is relaxed may give more answers than an examination Check feces for excessive hair, monitor cat for hair balls or constipation	

Table 2
(continued)

Test	Key points	Comments
Diagnostic tests if skin problem is identified		
Transparent cellulose adhesive scotch tape preparation	Identify lice, fleas, and fur mites	Train staff to save samples when there are questions about a parasite's identity
Hair pluckings	Mites, especially feline *Demodex*, may be seen microscopically among the hairs; on some cats, pluckings yield more mites than do skin scrapings	*Demodex cati* *Demodex gatoi* *Demodex* spp unknown
Impression smears	Pyoderma is a clinical diagnosis; impression smears are done to look for *Malassezia* organisms; if found, treat for yeast; remember, you are not sampling normal animals; if the animal is symptomatic, treat for it; if *Malassezia* is not present on impression smear, there is no need to include ketoconazole in the treatment plan or therapeutic trial; this is cost-effective, because ketoconazole is a relatively expensive drug	Heat fix slide for yeast Slide to be examined for cell integrity should not be heat fixed Yeast are often best found with scrape preparations made using a skin scraping spatula
Skin scraping	Use a skin scraping spatula; use of scalpel blades is less effective and risks laceration with difficult-to-restrain animals	
Ear cytology	Use this as a guide for therapy; treat for yeast using systemic antifungals; if rods are seen, culture the ear	If rods are seen, assume a worst case scenario and treat for *Pseudomonas*
Otic examination	Rule out polyps, occlusion, or neoplasia (rare)	May not be able to do examination until after animal is sedated and ear cleaned; collect diagnostic specimens first
Fine needle aspirate	Masses may have a wide range of influence on the potential to be adopted	

(continued on next page)

[13]. Oral daily ivermectin therapy is the easiest and least expensive therapy for most dogs in shelters. The recommended dose is 400 to 600 µg/kg administered orally once daily. The authors recommend starting therapy at 100 µg/kg and increasing the dose in increments of 100 µg/kg until the treatment dose is reached. If a dog is sensitive to ivermectin, clinical signs are usually seen at a dose of 100 to 200 µg/kg; if tremors, excessive salivation, or persistent pupil dilation is seen, the drug should not be used. Ivermectin-sensitive breeds or dogs are best treated with amitraz or milbemycin at a dose of 2 to 3 mg/kg administered orally once daily (Interceptor, Novartis Animal Health, Basel, Switzerland). Amitraz is often difficult to obtain, and there are special concerns about using it in shelter animals. Label recommendations for the use of amitraz stipulate that animals not be subjected to stress for at least 24 hours after treatment. Therefore, ivermectin-sensitive dogs requiring amitraz therapy should be treated in foster care. Treatment should be continued until there are two negative skin scrapings at weekly intervals. Dogs with generalized demodicosis may require 4 to 12 months of treatment before cure. Skin scrapings should be done weekly in the shelter to monitor therapy. Dogs with superficial pyodermas should be treated with oral cephalexin at a dosage of 30 mg/kg administered orally every 12 hours for 21 to 30 days. Dogs with deep pyoderma require treatment for at least 4 to 6 weeks. If impression smears reveal large numbers of rods or a mixed bacterial infection, generic ciprofloxacin at a dose of 20 mg/kg administered orally every 24 hours is recommended. The prognosis for dogs in shelters with generalized demodicosis and deep pyoderma is guarded, and potential owners should be aware that a cure may not be possible.

It is the clinical impression of one of the authors (KM) that the overall prevalence of generalized demodicosis has declined. There are many possible causes for this, including but not limited to widespread spay and neutering, education by breeders about the heritable predisposition for this form of the disease, and early and more aggressive treatment by private practice veterinarians. In shelters, it has been the same authors' experience that generalized canine demodicosis is common in American Pit Bull Terriers. We strongly recommend that these dogs be spayed or neutered before adoption.

Canine and Feline Bacterial and Yeast Pyoderma

In shelters, animals with superficial or deep pyoderma commonly have dual infections with bacteria (*Staphylococcus* spp) and *Malassezia* organisms. These infections represent an overgrowth of normal flora, and this occurs because of some predisposing factor (eg, stress, increased humidity, poor grooming, fleas, atopy). Dual infections are most common in the warm weather months or in humid conditions. In private practice, optimum therapy would be to treat for both diseases concurrently using systemic antimicrobials. This may not be possible in a shelter setting, and impression smears, ear swabs, and nail bed cytologic findings can help to guide therapy. In the authors' experience, *Malassezia* organisms from the skin are often smaller and rounder than what is commonly seen on ear cytology.

Bacterial pyoderma

There are many options, but for shelter dogs, cephalexin (30 mg/kg administered orally every 12 hours) or potentiated sulfas (15–30 mg/kg administered orally every 12 hours) are the most cost-effective therapies for bacterial pyoderma. Superficial pyodermas should be treated for 21 to 30 days. Deep pyodermas, including areas of pyotraumatic dermatitis and acral lick granulomas, should be treated for a minimum of 4 weeks. In cats, cephalexin liquid suspension (30 mg/kg administered orally every 12 hours) or amoxicillin and clavulanic acid (12.5–20 mg/kg administered orally every 12 hours) are quite effective.

Malassezia overgrowth

Ketoconazole administered orally at a dose of 5 to 10 mg/kg once daily is the drug of choice for dogs, and itraconazole administered orally at a dose of 5 to 10 mg/kg once daily is the drug of choice for cats. The use of ketoconazole in cats should be avoided because they do not tolerate this drug well and many become anorexic. Itraconazole is somewhat problematic to use because it comes in a 100-mg sized capsule and must be reformulated into smaller capsules. In a shelter, where resources are limited and systemic antifungals are expensive, some rules of thumb for use are helpful. Concurrent treatment is recommended in any animal in which yeast can be found on skin impression smears or nail bed cytology, in pruritic animals with oily skin or hair, in cases of severe pruritus with obvious bacterial pyoderma, in patients with concurrent yeast otitis, or in animals with severe pedal pruritus. If resources are limited, systemic antibiotic therapy combined with topical shampoo therapy every 2 to 3 days using an antifungal shampoo (Ketochlor Shampoo, Virbac Corporation; Malaseb, DVM Pharmaceuticals) may be effective. It is important to note that combined yeast and bacterial infections in dogs and cats are extremely pruritic and can mimic the severity of the pruritus of scabies in dogs. If in doubt, treat with ketoconazole at a dose of 5 to 10 mg/kg administered orally every 24 hours (dogs) or itraconazole at a dose of 5 mg/kg administered orally every 24 hours (cats) for 7 to 10 days; if there is a marked decrease in pruritus, continue treatment for the duration of antibiotic therapy. Topical therapy is always beneficial, but its use depends on whether or not staff or volunteers are available to bath animals.

Shelter Skin Diseases Worthy of Special Mention

Mad itchy cats

Over the last several years, both authors have seen cats from several shelters in south-central Wisconsin presenting with unusually intense pruritus. In addition, the authors have heard anecdotal reports from other shelters describing the same problem. In both presentations, the onset was acute and care staff often reported the cats to be normal one day and the cage full of hair the next. The source of the pruritus seems to be quite contagious, especially in multiple-cat housing areas. Contagion does not seem to require direct contact, because spread was noted even in caged wards, where there was no direct cat-to-cat contact or contact was limited to paws extended through cage bars. These presentations developed in housed cats in spite of treatment at the time of admission with spot-on flea control (selamectin). Initial diagnostics of these outbreaks have included skin scrapings, flea combings for fleas and *Cheyletiella* mites, retreatment with spot-on flea control, repeat fungal cultures, acetate tape preparations, and fecal flotations.

In our experience, we have seen two clinically different presentations of "mad itchy cats." In the first presentation, we often but not always found feline demodicosis. In cats in which mites were not found, the cats responded to treatment for feline demodicosis. Clinically, these cats were intensely pruritic, they pulled their hair out by the roots, the hairs were easily epilated in sheets with only gentle traction, the skin was erythematous and inflamed, and follicular plugging was common and often dramatic in appearance (Fig. 3). Although the cats were intensely pruritic, they never created areas of self trauma. Cats responded to weekly lime sulfur or weekly lime sulfur (8 oz/gal) in combination with daily ivermectin (200 μg/kg).

In the cats with feline demodicosis, mites were found via skin scrapings, hair pluckings, and/or fecal examination. In our shelter, we have noted three different appearances of feline *Demodex* mites: short stubby *Demodex gatoi* (Fig. 4), long thin *Demodex cati* (Fig. 5), and a third midlength *Demodex* mite (Fig. 6). The third mite form is rounded at the ends, and it is unclear if it is a developmental stage of *D gatoi* or a different species. *D gatoi* and this third form are often seen together on the same cat. Mites have been found on deep and/or superficial skin scrapings. In our experience, mites were found most commonly in hair pluckings collected from areas in which there was some degree of inflammation and easily epilated hairs. These sites are easy to find, because there is usual preexisting hair loss. Another interesting observation is that even in cats with large infestations, the mites may be found in large numbers in one site and not in another. In one instance with a gray and white kitten, mites were found exclusively and consistently in areas in which there were gray

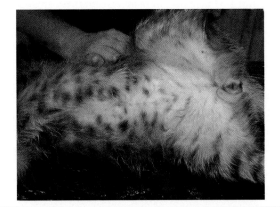

Fig. 3. Mad itchy cat caused by feline demodicosis.

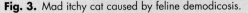

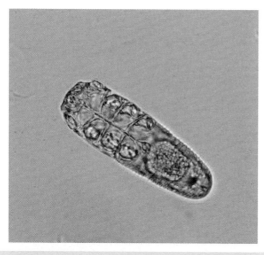

Fig. 4. *D gatoi* (original magnification, ×40).

hairs. After initial diagnosis, plucked hairs were placed in a sealed plastic bag for several days. On re-examination, mites were dead but were still found in the gray hairs only and not in the white hairs. One of the authors (KM) has found live mites on recently shed hairs collected from the cage of an affected cat. In some cats in which mites could not be found on the skin scraping, they were found on fecal examination. The presumption is that mites were removed via grooming. Because so little is known about the life cycle of feline *Demodex* mites, it is possible that mites spend part of their life cycle on the proximal immediate extrafollicular region of the hair shaft. If this is the case, it may explain why it is so hard to find mites in some cats. In the cats with definitively diagnosed demodicosis, the cats almost always responded to weekly lime sulfur (8 oz/gal), with an immediate notable reduction in pruritus and usually fast regrowth of hair. Cats were generally treated for 4 to 6 weeks. In our shelter, cats with severe pruritus, follicular plugging, and easily epilated hairs are considered likely suspects for demodicosis. Because the disease is contagious, these cats are isolated during treatment.

In the second group, we never found a cause. Affected cats were friendly, apparently healthy, and outgoing individuals that frequently interrupted their normal activities and suddenly and aggressively bit at their hair and skin.

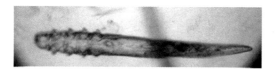
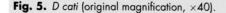

Fig. 5. *D cati* (original magnification, ×40).

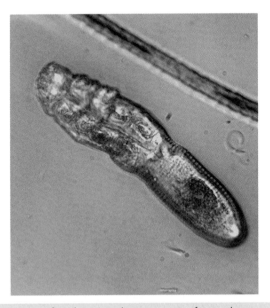

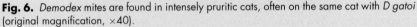

Fig. 6. *Demodex* mites are found in intensely pruritic cats, often on the same cat with *D gatoi* (original magnification, ×40).

During a 5-minute itch watch, these cats acted as if something was biting them. They nibbled at their skin, engaged in corn-cob biting behavior, and pulled out large clumps of hair. In addition to intense pruritus, these cats had thinning of the hair coat and barbering (Fig. 7). Two major differences between the two groups were that the hairs in the second group were not easily epilated and cats with the second presentation created areas of ulceration caused by self-trauma. These cats responded to weekly fipronil spray and oral daily ivermectin only after their hair coat was clipped. Before clipping of the hair coat, the cats were so agitated by the pruritus that they did not sleep. Within hours of clipping followed by topical fipronil spray, the cats were observed to be sleeping. The authors suspect that this second presentation may be caused by *Cheyletiella* infestations. In these cats, it is possible that the pruritus is similar to that of scabies in dogs, in which there is a strong hypersensitivity component triggered by a small number of mites. Anecdotally, there is some concern that the prolonged use of monthly spot-on flea control products may be resulting in populations of resistant *Cheyletiella* mites. Clinical signs of pruritus in people handling or caring for these cats were rare; one author (KM) developed a pruritic papular eruption on her arms only after spending the greater part of a day examining the hair coat of six cats.

In a shelter, cats with pruritus should be quarantined and treated as potentially contagious. Furthermore, cats biting and pulling out their hair coat should not be considered to have "psychogenic alopecia." It has been our experience that these cats have a treatable disease. A thorough investigation for external

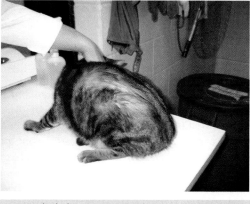

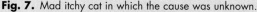

Fig. 7. Mad itchy cat in which the cause was unknown.

parasites is warranted, including treatment trials with lime sulfur or fipronil spray combined with ivermectin. It is also important to remember that dermatophytosis can mimic what has been classically pictured as psychogenic alopecia as well as bacterial and yeast infections of the skin and feline allergies. In short, if a cat is pruritic, the cause is in its skin rather than its head.

Effluvium

The authors routinely see cats at the Dane Country Humane Society with a nonpruritic and noninflammatory hair loss pattern characterized by massively easily epilated hairs. Close examination of the hair bulbs reveals that the hairs are in the telogen stage; this has been confirmed by histologic examination of skin biopsy specimens. Often, there is a history of these cats having been treated for upper respiratory infections, usually but not always with doxycycline. This nonpruritic alopecia resolves in almost every case with no treatment. The cause of this effluvium is unknown and could be the result of the viral infection or antibiotic therapy. Because some, presumably untreated, stray cats are presented to the shelter with this type of hair loss pattern and concurrent upper respiratory disease complex, we cannot help but hypothesize that it may be related more to the viral infection than to the medication used as treatment.

Happy tail

"Happy tail" is a common traumatic injury to the tail tip that is caused when kenneled dogs enthusiastically swing their hindquarters and tail wag. Dogs usually present with blood-splattered kennel walls and a distressed volunteer. Happy tail can be difficult to manage in large outgoing dogs. Repeated injuries and bleeding may become a chronic problem. Chronicity can make resolution difficult and, if left untreated, can necessitate amputation. Whenever possible, dogs with kennel wall abrasions to the tip of the tail should be moved to larger and wider housing. Alternatively, a protective bandage can be placed around the tip of the tail after cleaning. The bandage should be well secured. It can be quite difficult to keep these bandages in place without placing an Elizabethan collar on the dog simultaneously. One word of caution, a bandaged enthusiastic tail can really pack a wallop.

Kennel nose
Abrasions to the dorsum of the muzzle can be seen from cage bar-rubbing injuries. These abrasions often occur near the mucocutaneous junction and can mimic immune-mediated diseases. Abrasions are a sign of kennel stress and are best addressed by enrichment programs and placement in alternate housing whenever possible. Treatment is not usually necessary, but topical or systemic antibiotics may be indicated depending on severity. When large numbers of animals are in a shelter, it may be difficult to know when a lesion occurred. Digital pictures at the time of admission can be helpful with this problem.

Middle ear infections in cats
In most private and specialty dermatology practice, otitis media is not common in cats. It is usually associated with polyps, tumors, or *Malassezia* infections (C. Griffin, DVM, Animal Dermatology Clinic, personal communication, 2001). In shelter cats, this is not the case, and it is common to see cats with severe otitis media. It is important to recognize these infections quickly and to treat them aggressively (ear cleaning and systemic and topical therapy) to give the cat the best possible chance for recovery. On examination, the ear canal is visibly inflamed and palpably thickened, and the ear is malodorous and exudative. Self-trauma may be present, and depending on the severity of the infection, head tilting and, rarely, circling may be seen in severe cases. In some cases, there is obvious evidence of old aural hematomas, suggesting previous ear mite infestation, but this is not always the case. Ear cytology is a key to initial diagnosis and treatment. Rods are frequently found on ear cytology, and cultures have revealed a wide range of gram-negative bacteria, including but not limited to *Pseudomonas* spp, *Klebsiella*, *Escherichia coli*, and *Enterococcus* spp. Cleaning and otic examination are often difficult without sedation or anesthesia. Humane ear cleaning requires anesthesia, and otic examination under anesthesia is invaluable in determining whether or not the ear canal needs to be cleaned with deep lavage or if middle ear irrigation of the bulla is also needed. The latter is recommended if rods or large amounts of exudates are found in the ear canal. Often, the ear canal is filled with tenacious debris and impacted exudates. Polyps are seen but are the exception rather than the rule. When polyps are found, the most common treatment approach is to remove them via manual extraction by grasping the stalk and pulling them out. When polyps are seen, they must be removed to resolve the infection. Ideally, ear cultures should guide systemic therapy choices. If yeast organisms are seen, itraconazole at dosage of 5 mg/kg administered orally once daily for 21 days is recommended. Infections caused by cocci have responded well to amoxicillin and clavulanic acid (12.5–20 mg/kg administered orally every 12 hours). If rods are seen, a worst case scenario is assumed and marbofloxacin at a dose of 2.5 mg/kg administered orally once daily is prescribed pending culture sensitivity results.

Concurrent topical ear therapy is routine even when there is a ruptured tympanic membrane. Enrofloxacin-steroid ear drops are effective and have not resulted in any adverse effects to our knowledge. Silver sulfadiazine diluted 1:10 is also effective and safe to use. Treatment is normally scheduled for 21 days with a recheck several days after discontinuation of treatment. Detailed information is given to new owners on follow-up, and the importance of not missing treatment doses in preventing resistant bacterial infections is emphasized. Often, because of concerns about compliance and prognosis, cats with *Pseudomonas* otitis media are sent to reliable foster homes for treatment.

Yeast otitis
Malassezia spp otitis is common in dogs and cats. Most veterinarians are familiar with "yeasty ears"; less common presentations in shelters may include dogs presented for facial trauma because of rubbing of the ears, aural hematomas, and corneal ulcers secondary to self-trauma from rubbing of the ears. Cats are often reported as having itchy ears, ear twitching, facial pruritus, or just dirty ears. In cats, close examination of the nail beds often reveals black debris. If examined cytologically, this debris is often teeming with yeast organisms. There are several species of *Malassezia* in cats, and they are variable in size and may look like "miniature yeast" or "large cocci." The treatment of choice is systemic antifungal therapy for 14 to 30 days and topical glucocorticoids for immediate relief of the otitic pruritus. Yeast otitis is common in shelters year round because of the increased humidity.

Focal noninflammatory hair loss in the intrascapular region in cats
This is a common finding in shelter cats and is most commonly associated with the application of spot-on flea control products. Dermatophytosis should be ruled out, however.

Underlying Skin Diseases
In essence, there are two major groups of skin diseases seen in shelters: treat it, cure it, and forget about it diseases and "manageable but not curable" skin diseases. The manageable but not curable skin diseases most commonly include allergic skin diseases (atopy or food allergy), disorders of keratinization, seborrheic otitis, and endocrine disorders. Diagnostic endocrine testing may not be feasible in most shelters because of cost constraints. With that said, it has been our experience that many animals are surrendered because of underlying endocrine diseases that the owners are unable or unwilling to treat; however, another owner may be. The primary strategy for the management of an animal with allergic skin disease is to control secondary infections, address grooming issues that may be making the problem worse, and find a cost-effective antipruritic. In some cases, the latter is relatively inexpensive and may include otic ophthalmic glucocorticoids or topical steroid sprays (eg, Genesis, Virbac Animal Health). In obviously allergic animals, it is important to be aggressive in the treatment of secondary infections, and this is one time when systemic antibiotic and antifungal therapy may be helpful. The management of disorders of keratinization is difficult in shelters, because "control" requires antimicrobial

therapy and aggressive bathing (2–4 times per week) with medicated shampoos that can be expensive. Animals surrendered for seborrheic otitis are rewarding to treat. Cytology invariably reveals large numbers of yeast organisms. These animals respond well to ear cleanings, topical glucocorticoid therapy (in some cases, systemic therapy if the ear is proliferative), and systemic ketoconazole. Once the condition is "in remission," it can often be maintained that way with chronic ear steroids and ear cleanings. The authors commonly use a 1:1 dilution of injectable dexamethasone in propylene glycol for this purpose. This is inexpensive and quite effective.

Acknowledgments

The authors thank Kate Hurley, DVM, MS, for her contributions to this article.

References

[1] Hurley KF. Implementing a population health plan in an animal shelter: goal setting, data collection, and monitoring, and policy development. In: Miller L, Zawistowski S, editors. Shelter medicine for veterinarians and staff. Ames (IA): Blackwell Publishing; 2004. p. 211–34.
[2] Scarlet J. Pet population dynamics and animal shelter issues. In: Miller L, Zawistowski S, editors. Shelter medicine for veterinarians and staff. Ames (IA): Blackwell Publishing; 2004. p. 11–23.
[3] Fennell LA. Beyond overpopulation: a comment on Zawistowski et al and Salmon et al. J Appl Anim Welf Sci 1999;2:217–28.
[4] Moriello KA. Zoonotic skin diseases of dogs and cats. Anim Health Res Rev 2004;4: 157–68.
[5] Irwin PG. Overview: the state of animals in 2001. In: Salem DJ, Rowan AN, editors. The state of animals in 2001. Washington (DC): Humane Society Press, Humane Society of the United States; 2001. p. 75.
[6] Newbury S, Verbrugge M, Steffen T, et al. Management of naturally occurring dermatophytosis in an open shelter: part 1: development of a cost effective screening and monitoring program [abstract]. Vet Dermatol 2005;16:192.
[7] Kirkwood S. A prescription for better veterinary relations. Animal sheltering. Washington (DC): Humane Society Press, Humane Society of the United States; 1999.
[8] Jackson HA, editor. Dermatologic diagnostics. Clin Tech Small Anim Pract 2001;16(4).
[9] Scott DW, Miller WH, Griffin CE, editors. Mueller and Kirk's small animal dermatology. 6th edition. Philadelphia: WB Saunders; 2001.
[10] Foster A, Foil C, editors. BSAVA manual of small animal dermatology. Quedgeley Gloucester, United Kingdom; 2003.
[11] Medleau L, Hnilica K, editors. Small animal dermatology: a color atlas and therapeutics guide. Philadelphia: WB Saunders; 2001.
[12] Curtis CF. Current trends in the treatment of Sarcoptes, Cheyletiella and Otodectes mite infestations in cats and dogs. Vet Dermatol 2004;15:108–14.
[13] Mueller RF. Treatment protocols for demodicosis: an evidence-based review. Vet Dermatol 2004;15:75–89.

Recommendations for the Management and Treatment of Dermatophytosis in Animal Shelters

Karen A. Moriello, DVM[a],*, Sandra Newbury, DVM[b]

[a]Department of Medical Sciences, School of Veterinary Medicine,
University of Wisconsin–Madison, 2015 Linden Drive, West Madison, WI 53706, USA
[b]Dane County Humane Society, 5132 Voges Road, Madison, WI 53718–6941, USA

D ermatophytosis is a superficial fungal infection of hair, skin, and nails. In animals, it is most commonly caused by one of two genera: *Microsporum* and *Trichophyton*. Although it is highly contagious and infectious, it is associated with little mortality; if left untreated, the infection is normally eliminated by the skin's immune system. It can occur in any patient, but young, old, and debilitated animals are most at risk. The clinical presentation is variable in dogs and cats, but definitive diagnosis is not technically difficult and is easily done via fungal culture. Luckily, the fungal culture techniques are relatively simple and can be performed in-house. Dermatophytosis is treatable and curable, so why is this relatively benign skin disease so problematic in shelters? The answer to this question is complicated.

First and foremost, the disease is a zoonosis. Shelters have a responsibility to protect their staff, volunteers, and public from zoonotic diseases. Control of this zoonotic disease is complicated by the fact that the infective material is microscopic and easily spread on fomites and even air currents. Second, actively infected animals or fomite carriers adopted into homes are potential public health and public relations nightmares. Lesions can be difficult to find or absent, especially during the incubation period, and it is quite possible for a "healthy kitten or puppy" to be adopted and develop clinical lesions shortly after adoption. Some owners may accept this as "part of the deal" and seek private medical care. Other owners may return the newly adopted pet to the shelter or complain to the shelter, local newspaper, or public health department, for example. It does not take too many "ringworm complaints" or outbreaks for a shelter, rescue organization, or sanctuary to develop a reputation of adopting sick animals. Negative experiences or perceptions in the community about a shelter may have a significant negative impact on adoptions, fund-raising, and donations. Third, a combination of shelter resources and policies determines how

*Corresponding author.

0195-5616/06/$ – see front matter
doi:10.1016/j.cvsm.2005.09.006

any infectious disease is managed in a shelter. "Recognize and euthanize" (RE) polices are used in many animal shelters to control dermatophytosis. Although this approach may work for some diseases, it often does not work for dermatophytosis. From a purely medical perspective, the mere act of bringing an actively infected animal into the building spreads spores into the environment. Add to this the near impossibility of identifying animals that are mechanically carrying spores on their hair coat without fungal culture, and it is inevitable that an infectious animal enters the population. RE policies are only effective for disease control if staff and volunteers willingly comply and no exceptions are made. Dermatophytosis affects the most adoptable population in a shelter, kittens and puppies. RE policies would target this population, because the disease targets this population. Euthanizing kittens and puppies for treatable and curable diseases becomes emotionally and politically charged. RE shelter policies can be divisive and have a negative impact on volunteerism. Finally, little research has been done on the management and treatment of dermatophytosis in animal shelters. The physical facility and animal turnover and population density create a unique environment. Individual animal medicine practices do not always transfer to population medicine practices. The management of infectious diseases in production animal medicine has taught us that treatment and prevention protocols must be tested and refined in the field.

For veterinarians unfamiliar with control strategies for infectious diseases in an animal shelter, it is important know that RE policies are used in many shelters. RE approaches may be the only option for the control of many diseases during an acute outbreak. For shelters with limited resources, RE programs also may be the only way to protect the general population. It is often the case that because of the mathematic difference between the numbers of animals coming into a shelter and the numbers of animals being adopted, euthanasia is an inevitable and responsible choice for some animals. By limiting the population density within a shelter, the health of the individuals making up the group may be protected. When making such difficult decisions, it may be best to focus treatment efforts on those diseases that, like dermatophytosis, (1) affect otherwise adoptable animals, (2) have a generally good prognosis for complete resolution and, (3) have no impediment to adoption after treatment. RE programs work best when the clinical signs of the disease are pathognomonic and lay staff can be trained to recognize the clinical signs or confirm the diagnosis at the point of entry. One example, although still complex, is the testing of dogs with diarrhea with the fecal parvovirus test. RE policies are emotionally and politically charged in shelters even when disease recognition and confirmation of diagnosis are relatively easy and rapid, respectively.

With respect to dermatophytosis, RE programs are used by many shelters to control this disease. In this article, we describe the collaborative findings of field studies from a shelter where the shelter veterinarian (SN) decided to abandon this approach and instead institute a screening, treating, and monitoring program [1–3]. It is not within the scope of this article to review all aspects of dermatophytosis in detail. We review the most important points as they relate to control and treatment. Comprehensive discussions can be found in textbooks or recent reviews [4,5].

ETIOLOGY

Dermatophytosis is a superficial fungal skin disease involving the hair, skin, and nails or claws of people and animals. In small animals, dermatophytosis is the most common infectious and contagious skin disease of cats, and if parasites are excluded, dermatophyte infections are probably the most common contagion of all small animals. The disease is a zoonosis and, again, if parasites are excluded, probably the most common zoonotic skin disease of small animals. More than 20 different species of dermatophytes have been isolated from dogs and cats [4,5]. It has been well established that the most commonly isolated dermatophytes are *Microsporum canis*, *Microsporum gypseum*, and *Trichophyton* spp. These three organisms are the most commonly encountered dermatophytes in our shelter research.

There are two important groups of studies on the fungal flora of animals, and they have been summarized elsewhere in detail [6]. The first group is those studies that established the normal fungal flora of dogs and cats [7,8]. These studies have shown that the pathogenic fungi are not part of the normal fungal flora of dogs and cats. This is important, because it means that the isolation of a dermatophyte from the hair coat is the result of an active or incubating infection or of mechanical carriage. The second group is those studies that surveyed the fungal flora of large numbers of animals that were free-roaming or held in confinement (eg, catteries). Prevalence in these studies varied from 6.5% to 88%, and the following conclusions can be made. Dermatophytosis is most common in tropical and subtropical climates and in the warm weather months in temperate climates, prevalence is higher in underdeveloped countries or in countries in which there are large numbers of free-ranging dogs and cats, prevalence is more common in countries in which the custom is to allow pet cats to be indoor or outdoor cats, and dermatophytosis can become endemic in catteries or homes once it is introduced [9–15].

PATHOGENESIS OF INFECTION

The infective stage of a dermatophyte is called an arthrospore. These spores are formed via segmentation and fragmentation of fungal hyphae. Infective spores are deposited on a susceptible host's skin or hair coat after contact with another infected animal or via contact with a contaminated environment or fomite. Once on the hair coat, the spores must reach the skin or hair follicles to establish a foothold. Spores must compete with normal flora, fungistatic effects of sebum, and the dry humidity of the hair coat, for example. They may also fall off or be groomed off the hair coat. Under optimum conditions, infective spores may germinate within 6 hours of adherence to keratinocytes [16]. Arthrospores adhere strongly to keratin, and the presence of keratinocytes produces favorable conditions for germination. These spores cannot penetrate healthy skin, so some type of microtrauma is needed to facilitate infection;

experimental infections have been established with trauma equivalent to that of grooming. Germination of spores is temperature dependent, with warm temperatures favoring germination. The need for moisture and warmth explains why dermatophytosis is more common in tropical and semitropical climates and during the warm months in temperate climates.

Shelter Life: Factors That May Affect Pathogenesis of Infection

Infection requires a source of exposure, compromised host defenses, increased warmth and humidity, and a source of microtrauma. All these are present in shelters. Admittedly, the critical mass of spores needed to establish an infection is unknown. Shelter life may decrease the number of spores needed to cause clinical disease in a susceptible host, however. Animals that may otherwise be able to defeat a dermatophyte infection via natural host defenses may not be able to do so in a shelter. Because of the high traffic of animals in a shelter, there is increased exposure to infective spores. One of the most infectious places for fungal spore contamination is the admission area, even with staff cooperation with cleaning and disinfection (K.A. Moriello, DVM, S.N. Newbury, DVM, unpublished data, 2004). Animals surrendered to shelters are stressed, and stress is known to have a negative influence on the immune system. This would compromise the skin's immune system. Because of stress, cats that normally would groom themselves may not groom as well or at all in a shelter. Mechanical removal of spores is an important protective mechanism for this species. The first signs of disease in kittens often develop on the face, a place that is difficult for young kittens to groom. Admission to a shelter may occur at the same time as separation from the queen. Cleaning practices increase the humidity in animal shelters, and confinement to cages or enclosures may increase the skin's ambient temperature, favoring establishment of an infection. Additionally, ectoparasites, such as lice, fleas, ticks, *Cheyletiella* mites, *Otodectes* mites, and pruritus from secondary infections, are some of the many sources of microtrauma that can predispose animals to dermatophytosis.

Any aged animal, sex, or breed is susceptible to infection; however, the disease tends to be more common in young, old, or debilitated animals. As mentioned previously, the disease is more common in free-roaming animals. Viral infections may play a role in making hosts more susceptible to infection. In one study, dermatophytosis was three times more common in cats with feline immunodeficiency virus (FIV) than in uninfected cats [17], but in another, no association was found between FIV or feline leukemia virus (FeLV) and dermatophyte infections [15]. Development of dermatophytosis in FIV- or FeLV-infected cats may have more to do with overall health than with the simple "positive" or "negative" viral status.

> Control of dermatophytosis in a shelter begins with the admission point. This room should be arranged so that it is clutter-free and easily cleaned and decontaminated on a daily basis. Mechanical removal of organic material (vacuuming and removal of dust using a Swiffer cloth [Procter and Gamble, Cincinnati, Ohio]) followed by triple cleaning (detergent, scrub,

and rinse three times) is efficacious. A dilution of 1:10 household bleach can be used on nonporous surfaces. This room is monitored weekly for environmental contamination via culturing with a Swiffer cloth.

Key Points Regarding Common Clinical Presentations

The clinical signs of dermatophytosis are related to the pathogenesis. Dermatophytes invade hair shafts and cornified epithelium. This results in destruction of the hair shaft and disruption of normal keratinization. Clinically, this results in hair loss and scaling; however, feline dermatophytosis is pleomorphic and may present with any combination of the following [4–6,18]:

- Pruritus: the disease may be pruritic or not pruritic. The severity of the pruritus can vary from mild to severe, resulting in self-mutilation.
- Hair loss: the hair loss may be subtle or dramatic, symmetric or asymmetric, or inflammatory or noninflammatory. In dogs, circular areas of alopecia are most likely to be signs of bacterial pyoderma and not signs of dermatophytosis. Bacterial pyoderma is commonly misdiagnosed in dogs as dermatophytosis. In dogs, bacterial pyoderma tends to be most common from the neck caudally. If a dog presents with areas of hair loss on the face, dermatophytosis and demodicosis should be considered.
- Crusting and scaling: lesions of dermatophytosis are usually exfoliative at some stage in their existence. In some cats, the scaling may be severe and resemble that of pemphigus foliaceus. Mounds of thick adherent crusting can develop on the face, ears, and nail bed regions, especially in long-haired cats.
- Comedones: M canis can cause comedone-like lesions (ie, "chin acne") in young cats. Other considerations are Malassezia dermatitis and feline demodicosis. Comedones are not common in dogs.
- Hyperpigmentation: hyperpigmentation is an uncommon clinical finding in cats with skin disease. In the authors' experience, however, the most common cause of hyperpigmentation in cats is dermatophytosis.
- Paronychia: in some cats, crusted or exudative paronychia may be the only dermatologic finding of M canis infection. The other major differential diagnosis in cats is pemphigus foliaceus. In dogs, paronychia dermatophytosis is most commonly caused by M gypseum or Trichophyton spp. If left untreated, nails have a corkscrew appearance; the nails resemble tree trunk roots when they are seen above ground. In dogs, nails that easily break off or split are more likely to have other causes, including trauma and lupoid onychodystrophy.
- Erythema: erythema is a common clinical finding in early lesions of dermatophytosis. It often accompanies the development of hair loss. Erythema can be difficult to see in cats and is most common in cats with light hair coats, especially orange cats. Erythema is most likely to be seen in the periocular and preauricular areas.
- Lesion distribution: dermatophytosis is not a "localized disease." Clinical lesions may be focal or multifocal, but spores are present throughout the hair coat via the cat's grooming behavior.
- In kittens and puppies, the scaling and alopecia on the face, muzzle, ears, and front legs are the most common clinical presentations.

- In older kittens and young cats, irregular patches of alopecia with or without crusting are a common presentation.
- Focal areas of hair loss or crusting are difficult to find in long-haired cats or dogs. Often, the most obvious clinical sign is excessive shedding.
- Cats with generalized dermatophytosis often ingest large amounts of hair while grooming, and shelter staff may report vomiting, constipation, anorexia, or hairball problems.
- In dogs, lesions of bacterial pyoderma on the face are uncommon. If such lesions are present, consider dermatophytosis.
- Reaction patterns: cats with skin disease often present with one of many "skin problems" or, more appropriately, reaction patterns. M canis should be included in the differential diagnosis of the following:
  - Miliary dermatitis: miliary dermatitis is a papular-crusted reaction pattern most commonly associated with flea allergy dermatitis. It is a type of folliculitis, however. M canis–induced miliary dermatitis–like lesions are commonly observed after clipping.
  - Eosinophilic plaques: allergies are the most common cause of eosinophilic plaques in cats; however, we have seen "eosinophilic plaque"–like lesions in cats with pruritic M canis infections.
  - Indolent lip ulcers: the etiology of indolent lip ulcers is multifactorial. In a recent study conducted by one of the authors (KAM), several cats developed indolent ulcers on their lips, where there had been one or more M canis–infected hairs. The hairs at these sites were rapidly shed; the etiology of the lesions in these research cats would have been recorded as "unknown" had knowledge of the M canis infection not been available. It is possible that M canis is an underrecognized cause of indolent lip ulcers in young cats. In a shelter, cats with unilateral lip ulcers should be cultured for dermatophytosis.
- Symmetric alopecia and/or overgrooming: M canis can present as symmetric alopecia in cats. In the cases seen by one of the authors (KAM), the cats were all adults that had received glucocorticoid injections as part of the therapy for symmetric alopecia. This information may not be available to shelter operators. Cats with presumed psychogenic grooming should be screened for dermatophytosis and feline demodicosis. Regarding the latter, response to treatment may be the diagnostic test of choice.
- Pruritic pinnae: unilateral or bilateral pinnal pruritus is another underrecognized presentation of M canis. In the cats, infected hairs are often limited to the ear margin or long hairs within the "bell" of the ear. Erythema and scaling of the inner or outer pinnae represent another presentation that seems to be common in shelter cats with Trichophyton dermatophytosis.
- Granulomatous lesions: granulomatous skin lesions may occur in some cats, particularly long-haired cats. These lesions may present as nonhealing wounds or nodules. These are referred to as "pseudomycetomas" and are diagnosed via skin biopsy. Dogs develop focal granulomatous reactions, especially on their face and extremities, and these are referred to as "kerion" reactions. Diagnosis is usually via skin biopsy.
- Miscellaneous: in some cases of chronic dermatophytosis, there are "anatomic reservoirs" of infection on the body. The most common areas are facial folds and periocular hairs. This has been most commonly observed in cats

with generalized dermatophytosis treated with topical therapy alone because of concerns about applying therapy to the face. These cats presented not only with chronic dermatophytosis but with facial fold pyoderma, conjunctivitis, and blepharitis.

Newly Recognized Clinical Presentations

Trichophyton *spp dermatophyte infections in cats*

Surveys on the fungal flora of pet cats and stray cats in the United States have reported isolating *Trichophyton* spp [7,19,20]. In a survey of the fungal flora of pet cats from the midwestern United States, *Trichophyton* spp were isolated from 14 of 172 cats. Interestingly, *M canis* was never isolated from any of the cats. In another study conducted in the United States on the prevalence of dermatophytes from stray cats in animal shelters from northern regions (New York, Pennsylvania, and Wisconsin) and cats from Florida, *Trichophyton* spp were again isolated. For unknown reasons, in all studies, *Trichophyton* spp isolates were significantly more common in cats from colder climates (13 of 100 cats) than from southern climates (3 of 100 cats). In this latter study, surveys were conducted in the fall months. *M canis* was not isolated from any of the northern shelters and was isolated in 8 of 100 cats in the Florida shelter.

Recently, there is some emerging clinical evidence to suggest that *Trichophyton* spp infections may be an underdiagnosed cause of skin disease in cats. This is based on field studies conducted in two shelters in the Midwest. Beginning in the late summer of 2003, the Dane County Humane Society abandoned an RE approach to managing dermatophytosis in the shelter. A screening and treating program in which all cats are routinely screened for dermatophytosis via clinical examination and toothbrush culture of the hair coat at the time of admission replaced it. This is an open shelter that admits more than 3000 cats per year. Data from the first 12 months of this program suggested that *Trichophyton* spp infections may be an underrecognized skin disease (S.N. Newbury, DVM, K.A. Moriello, DVM, R.D. Schultz, PhD, University of Wisconsin–Madison School of Veterinary Medicine, unpublished data, 2003–2005). In the late summer and early fall months, the predominant pathogen was *M canis*; culture-positive cats were clinically infected or mechanical carriers. In the early winter months, *M canis* isolation dropped to almost zero and was rarely isolated from cats entering the shelter. This was somewhat expected, because the total number of kittens and juvenile cats admitted to the shelter decreased. What was unexpected was the rise in the isolation of *Trichophyton* spp from cats. Before the sharp decline in *M canis* isolates, this organism had not been isolated from cats entering the shelter. This trend continued until late spring, when *M canis* again became the predominant pathogen. This trend was also noted in fungal culture data from another shelter screening all cats at the time of admission (K.A. Moriello, DVM, D.J. DeBoer, DVM, University of Wisconsin–Madison School of Veterinary Medicine, unpublished data, 2001–2003). What was interesting clinically was that most of the *Trichophyton*-infected cats at both shelters had lesions limited to their ears, consisting of pruritus or crusted scaling, and hair loss on the ear margins. The lesions were mild and easily overlooked; at their worst, they resembled mild insect bite hypersensitivity. Generalized *Trichophyton* infections did occur in kittens. All the cats responded to a combination of itraconazole and lime sulfur topical rinses. Although no treatment data were recorded, it is interesting to note that *Trichophyton* spp isolates were significantly more common in northern shelters in the study on fungal flora of shelter cats [20].

It is unclear why this seasonal occurrence of *Trichophyton* spp was noted. It is possible that these infections may simply have been missed during the warm weather months. *Trichophyton* spp fungi grow slowly and require warmer incubation temperatures. It is possible that this pathogen was missed because of contaminant overgrowth; in the case of dual infection, it is possible that *M canis* dominated the plate and the second pathogen was never isolated. Another possible explanation is that the population of cats being surrendered to the shelter may be a factor. Early in the summer and fall months, most cats were young, and during the winter months, the population was predominantly older cats, strays, or feral cats. *Trichophyton* spp is common in large animals, and the natural reservoir for infection is rodents. In the Midwest during winter, free-ranging cats are frequently trapped by farmers, landowners, and other concerned individuals to prevent them from dying as a result of exposure to the elements. This may have selected for a population of cats with increased exposure to *Trichophyton* spp. Another reason why this may not have been previously noted was that these infections were markedly less severe than *M canis* infections and limited in their lesion distribution for reasons that are unknown. Studies are continuing to determine if this seasonal occurrence is unique to the geographic region or not. It is not likely that *Trichophyton* spp infections are limited to shelters, just that they may be easily overlooked. There is a recent case report of *Trichophyton mentagrophytes* infection in a cat from France. In that case, the cat was presented for scaling and crusting of the ear pinnae, but unlike the cats we have seen, lesions rapidly became diffuse with severe scaling and erythema [21].

Microsporum canis *infections in Yorkshire Terriers*
Yorkshire Terrier dogs are increasingly being reported as the most common dog breed with a predisposition to *M canis* dermatophytosis [9,22,23]. In this breed, the disease has been reported alone or concurrently with other systemic diseases, such as diabetes mellitus, demodicosis, ehrlichiosis, and leishmaniasis. In the reported cases, only partial resolution of the dermatophytosis was possible. It is unknown why this particular small breed of dog seems uniquely predisposed to dermatophytosis. Hair length cannot be the only explanation; otherwise, dermatophytosis would be problematic in other long-haired small- and large-breed dogs, particularly those breeds that are commonly taken to dog grooming salons. Grooming salons are ideal places for exposure to dermatophytosis, and grooming procedures (bathing, clipping, and hair coat stripping) would provide the ideal conditions for establishment of infection. The

popularity of the breed and possibility of a heritable defect in cell-mediated immunity are other explanations. Consideration should be given to routine screening of this breed for dermatophytosis when Yorkshire Terriers are presented for any skin disease. Also, newly acquired puppies or adult dogs should be screened for dermatophytosis. In shelters, this breed may represent an unrecognized source of dermatophytosis.

Shelter life: how often do clinical signs predict infection?
Some RE programs rely heavily, if not solely, on the presence or absence of lesions as a "diagnostic criterion" for dermatophytosis, especially in cats. The assumption is that because dermatophytosis is the most common infectious and contagious skin disease of cats, it is the most common skin disease. Therefore, if a cat has skin lesions, odds are that it is caused by dermatophytosis, and not allowing entry of cats with skin disease into a shelter should prevent outbreaks and contamination of the shelter. The admitting staff of the Dane County Humane Society were trained by one of the authors (SN) to look for and find skin lesions on cats at the time of admission. This information was recorded and accompanied fungal culture samples processed at the University of Wisconsin–Madison School of Veterinary Medicine Dermatology Research Laboratory. When we examined data from a 15-month period during which 4274 cats were cultured at the time of admission, staff recorded lesions in 304 cats (7%). Of these 304 cats, only 55 (18%) had positive fungal cultures and 249 (82%) had negative fungal cultures. If the presence or absence of skin lesions was used alone, 249 cats would have been misdiagnosed and unjustly euthanized. When we looked at culture data from the same 15-month period, we found that there were 397 culture-positive cats. Of these, only 55 (14%) of culture-positive cats had skin lesions; the remaining 342 (86%) did not. Again, if lesions were used as the sole criterion to screen cats for dermatophytosis, we would have missed 342 culture-positive cats. Removing cats with skin lesions at the time of admission is no guarantee that the general population and facility are being protected from the introduction of dermatophytosis.

> The control of dermatophytosis in a shelter cannot rely on the culling of lesional animals at the time of admission. Removing cats with lesions at admission does not protect the general population from exposure to dermatophytosis, it does not protect against outbreaks, and it does not protect the facility from environmental contamination. It also results in the unjust euthanasia of cats that have other treatable conditions.

SHELTER-FOCUSED DIAGNOSTIC TESTING
Diagnostic testing for dermatophytosis has been reviewed elsewhere [24]. The goal of this section is to discuss cost- and time-effective use of the Wood's lamp examination, direct examination of hairs, fungal culture, and skin biopsy.

Take-Home Points About Diagnostic Tests for Dermatophytosis
- Clinical signs: dermatophytosis cannot be diagnosed definitively based on clinical signs alone. In a shelter, dermatophytosis can look like "nothing" or it can look like "anything."
- Wood's lamp: a Wood's lamp is an ultraviolet light filtered through a cobalt or nickel filter. It is used to screen lesions for the presence of fungal metabolites that fluoresce an apple-green color when exposed to the light. The only pathogen of veterinary importance that fluoresces is *M canis*, and not all strains glow. It has been estimated that only 50% of strains glow; however, the truth is that we do not know how many strains glow and what factors influence the development of fluorescence. Both authors have seen cats in which one lesion on the cat glows but others do not. The explanation of this is unknown, but it is possible that cats are infected by more than one strain or isolate. In addition, topical drugs or shampoos can change or alter the color of the fluorescence. Sebum can give a false-positive test result, as can many bacterial infections of the skin. Many drugs commonly used in a shelter, such as doxycycline and terramycin, falsely fluoresce. A positive test is only suggestive of an infection and is not diagnostic. The primary use of this tool is for the selection of hairs for culture or microscopic examination. Battery-operated Wood's lamps are not reliable and should not be used.
- Direct examinations: direct examination of hair and scales may show evidence of fungal spores growing in cuffs on the outside of hairs or fungal hyphae invading hair shafts. It is often positive in human patients but is not no so in veterinary patients. Because of the density of the hair coat of dogs and cats and the difficulty associated with finding lesions, it can be difficult for the shelter staff to find actively infected hairs for examination. The chance of finding infected hairs is increased if Wood's lamp-positive hairs are examined; unless the patient has active lesions that are Wood's lamp-positive, this test is not cost-effective to perform.
- Skin biopsy: the diagnosis of dermatophytosis via skin biopsy in a shelter is almost always going to be a "surprise." Biopsy specimens most likely have been submitted on an unusual skin lesion to rule in or out a tumor, immune-mediated disease, or other disease. Unfortunately, the identity of the pathogen cannot be determined from the tissue specimen.
- Fungal culture: this is the diagnostic test of choice; however, in a shelter situation, a "positive fungal" culture could indicate one of two things: true infection or fomite carriage. Guidelines for discriminating between these two situations are discussed later in this article.

Direct Examination of Hair for Spores and Hyphae Practice Tips for
Making This a User-Friendly Diagnostic Tool
Wood's lamp-positive hairs can be used for culture, although it is important to remember that not all Wood's lamp-positive hairs are culture-positive. This is especially true of hairs collected from animals that are being treated with drugs for upper respiratory infections, because tetracycline and related compounds can cause hairs to fluoresce. These hairs can also be used for immediate microscopic examination to look for spores and hyphae. Finding these spores is definitive evidence of an active fungal infection, and treatment can be started immediately

pending confirmation via the "gold standard," (ie, fungal culture). There are several major obstacles that are commonly encountered when performing direct examinations. The first is finding an appropriate sample. Although fungal spores can be found in *M gypseum* and *Trichophyton* infections, for all practical purposes, this technique is only time- and cost-effective when you can find a Wood's lamp-positive hair. Hairs should be plucked in the direction of growth, and every effort should be made to obtain the hair root. The next obstacle is the "clearing agent" (eg, potassium hydroxide, chlorphenolac). Clearing agents are chemical compounds that cause background debris to swell, making hair shafts and fungal spores more refractile. Contrary to popular belief, clearing agents are not absolutely necessary to perform this technique. If necessary, plain mineral oil can be used for what is essentially a hair trichogram or hair shaft examination. The trick is to use a small amount of mineral oil for mounting the hair specimen and a large glass coverslip (Fig. 1). This helps to "secure" the specimen to the slide and minimizes "streaming" of mineral oil across the slide. In *M canis* infections, the fungal spores are present on the outside of the hair shaft in a "cuff." They can easily be lost in the mounting fluid if too much is used. The final obstacle is finding the suspect hair once it is placed on the slide in a clearing agent or tiny drop of mineral oil. More often than not, many normal hairs are obtained when collecting the Wood's lamp-positive hairs. At this step, the easiest thing to do is to place the glass slide with the hair sample on the microscope stage and turn off the lights in the laboratory. Shine the Wood's lamp over the glass slide until the glowing hair is located, and then position it under the microscope lens (magnification, ×10). Continue shining the Wood's lamp on the slide from the slide or from underneath the stage as you look into the microscope and locate the Wood's lamp-positive hair (Figs. 2 and 3). It should appear blue green in color. When you turn off the Wood's lamp and turn on the microscope light, the infected hair should be visible. Infected hairs can usually be identified at

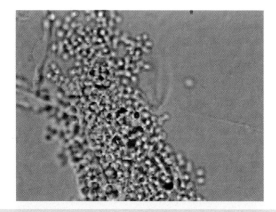

Fig. 1. Fungal spores (original magnification, ×40) from a Wood's lamp-positive hair. These hairs were mounted in mineral oil.

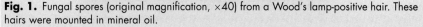

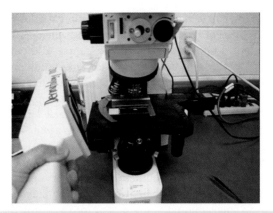

Fig. 2. Placement of Wood's lamp next to the microscope to aid in finding Wood's lamp-positive hairs.

a magnification ×10, and cuffs of spores can be easily seen at a magnification ×40.

Comments on fungal culture techniques

Fungal culture is still the gold standard for the diagnosis of dermatophytosis, and there are basically two techniques that can be used: the toothbrush culture technique and the hair-plucking technique. The toothbrush technique is recommended for culturing of cats and individual lesions. Toothbrush samples collect debris from the surface and, because of the comb-like bristles, also obtain samples from the surface of the skin.

Even though toothbrush fungal cultures are superior to random hair pluckings when screening cats for dermatophytosis, false-negative fungal culture

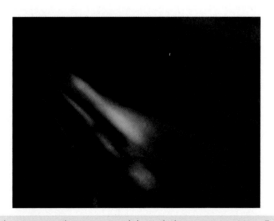

Fig. 3. Wood's lamp-positive hair as viewed through the microscope (see Fig. 2).

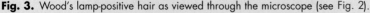

results are still possible. Based on our experience with shelter screenings, the most common reasons for this are poor technique in culturing, rapid over-growth of the plate because of contaminants, or poor handling of the tooth-brush culture before inoculation. Excluding inexperience in reading fungal culture plates, false-positive results can occur from cross-contamination of test-ing materials; if fungal culture plates are inoculated in the admission area, where there may be airborne infective spores; and cross-contamination of plates during incubation. These problems can be avoided if the following points are kept in mind when culturing cats (especially kittens):

- Be sure to toothbrush culture the entire hair coat thoroughly until the bristles are full of hair or the cat has been combed for at least 1 minute.
- Early infections often occur on the face and ears. Be sure the last place sam-pled is the face and inside of the bell of the ear. Care must be taken when combing around the eye. The tip of most toothbrushes is small enough to comb inside the bell of the ear of most kittens. When large numbers of animals are being cultured, it is easy to "give the coat a few swipes" and move on to the next cat; workers should avoid this temptation.
- Early lesions in kittens are most common periocularly, in and around the ears, on the muzzle, and on the paws. These areas should get extra attention during culturing.
- If obvious lesions are present, culture the nonlesional part of the body first and the lesion last. This serves two purposes. First, it minimizes the chance that toothbrushing mechanically spreads spores over the body. Dermatophyte lesions start locally and then spread, and the veterinarian does not want to facilitate the spread of infection. Second, if cultured last, spores are present in the largest numbers on the tips of the bristles.
- Pending inoculation of culture plates, keep toothbrush cultures at room temper-ature and protect them from heat extremes, especially high temperatures (eg, inside of a car during the summer months).
- Toothbrush cultures should be inoculated in the clinic laboratory or at a site where animals are not housed. Dermatophyte spores are small and can be carried on air currents. Plates should never be inoculated in the admissions area. Fungal culture kits (toothbrushes packaged in plastic bags) should be made off-site in a sterile or clean environment known to be free of dermato-phyte spores. This is good activity for a volunteer, but that person needs to be selected with care. If Petri dishes are used for culture, care should be taken to make sure the plates do not open accidentally and contaminate other plates. This can be done by sealing the plates with tape or simply putting each plate into a small plastic bag. These measures should minimize cross-contamination.

Hair pluckings are best used for Wood's lamp-positive hairs or for sampling hairs at a lesion's margin. If an individual lesion is heavily contaminated with organic debris or plant material, it should be wiped with alcohol before sam-pling to aid in minimizing contaminant growth on the fungal culture plate. It is important to pluck the hair in the direction of growth and to obtain hair bulbs or roots for culture, because dermatophyte spores are most common and viable at this level of the hair.

Toothbrush cultures cannot be inoculated if glass culture jars are used. If toothbrush samples are sent to a diagnostic laboratory, be sure the laboratory knows how to inoculate the specimen onto a fungal culture plate. Many human laboratories are not familiar with this culture technique and attempt to pull individual hairs from the bristles instead of stabbing the bristles onto the surface of the plate. New toothbrushes in their original packaging are mycologically sterile. The most inexpensive source of toothbrushes is an on-line hotel supply store, where they can be purchased for $0.05 to $0.10 each. Shelters may be able to obtain donated toothbrushes from dental supply stores or local dentists.

Fungal culture media and incubation temperatures

There are many commercially available fungal culture media for in-house laboratory use, and the question always arises as to what is the "best medium." In one unpublished study (abstract), five different fungal culture media were evaluated [25]. The investigators compared Rapid Sporulation Medium (RSM; Bacti-Labs, Mountain View, California), two commercial brands of Sabouraud's dextrose agar, and two commercial brands of dermatophyte test medium (DTM) for growth, sporulation, and identification characteristics of *M canis*. The study found all five diagnostic media to be adequate for growth and identification of *M canis*. Despite its name, RSM did not produce macroconidia faster than the other media. Based on the findings of this study, the authors recommend that cost, shelf life, and ease of inoculation be the most important criteria when considering what culture medium to purchase. Fungal culture plates should be at least three times as large as the head of a toothbrush to allow for adequate nutrients and inoculation space.

In another study reporting on the efficacy of a commercial fungal culture medium developed for animals (Rapid Vet D; DMS Laboratories, Flemington, New Jersey), the authors found that incubation temperature may be an important but overlooked factor in sporulation. Currently, it is recommended that fungal cultures be incubated at "room temperature." This is a vague recommendation, and room temperature can vary considerably depending on the outside ambient temperature. In this study, the authors found that increased incubation temperatures (24°C–27°C or 75°F–80°F) resulted in more rapid sporulation of fungi [26]. This is an important finding, because room temperature in many veterinary clinics is rarely this warm in the winter and clearly nowhere near this ideal temperature in the summer when air conditioning is used. In the authors' experiments with temperature and fungal culture sporulation, less than optimum temperatures resulted in colony growth that grossly resembled *M canis*, but microscopic examination revealed only unsporulated hyphae (Fig. 4). This was true for DTM and Sabouraud's dextrose agar. This is frustrating, because the gross colony characteristics are often "classic," yet macroconidia are absent.

The authors recommend keeping fungal cultures in a warm location away from air-conditioning ducts, relocating the cultures to plastic box placed inside

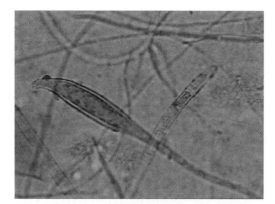

Fig. 4. Early sporulation of M canis. Note that the classic cell divisions are absent and that many of the hyphae appear as thick finger-like projections. This appearance is common when cultures are incubated in an air-conditioned room.

a cabinet or drawer, using a light bulb incubator, or purchasing a tabletop incubator. The latter is only practical if the practice performs large numbers of cultures. Isolation of *Trichophyton* spp requires increased temperatures and, often, special media, and use of a diagnostic laboratory may be needed in some cases. If the fungal culture medium is dehydrating too quickly, place the individual plates in self-closing plastic bags. Another advantage of this is that it prevents or minimizes cross-contamination.

Practical use of InTray DM culture medium. The InTray DM (IVD Biomed Diagnostics, White City, Oregon) fungal culture medium was originally designed for use in people rather than animals. The major advantages of this system are that the fungal culture tray fits on a microscope stage and colony growth occurs without opening the culture well and without the use of special stains. It is essentially an all-in-one "culture/slide mount" test kit. The disadvantages are that laboratory personnel need to be familiar with examining slide mounts and cultures in situ, the surface area is too small for toothbrush culture inoculations, and the small surface area is rapidly overgrown by contaminants. In veterinary medicine, the commercial medium is best used for subculturing suspect colonies or for culturing individual glowing hairs. These plates must be examined daily, because the medium volume is small and rapid color change occurs.

Microscopic Examination of Fungal Cultures: Making It Easier
Microscopic examination of fungal cultures can be simplified if the following points are kept in mind when deciding which colonies to target for examination:

- Pathogens are pale or buff in color.
- Heavily pigmented gross or microscopic colonies are not pathogens.

- Examination of fungal culture plates daily aids in the identification of fungal pathogens, because highly suspect colonies to watch are pale colonies producing a red color change in the medium as it is growing.
- In most cases, *Microsporum* pathogens grow within 7 to 14 days; however, *Trichophyton* colonies are more problematic and may take up to 21 days to grow.
- A red color change in the medium is not diagnostic for a pathogen.

Microscopic examinations using clear or frosted tape

The most simple method for examining fungal culture colonies is to use a transparent cellulose adhesive tape preparation. The most commonly recommended stain is lactophenol cotton blue; however, one of the authors (SN) routinely uses new methylene blue stain (NMB) with good success. The major advantage of NMB stain is its ready availability and the minimal risk of damage to the microscope lens. Phenol is a caustic agent. One disadvantage is that it does not kill the specimen, and care should be taken when handling preparations made with this stain. Samples can be collected from a target colony using a tease technique that transfers a small amount of colony growth to a drop of stain on a glass slide via a wooden stick or inoculation loop. The easiest and most practical method is to collect a specimen using sticky tape, however. Tape preparations can be made using clear or frosted tape (L. Sigler, PhD, Microfungus Collection and Herbarium, University of Alberta, personal communication, 2005). For both techniques, a small drop of stain is placed on a glass microscope slide. The sticky side of the tape is pressed to the edge of the target colony to collect a specimen. If clear tape is used, place the sticky side down over the drop of stain. The preparation can be examined at this step, but the quality of the preparation is improved if a second drop of stain is placed over the tape and the specimen is then coverslipped. If frosted tape is used, place the tape sticky side up over the drop of stain. Place a second drop of stain on the tape and coverslip before examination. When frosted tape is used, the second drop of stain and coverslip are mandatory.

Shelter life: minimizing the cost of fungal cultures

In the authors' program, all cats are screened for dermatophytosis via toothbrush fungal cultures. In addition, any animal with skin disease in which dermatophytosis is a possible differential diagnosis is screened with a fungal culture. This is only possible because we prepare our own media and pour our own fungal culture plates. The cost of commercially prepared fungal culture medium may be cost-prohibitive for most shelters; however, this obstacle can be overcome by preparing fungal plates in-house. Although this task is not difficult, it is time-consuming and does require someone with training and experience in sterile laboratory procedures. Many individuals in the community have these skills or facilities, including veterinary technicians, veterinarian medical technicians, biology teachers, and laboratory technicians, for example. Media plates should be prepared off-site in a clean facility (eg, high school chemistry laboratory, meticulously clean kitchen) that is free of animal exposure. The preparation of fungal culture plates in a volunteer's kitchen is not an unreasonable activity, nor is it a "first." One of the founding fathers of dairy cow mastitis screening and control started his work in practice and used blood agar plates prepared by his mother-in-law in her kitchen (J. Dahl, DVM, Production Animal Medicine, University of Wisconsin–Madison School of Veterinary Medicine, personal communication, 2003). Essentially, if there is a will, there is a way.

> The most effective way to control dermatophytosis in a shelter is to culture all cats and suspect infected dogs at the time of admission. The major obstacle to this is the cost of commercially prepared fungal culture plates. Shelters should survey volunteers for people with laboratory skills needed to make fungal culture plates.

USING FUNGAL CULTURE RESULTS FOR MAKING TREATMENT DECISIONS

Typically, cultures are interpreted as "culture-positive" or "culture-negative." In our experience with screening and treating for control, this is an inadequate amount of information. The following is a summary of how we report and use fungal culture results to make treatment decisions:

- All samples must be adequately identified, and the key information other than the animal's name or booking number includes the animal's age, hair length, and whether or not lesions are present. It is helpful sometimes to know if the animal is a surrendered house pet or stray, but this information is often unreliable in shelters if there is a fee for surrendering a pet cat and no fee for surrendering a "stray."
- Samples are inoculated onto modified Mycosel Medium (BD, Franklin Lakes, NJ) with phenol red, which is essentially equivalent to DTM but much easier to make in large quantities.
- All samples are held for 21 days, and culture results are recorded once weekly in columns labeled "wk1, wk2, and wk 3." Results are reported to the shelter as no growth (NG), contaminant growth (C), or heavy contaminant growth (HC), or the pathogen is identified and the number of colony-forming units recorded. The significance of the latter is discussed in detail elsewhere in this article.
- Plates that are rapidly overgrown with contaminants in the first 7 to 10 days are reported as HC. These plates are of particular concern, because rapid overgrowth of the plate may result in a false-negative fungal culture. We have seen this most commonly in kittens and stray cats, and it is prudent to reculture these cats as soon as the overgrown plate is noted. Rapid overgrowth of the plate usually results in the entire surface of the plate turning red, making it impossible to watch for pale colonies with a ring of red around them as they grow.
- In our experience, all M canis-positive cats have been identified within 7 to14 days of culture. Plates are held for 21 days, because Trichophyton spp dermatophytes take longer to grow. From a practical perspective, if cats are culture-negative for M canis after 14 days, they can be considered culture-negative at the time of admission.

- The key to early and fast identification of pathogens is daily examination of fungal culture plates. Contrary to popular belief, this is not a time-consuming activity. One hundred or more plates can be quickly scanned in less than 7 to 10 minutes. What you are looking for are small white colonies with a red ring of color change around them as they are growing. Often, the colonies may be too young for definitive identification, but once a plate is identified as "suspect," it can be watched more closely. An organized approach to reading plates should make this process fast and easy.
- The number of colony-forming units is an important aid in determining if the animal is infected or merely a fomite carrier.

Using Colony-Forming Units to Aid in Treatment Decisions

In our shelter work, we have found that simply reporting a fungal culture as positive or negative is not helpful to the staff, because toothbrush cultures cannot distinguish fomite carriers from truly infected cats. To help do this, we incorporate the number of colony-forming units found on the plate in the report via something we call a pathogen score, or "P-score." If a culture has been properly obtained, the number of colony-forming units per plate generally corresponds to the severity of infection or degree of contamination when evaluating environmental cultures. The system is simple: a score of P-1 is equivalent to 1 to 4 colony-forming units per plate, P-2 equals 5 to 9 colony-forming units per plate, and P-3 equals 10 or more colony-forming units per plate. This information, along with the recorded age and presence or absence of lesions at the time of culture, can help to speed identification of culture-positive cats and differentiate fomite carriers. When the laboratory alerts the shelter that a positive animal has been identified, the animal is immediately examined.

Cats with a score of P-1 fall into two categories. The first category is cats that are fomite carriers. These cats are lesion-free and Wood's lamp-negative when examined. All repeat cultures of these cats have been negative, and it is hypothesized that the cats were mechanically carrying spores on their hair coat that were removed during grooming. As just mentioned, these cats are recultured as a safeguard and treated with one topical application of lime sulfur. We refer to these in-house as "dip and go" cats. The second category is cats that were incubating infections at the time of admission. Lesions in these cats are subtle, and the face and hairs of bell of the ear and the ear canal should be carefully examined. Wood's lamp examinations may or may not be positive depending on the strain of *M canis*; *Trichophyton* infections do not fluoresce.

Cats with a score of P-2 can fall into the fomite carrier group or the "infected group." The major difference with these cats is that if lesions are found, they tend to be more noticeable. Shelter staff often report these lesions almost simultaneously with the reporting of the fungal culture.

Cats with a score of P-3 are immediately removed from the general population regardless of whether or not they have lesions. In general, the admitting staff are often suspicious of these cats, and such cats are usually placed in quarantine pending the results of their fungal culture. Cats with a score of P-3 are considered a risk to the population and are removed from the general population.

The P-scoring system is also useful when monitoring treatment. Animals under treatment in our program are cultured once weekly, and the P-scores are reported. As animals are cured, the P-score becomes lower. Another area in which we have found colony-forming units to be helpful in managing disease in the shelter is in the reporting of environmental cultures. Reporting a site as culture-positive is not helpful to staff charged with the task of cleaning and disinfecting the site. The P-score system has resulted in "buy-in" by the staff; no one wants there to be a positive culture, let alone a score of P-3.

> Control of dermatophytosis in a shelter cannot rely solely on results being reported as "positive" or "negative" for pathogens. Colony-forming unit counts along with clinical examination can help to differentiate fomite carriers from infected cats and help to control treatment costs.

TREATMENT RECOMMENDATIONS FOR INFECTED ANIMALS

The reader is referred to a recently published article on a review of published studies on the treatment of dermatophytosis [27]. It is important to note that all the topical treatment studies have been conducted using isolated infected hairs in the laboratory, experimental infections, pet cats, or cattery cats [28–39]. Systemic treatment studies are reports of cases or experimentally infected cats that were treated or field studies on cattery cats [32,34,36–38,40–53]. Based on the findings of these studies and our work with shelter animals [1,2], the following are our recommendations regarding the treatment of animals with dermatophytosis in animal shelters.

Cage Confinement

Infected animals should be confined to a cage or kennel until cured. Cage comforts should be limited to items that can be washed daily, and all cage toys should be plastic. Care staff must be educated about the risk of fomite transmission and proper handling of these animals. Staff should wear protective coats that are changed daily, and these animals should be cleaned and fed last or by someone who is not circulating in the general population. In our shelter, cats are housed in an annex building and cared for by volunteers. In other shelters, a room should be designated for these animals. The room should be furnished with the bare essentials for the care of these animals. Staff should wear disposable gowns, and traffic into and out of this room should be minimized.

Clipping of the Hair Coat

Cats with severe generalized infections or long hair should be clipped to remove infective material and prevent it from contaminating the environment. Focal lesions can be clipped. If infected hairs can be identified via a Wood's lamp, they should be removed. This is critical in shelters to minimize contamination and protect staff. Not clipping severely infected cats is equivalent to not removing feces from the kennel of dogs with parvovirus.

Antifungal Treatment

The goal of treatment is to cure these animals as rapidly as possible and minimize the risk of contamination of the shelter or spread to other animals. Clipping of the hair coat can accomplish part of this goal by "debulking" and removing infective material. Optimum treatment requires the use of a topical agent and a systemic antifungal agent. It is our opinion that dermatophytosis is a treatable and curable disease in an animal shelter; however, not all animals are candidates for treatment. For animals to be treated, they must be tame enough to be handled on a daily basis. The most effective treatment is a combination of topical and systemic therapy. Effective topical agents include lime sulfur, miconazole shampoo and/or rinse, and enilconazole. Currently, the authors recommend the use of twice-weekly topical therapy until mycologic cure, coupled with short-term itraconazole therapy (5–10 mg/kg administered orally every 24 hours for 21–28 days). Our topical treatment of choice is lime sulfur administered twice weekly at a rate of 8 oz/gal. This is easily applied with a watering can held close to the skin or a commercial rose garden sprayer (Fig. 5). One-half gallon of rinse applied by this method can treat 10 to 15 cats depending on hair length. It is important to hold the sprayer close to the skin and allow the coat to be soaked proximally (skin and hair follicle) to distally (hair tip) (Fig. 6). The face and ears

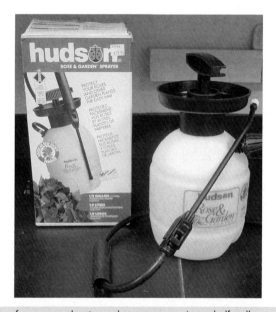

Fig. 5. Example of a sprayer that is used to treat cats. A one-half gallon sprayer is recommended because it is easy to handle.

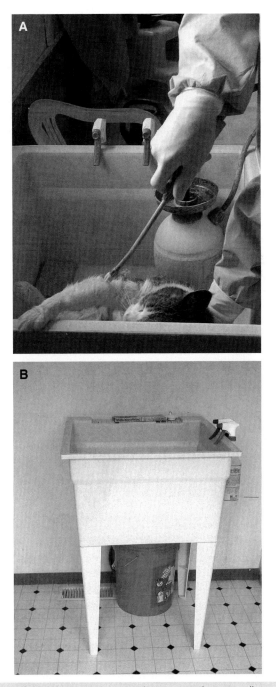

Fig. 6. (A) Lime sulfur applied to a cat using the sprayer. The cat is allowed to "grasp" the end of the dip sink. Cats tolerate procedure well. (B) Portable dip sink used for topical therapy.

should be treated with a sponge. Lime sulfur diluted in warm water applied by these methods is well tolerated by cats. The authors have used this product extensively and have found it to be safe and effective even in young cats. Cats can be collared to prevent them from licking the solution; however, we do not do this. Oral ulceration has been anecdotally reported as a possible adverse effect; however, this has not been the authors' experience when treating cats. Lime sulfur can be used at a rate of 4 or 8 oz/gal. Early use in our shelter revealed that the higher concentration was more effective. Itraconazole is the preferred drug of choice over griseofulvin, fluconazole, and terbinafine because it is consistently effective, associated with few adverse effects, does not require hematologic or biochemical monitoring, and is known to exhibit antifungal activity for several weeks after discontinuation of therapy.

Monitoring Therapy

Previous recommendations for monitoring recommended starting posttreatment fungal cultures after 4 weeks of therapy. We recommend weekly cultures for monitoring. The treatment end point is two negative fungal cultures at weekly intervals. Based on our studies to date, cultures can be finalized after 14 days. Shelter operators may argue that the cost of weekly fungal cultures is prohibitive, but the shelter must weigh the cost of an individual fungal culture versus the cost of animal care per day when making this decision.

Efficacy of Itraconazole and Lime Sulfur

In a recent field study, when data were retrospectively evaluated to exclude additional days for finalization of fungal cultures, the mean number of days to cure was 18 ± 8.5 days and the mean number of lime sulfur treatments was six $\pm$ three treatments [2]. Adverse effects of the lime sulfur treatments were uncommon and limited to hair loss on the ear pinnae and drying of the hair coat. Oral ulcerations did not occur.

Lufenuron and Fungal Vaccines

Lufenuron has repeatedly been found to be ineffective in the treatment and prevention of dermatophytosis, and it is not recommended for the treatment of dermatophytosis [52,53]. Fungal vaccines have been shown to be ineffective in the treatment or prevention of dermatophytosis, and the only commercial fungal vaccine for *M canis* has been withdrawn from the market [54–59].

> Treatment of dermatophytosis in a shelter must be aggressive to minimize contamination of the environment and spread to other animals. This is best facilitated by restriction of animals in cages or runs until they are cured, clipping of the hair coat to remove infective material, and twice-weekly topical therapy until animals are cured, coupled with short-term daily antifungal therapy.

ENVIRONMENTAL CONTAMINATION

Extent of Environmental Contamination and Efficacy of the
Triple-Cleaning Technique in Homes Exposed to *Microsporum canis*
Arthrospores

Environmental contamination is of major concern in animal shelters. Investigations into the extent of contamination after exposure are limited. In a recent study, investigators sampled the air and physical environment of the homes of 30 animals infected with *M canis* (9 dogs and 21 cats) [60]. Contact plates were used to sample environmental surfaces, and the air was sampled using a Sas-Super-100 Air sampler (Bioscience International, Rockville, Maryland). Contamination of the homes and air was found in all the homes in which infected cats were present and in four of nine homes in which infected dogs were present. Homes with kittens were found to be heavily contaminated. In eight of the homes in which infected cats or kittens were present, people had also contacted dermatophytosis. In another environmental study, 400 samples form the floors of 50 veterinary clinics were sampled using contact plates [61]. In this study more than 11 different pathogenic fungi were found in the environment, presumably from patients entering the facility.

In another study, the investigators reported not only on the extent of environmental contamination of homes housing infected cats but on the efficacy of decontamination practices [3]. In this study, 5-in × 5-in pieces of commercial Swiffer cloths were found readily and consistently to collect infected spores and debris when wiped over the target area until visibly soiled. Fungal culture plates were inoculated by pressing the soiled sample five times onto the surface of the plate. This technique was found over and over again to be a reliable method for sampling homes for contamination and for monitoring contamination in the home during the treatment period. During treatment, owners were asked to clean homes twice weekly using the triple-cleaning technique: mechanically remove spores and hairs via vacuuming, wash and rinse surfaces three times using a detergent solution, and disinfect target areas with 1:10 bleach. As expected, homes were easily contaminated when infected cats were present. Contamination was heaviest in homes in which infected cats were allowed to roam freely and owners made no effort to clean thoroughly during the treatment period. Using the triple-cleaning technique and Swiffer cloth sampling to monitor for contamination, homes were found to culture negative after one to three cleanings.

Shelter Life: Monitoring the Environment for Contamination

The easiest way to monitor the environment for contamination is with the Swiffer cloth cultures. These can be used to identify areas of contamination and monitor postcleaning efforts by staff. Cleaning and disinfecting are tedious and often thankless jobs. Staff can become more engaged and take a sense of "ownership" if they participate in the culture collection, inoculation, and monitoring.

References

[1] Newbury S, Verbrugge M, Steffen T, et al. Management of naturally occurring dermatophy-
    tosis in an open shelter: part 1: development of a cost effective screening and monitoring
    program [abstract]. Vet Dermatol 2005;16:192.
[2] Newbury S, Verbrugge M, Steffen T, et al. Management of naturally occurring dermatophy-
    tosis in an open shelter: part 2: treatment of cats in an off site facility [abstract]. Vet Dermatol
    2005;16:192.
[3] Heinrich KA, Newbury S, Verbrugge M, et al. Detection of environmental contamination in
    homes exposed to Microsporum canis arthrospores and efficacy of the triple cleaning tech-
    nique [abstract]. Vet Dermatol 2005;16:192.
[4] Foil CS. Dermatophytosis. In: Greene CE, editor. Infectious diseases of the dog and cat. Phil-
    adelphia: WB Saunders; 1998. p. 362–70.
[5] Scott DW, Miller WH, Griffin CE. Fungal skin diseases. In: Muller and Kirk's small animal
    dermatology. 6th edition. Philadelphia: WB Saunders; 2001. p. 336–61.
[6] Moriello KA, DeBoer DJ. Feline dermatophytosis: recent advances and recommendations
    for therapy. Vet Clin North Am Small Anim Pract 1995;25:901–21.
[7] Moriello KA, DeBoer DJ. Fungal flora of pet cats. Am J Vet Res 1991;52:602–6.
[8] Philpot CM, Perry AP. The normal fungal flora of dogs. Mycopathologia 1984;87:155–7.
[9] Cafarchia C, Romito D, Sasanelli M, et al. The epidemiology of canine and feline dermato-
    phytosis in southern Italy. Mycoses 2004;47:508–13.
[10] Khosravi AR, Mahmoudi M. Dermatophytes isolated from domestic animals in Iran. Myco-
    ses 2003;46:222–5.
[11] Mancianti F, Nardoni S, Cecchi S, et al. Dermatophytes isolated from symptomatic dogs
    and cats in Tuscany Italy during a 15 year period. Mycopathologia 2003;156:13–8.
[12] Gradzki Z, Boguta L, Winiarczyk S. Canine dermatophytosis as a hazard to people. Med
    Weter 2001;57:815–8.
[13] Cababes FJ, Abarca ML, Bragulat MR. Dermatophytes isolated from domestic animals in
    Barcelona, Spain. Mycopathologia 1997;137:107–13.
[14] Khosravi AR. Fungal flora of the hair coat of stray cats in Iran. Mycoses 1996;39:241–3.
[15] Mignon BR, Losson BJ. Prevalence and characterization of Microsporum canis carriage in
    cats. J Med Vet Mycol 1997;35:249–56.
[16] Aljabre S, Richardson MD, Scott EM. Adherence of arthroconidia and germlings of anthro-
    pophilic and zoophilic species of Trichophyton mentagrophytes to human corneocytes as an
    early event in the pathogenesis of dermatophytosis. Clin Exp Dermatol 1993;18:231–8.
[17] Mancianti F, Giannelli C, Bendinelli M, et al. Mycological findings in immunodeficiency in-
    fected cats. J Med Vet Mycol 1992;30:257–9.
[18] Moriello KA, DeBoer DJ. Dermatophytosis: advances in therapy and control. In: August J,
    editor. Consultations in feline internal medicine. 3rd edition. Philadelphia: WB Saunders;
    1997. p. 177–90.
[19] Moriello KA, DeBoer DJ. Fungal flora of cats with and without dermatophytosis. J Vet Med
    Mycol 1991;29:285–9.
[20] Moriello KA, Kunkle G, DeBoer DJ. Isolation of dermatophytes from the hair coats of stray
    cats from selected animal shelters in two different geographic regions in the United States.
    Vet Dermatol 1994;5:57–62.
[21] Carlotti DN, DeBarbeyrac P, Mignon B, et al. A case of sylvatic dermatophytosis due to Tri-
    chophyton mentagrophytes in a cat [abstract]. Vet Dermatol 2005;16:192.
[22] Sparkes AH, Gruffydd-Jones TJ, Shaw SE. Epidemiological and diagnostic features of ca-
    nine and feline dermatophytosis in the United Kingdom from 1956 to 1991. Vet Rec
    1993;133:57–61.
[23] Cerundolo R. Generalized Microsporum canis dermatophytosis in six Yorkshire terrier dogs.
    Vet Dermatol 2004;15:181–7.
[24] Moriello KA. Diagnostic techniques for dermatophytosis. Clin Tech Small Anim Pract
    2001;16:219–24.

[25] Elliot C, Plant J. A comparison of the performance of five growth media used to culture and identify Microsporum canis [abstract]. In: Proceedings of the Annual Members Meeting of the American Association of Veterinary Dermatology and American College of Veterinary Dermatology. Sante Fe (NM): AAVD/ACVD; 1995. p. 28.

[26] Guillot J, Latié L, Manjula D, et al. Evaluation of the dermatophyte test medium Rapid Vet-D. Vet Dermatol 2001;12:123–7.

[27] Moriello KA. Treatment of dermatophytosis in cats and dogs: review of published studies. Vet Dermatol 2004;15:99–107.

[28] Rycroft AN, McLay C. Disinfectants in the control of small animal ringworm due to *Microsporum canis*. Vet Rec 1991;129:239–41.

[29] Moriello KA, DeBoer DJ. Environmental decontamination of *Microsporum canis*: in vitro studies using isolated infected cat hair. In: Kwochka KW, Willemse T, von Tscharner C, editors. Advances in veterinary dermatology, vol. 3. Oxford, United Kingdom: Butterworth Heinemann; 1998. p. 309–18.

[30] White-Weithers N, Medleau L. Efficacy of topical therapies for the treatment of dermatophyte-infected hairs from dogs and cats. J Am Anim Hosp Assoc 1995;31:250–3.

[31] Perrin N, Bond R. Synergistic inhibition of the growth in vitro of *Microsporum canis* by miconazole and chlorhexidine. Vet Dermatol 2003;14:99–102.

[32] Paterson S. Miconazole/chlorhexidine shampoo as an adjunct to systemic therapy in controlling dermatophytosis in cats. J Small Anim Pract 1999;40:163–6.

[33] Moriello KA, DeBoer DJ, Volk L, et al. Development of an in vitro, isolated, infected spore testing model for disinfectant testing of *Microsporum canis* isolates. Vet Dermatol 2004; 15:175–80.

[34] Mason KV. Treatment of a *Microsporum canis* infection in a colony of Persian cats with griseofulvin and a shampoo containing 2% miconazole, 2% chlorhexidine, 2% miconazole and 2% chlorhexidine or placebo [abstract]. Vet Dermatol 2000;12(Suppl 1):55.

[35] DeJaham C. Enilconazole emulsion in the treatment of dermatophytosis in Persian cats; tolerance and suitability. In: Kwochka KW, Willemse T, von Tscharner C, editors, Advances in veterinary dermatology, vol. 3. Oxford, United Kingdom: Butterworth Heinemann; 1998. p. 299–307.

[36] Guillot J, Malandain E, Jankowskin F, et al. Evaluation of the efficacy of oral lufenuron combined with topical enilconazole for the management of dermatophytosis in catteries. Vet Rec 2002;150:714–8.

[37] Hnilica KA, Medleau L. Evaluation of topically applied enilconazole for the treatment of dermatophytosis in a Persian cattery. Vet Dermatol 2002;13:23–8.

[38] Sparkes AH, Robinson A, MacKay AD, et al. A study of the efficacy of topical and systemic therapy for the treatment of feline *Microsporum canis* infection. J Feline Med Surg 2000;2: 135–42.

[39] DeBoer DJ, Moriello KA. Inability of topical treatment to influence the course of experimental feline dermatophytosis. J Am Vet Med Assoc 1995;205:52–7.

[40] Mancianti F, Pedonese F, Zullino C. Efficacy of oral administration of itraconazole to cats with dermatophytosis caused by *Microsporum canis*. J Am Vet Med Assoc 1998;213: 993–5.

[41] Moriello KA, DeBoer DJ. Efficacy of griseofulvin and itraconazole in the treatment of experimentally induced dermatophytosis in cats. J Am Vet Med Assoc 1995;207:439–44.

[42] Balda AC. Comparative efficacy of griseofulvin and terbinafine in the therapy of dermatophytosis in dogs and cats [abstract]. In: Proceedings of the World Small Animal Veterinary Association Congress. 2002.

[43] Colombo S, Cornegliani L, Vercelli A. Efficacy of itraconazole as combined continuous/pulse therapy in feline dermatophytosis: preliminary results in nine cases. Vet Dermatol 2001;12:347–50.

[44] Shelton GH. Severe neutropenia associated with griseofulvin therapy in cats with feline immunodeficiency virus. J Vet Intern Med 1990;4:317–8.

[45] Chen C. The use of terbinafine for the treatment of dermatophytosis [abstract]. Vet Dermatol 2000;12(Suppl 1):41.

[46] Mancianti F, Pedonese F, Millanta F. Efficacy of oral terbinafine in feline dermatophytosis due to *Microsporum canis*. J Feline Med Surg 1999;1:37–41.

[47] Kotnik T. Drug efficacy of terbinafine hydrochloride (Lamisil®) during oral treatment of cats experimentally infected with *Microsporum canis*. J Vet Med B Infect Dis Vet Public Health 2002;49:120–2.

[48] Castañón-Olivares LR, Manzano-Gayosso P, et al. Effectiveness of terbinafine in the eradication of *Microsporum canis* from laboratory cats. Mycoses 2001;44:95–7.

[49] Kotnik T, Erzuh NK, Kuzner J, et al. Terbinafine hydrochloride treatment of *Microsporum canis* experimentally-induced ringworm in cats. Vet Microbiol 2001;83:161–8.

[50] Ben-Ziony Y, Arzi B. Use of lufenuron for treating fungal infections of dogs and cats: 297 cases (1997–1999). J Am Vet Med Assoc 2000;217:1510–3.

[51] Ben-Ziony Y, Arzi B. Update information for the treatment of fungal infections in dogs and cats [letter to the editor]. J Am Vet Med Assoc 2001;218:1718.

[52] DeBoer DJ, Moriello KA, Blum JL, et al. Effects of lufenuron treatment in cats on the establishment and course of *Microsporum canis* infection following exposure to infected cats. J Am Vet Med Assoc 2003;222:1216–20.

[53] Moriello KA, DeBoer DJ, Volk L, et al. Efficacy of pretreatment with lufenuron for the prevention of *Microsporum canis* infection in a feline direct topical challenge model. Vet Dermatol 2004;15:357–62.

[54] DeBoer DJ, Moriello KA. The immune response to *Microsporum canis* induced by a fungal cell wall vaccine. Vet Dermatol 1994;5:47–55.

[55] DeBoer DJ, Moriello KA. Investigations of a killed dermatophyte cell-wall vaccine against Microsporum canis infection with *Microsporum canis* in cats. Res Vet Sci 1995;59:110–3.

[56] Manoyan MG, Panin AN, Letyagin KP. Effectiveness of Microderm vaccine against dermatophytosis in animals [abstract]. Vet Dermatol 2000;12(Suppl 1):59.

[57] Bredah LK, Bratberg AM, Solbakk T, et al. Efficacy of an experimental *Microsporum canis* vaccine in farmed foxes [abstract]. Vet Dermatol 2000;12(Suppl 1):39.

[58] Bredahl LK, Bratberg AM, Solbakk IT, et al. Safety of an experimental *Microsporum canis* vaccine in famed foxes [abstract]. Vet Dermatol 2000;12(Suppl 1):45.

[59] DeBoer DJ, Moriello KA, Blum JL, et al. Safety and efficacy and immunological effects after inoculation of an inactivated and combined live-inactivated dermatophytosis vaccines in cats. Am J Vet Res 2002;63:1532–7.

[60] Mancianti F, Nardoni S, Corazza M, et al. Environmental detection of *Microsporum canis* arthrospores in the households of infected cats and dogs. J Feline Med Surg 2003;5:323–8.

[61] Mancianti F, Papini R. Isolation of keratophilic fungi from the floors of private veterinary clinics in Italy. Vet Res Commun 1996;20:161–6.

Feline Facial Dermatoses

Cecilia Friberg, DVM

Animal Dermatology Center of Chicago, 3123 North Clybourne Avenue, Chicago, IL 60618, USA

C ats have become ever more popular as pets and family members and are being presented to veterinary clinics for diagnostic workup of diseases. Many new disorders have been described in the past decade, many of which affect the skin of the face, head, and ears. This review of these disorders is divided into taxonomic categories. Disorders associated with feline facial dermatoses may present at various times during the clinical course of the disease; thus, lesions may not correspond to traditional problem-oriented categories for a specific disease. Despite this, problem-oriented approaches are important for diagnosis; lesions have been recategorized using this scheme in Table 1. This review summarizes current information about diseases that may manifest on the face, head, and ears; however, it is important to remember that most diseases are not exclusive to this region of the body.

Because of their inquisitive nature and their tendencies toward hunting, cats may acquire various disorders on the head while pursuing predatory behaviors. Cats are likely to incur wounds during hunting, and disease transmission is then increased. Compared with other regions of the body, the hair is also sparser on the head (eg, preauricular, dorsal muzzle, pinnae regions) than on other areas of the body; thus, environmental insults have more access to the skin in these regions. Cats also tend toward being secretive; thus, client history may be misleading in some cases. Alopecia, for example, is often traumatic in nature, but many owners do not see their cats overgrooming because this behavior may take place out of sight or when the owner is not at home. Lesions may also not be obvious until some time has passed and the lesions have progressed. The primary lesions are therefore often missed, and we are left with only pieces of the puzzle to backtrack through our diagnostics to determine what disease we are seeing and then how to manage it.

VIRAL AGENTS

Calicivirus

Oral ulceration is common with calicivirus infection; however, infection of the haired skin is less common. Feline calicivirus is not a common cause of feline acne but can be isolated from some cats [1].

E-mail address: cfriberg@att.net

0195-5616/06/$ – see front matter
doi:10.1016/j.cvsm.2005.09.002

Table 1
Facial lesions categorized by problems

Oral ulcers and/or plaques
Calicivirus	Dermatophilus	Junctional epidermolysis bullosa[a]
Erythema multiforme[a]	Papillomavirus	

Crusting and/or scaling
FeLV dermatitis	Demodex gatoi (with erythema/pruritus)	Lymphocytic mural folliculitis (underlying erosions)
Notoedres cati	Sarcoptes scabiei	Dermatophytosis[a]
Pediculosis	Leishmaniasis[a]	Solar keratosis/actinic dermatitis[a]
Junctional epidermolysis bullosa[a]		

Crusting and/or scaling followed by alopecia
Pemphigus foliaceus	DLE	Follicular mucinosis
Pemphigus erythematosus	SLE	
MF[a]	Pseudolymphoma[a]	

Papules
Feline pox	Apocrine nevus[a]	Staphylococcal folliculitis

Papules developing into crusts
Trombiculosis/chiggers	Chin acne[a]	Urticaria pigmentosa
Feline pox lesions		

Papules/nodules that ulcerated and drain
Cryptococcus	Exophiala spinifera	Pseudolymphoma[a]
Histoplasmosis	Mycobacteria/tuberculosis	MF[a]

Plaque
Feline collagenolytic granuloma	Eosinophilic plaque	Xanthoma[a]
Solar keratosis/actinic dermatitis[a]	Multicentric Squamous cell carcinoma (later crusts)	

Nodules
Other fungi	Dilated pore of Winer (cystic, filled with wkeratin)	Metastatic calcification
Algae: Prototheca	Cuterebra	Foreign body reactions, nodules that ulcerate
Feline multisystemic granulomatous mycobacteriosis	Leishmaniasis	MF[a]
Dirofilaria immitis	Basal cell tumor (also alopecic)	Mast cell tumor (may ulcerate)
Melanoma	Pseudolymphoma[a]	Squamous cell carcinoma (later may ulcerate)
Fibropapilloma/feline sarcoid	Xanthoma[a]	Feline leprosy (also ulcerated nodules)
Apocrine nevus[a]		

Abscesses
Sporotrichosis	Actinomycosis	Yersinia pestis

Table 1
(continued)

Ulceration, erosions		
Herpesvirus (also crusts)	Feline indolent ulcer	Erythema multiforme[a]
Mosquito bite hypersensitivity (papule/plaque, then ulcer)	MF[a]	Idiopathic nasal scaling in Bengal cats (crust/scale, erosion)
Intertrigo		Vasculitis (crust, then erosions/ulceration)
Alopecia		
Dermatophytosis[a]	Preauricular alopecia	Feline multisystemic granulomatous mycobacteriosis[a]
Pigmentation disorder		
Leishmaniasis (hypopigmentation)[a]	MF (depigmentation)[a]	Periocular leukotrichia
Lentigo simplex		
Folliculitis/comedones		
Chin acne	Dermatophytosis[a]	
Pruritus		
Food allergy	Atopy	Methimazole drug reaction
Exudative		
Idiopathic facial dermatitis of Persian cats		
Trauma/bite wound		
Feline pox (rodent bite)		

Abbreviations: DLE, discoid lupus erythematosus; FeLV, feline leukemia virus; MF, mycosis fungoides (epitheliotropic lymphoma); SLE, systemic lupus erythematosus.
[a]Diseases that fall into more than one problem category.

Papillomavirus

Oral papillomas have been described in domestic cats as well as in exotic felids. Lesions are described as multifocal, small, soft, light pink, oval, slightly raised, flat, sessile lesions located on the ventral lingual surfaces. Truncal lesions are also described as rough, raised, nonpigmented to heavily pigmented (depending on the skin color of the cat), scaly, greasy plaques that are 3 to 5 mm in greatest diameter. On histopathologic examination, keratohyalin-like cytoplasmic granules and cytoplasmic inclusion bodies were noted in keratinocytes. Polymerase chain reaction (PCR) and immunohistochemical analysis confirms papillomavirus being present in these lesions [2].

Feline Herpes Virus

Vesicular, crusting, ulcerative, and necrotizing facial dermatitis affecting haired skin of the face or nasal planum or stomatitis has been associated with feline herpesvirus 1 infection. Usually, crusted skin lesions involve the nasal planum, bridge of the nose, or periocular skin. Under the crusts, the skin is inflamed and ulcerated. Ocular or respiratory signs or a history of these signs may or may not be present. The presence of concurrent respiratory signs is supportive of herpes virus infection.

Diagnosis is confirmed by a biopsy, which shows ulcerative and often necrotic dermatitis with suppurative folliculitis and furunculosis as well as perivascular to interstitial mixed inflammatory cell dermatitis with many eosinophils. The surface and follicular epithelium have multinucleated keratinocytic giant cells containing amphophilic intranuclear inclusion bodies. Necrosis of epitrichial sweat glands seems to be a unique feature of this disease. PCR is of limited diagnostic value because of the occurrence of herpesvirus DNA in healthy carriers. In adult cats, reactivation of disease can be triggered by stress or steroid use [3].

Feline Pox Virus

Feline cowpox is an orthopox virus whose natural reservoir is small wild mammals. The virus circulates in different rodent species, especially voles and wood mice, and cats are usually infected through wounds occurring while hunting these rodents. The primary lesion noted is a bite or scratch wound on the head, neck, or forelimb. Local viral replication worsens the primary lesion, and subsequent viremia develops. During the viremic phase, mild pyrexia, inappetence, and depression are usually noted. Secondary lesions develop over the entire body 10 to 14 days after the primary lesion. Pox lesions progress from macules to ulcerated papular to nodular lesions that form into crusts with variable pruritus. Oral vesiculation or ulcerations may also develop. Lesions heal slowly over 3 to 4 weeks, and permanent scarring may result. Definitive diagnosis is made via a skin biopsy, serology, and viral isolation [4]. There is no specific therapy, although secondary bacterial infections often occur and should be treated with drainage and antibiotics. Cat-to-cat, cat-to-human, and cat-to-dog transmission can occur.

Feline Leukemia Virus Infection

Feline leukemia virus (FeLV) can produce scaly, hyperplastic, crusted, and erosive focal lesions that most commonly involve perioral and preauricular skin and pinnae. Moderate to severe pruritus has been reported. Cats seem otherwise healthy; however, over time, most progress to show signs suggesting systemic disease, such as anorexia and lethargy. Positive serologic findings for FeLV and a skin biopsy are required to confirm a viral etiology of lesions. Histopathologic examination shows an epidermis that is irregularly hyperplastic and usually heavily crusted. Syncytial type giant cells are found in the epidermis and outer root sheath of the hair follicles to the level of the isthmus. Keratinocytes within and around the giant cells often are apoptotic. There is poor response to therapy, and the disease is progressive as FeLV becomes further manifested [5].

FUNGAL AGENTS

Cryptococcosis

Cryptococcus neoformans is a ubiquitous saprophytic fungus frequently associated with droppings and accumulated debris of pigeon roosts. In many cases (up to 42%) in which cats live indoors, however, the source of infection remains undetermined. This is an uncommon disease in cats. Male cats may be over-represented, and Abyssinian and Siamese cats may be at increased risk. Most cats present with papules, nodules, ulcers, abscesses, and draining tracts, with the nose and lips commonly involved. Large fluctuant swellings on the bridge of the nose or intranasal polyps are present in 70% of cats. The establishment and spread of infection are highly dependent on host immunity, and disease severity is accelerated or worsened by glucocorticoid therapy. Cryptococcosis is often associated with FeLV or feline immunodeficiency virus (FIV) infection [6,7]. Diagnosis involves examination of aspirates or direct smears of exudate, which show pyogranulomatous to granulomatous inflammation with numer-ous pleomorphic yeast-like organisms (narrow-based budding) surrounded by a mucinous capsule of variable thickness, forming a clear or refractile halo. A biopsy of lesions may show cystic degeneration or vacuolation of the dermis and subcutis that is often acellular or may consist of a nodular to diffuse pyogranulomatous to granulomatous dermatitis and panniculitis, con-taining organisms. Latex agglutination tests are available to detect cryptococcal capsular antigen and may be used to monitor response to therapy; however, titers may persist for months or years after diagnosis and treatment [8].

Histoplasmosis

Histoplasma capsulatum is a dimorphic saprophytic soil fungus, preferring moist humid conditions and soil with nitrogen-rich organic matter, such as bird or bat excrement. In most cases, the disease is disseminated with systemic signs, such as depression, weight loss, fever, anorexia, dyspnea, ocular disease, and skin disease. Skin lesions are extremely rare in cats; when they do occur, they are usually multiple and may be located anywhere on the body but are likely to be present on the face, nose, and pinnae in the form of papules, nod-ules, ulcers, or draining tracts [9]. Diagnosis is supported by travel to endemic area (Ohio, Missouri, and Mississippi River Valleys). Cytology reveals pyogra-nulomatous to granulomatous inflammation with numerous small round yeast bodies with a basophilic center and lighter halo (from shrinkage of the yeast during staining). A biopsy shows a nodular to diffuse pyogranulomatous to granulomatous dermatitis with numerous intracellular organisms. No reliable serologic test is available [10]. Many cats in endemic areas have positive titers; however, these are simply indicative of exposure to the organism.

Other Fungi

Paecolymyces spp are saprophytic opportunistic yeast-like fungi found in soil and decaying vegetation. A 5-year-old cat presented with a nonulcerated, 6-mm, cu-taneous mass on the upper lip. The cat had a previous lesion on a lateral meta-carpus. Mass removal, macerated fungal tissue culture, and histopathologic examination revealed the presence of *Paecilomyces lilacinus* [11].

Trichosporon spp are soil saprophytes that may also be a minor component of normal skin flora. Infection is extremely rare. *Trichosporon* infection has pre-sented as a solitary papular to nodular lesion on the nostril. Diagnosis is via histologic identification of organisms invading tissue and isolation from culture [12,13].

Phaeohyphomycosis (fungi that are grouped together because they form pigmented hyphae in tissues) are subcutaneous mycoses and are uncommon in cats. Infection is caused by several ubiquitous saprophytic fungi normally found in soil or organic material that are inoculated into tissue via wound contamination. Underlying immunosuppressive diseases may not be present, and relapses may occur. Diagnosis is based on biopsy findings of fungal elements in tissue and culture of the organisms.

Exophiala jeanselmei has been reported in a cat as an irregular, painless, nonulcerated, 1-cm mass involving the subcutaneous tissues of the nose [14].

Exophiala spinifera has been described in a cat in Australia in which granulomatous tissue appeared in the nostril and abscess formation and rupture developed on the bridge of the nose [15].

Alternaria alternate presented as a bulbous enlargement of the dorsal nose; a fleshy mass was also seen occluding the nostril [16].

Fonsecaea pedrosoi was confined to the skin and appeared as a firm swelling on the bridge of the nose. Diagnosis was based on histologic examination of a cutaneous biopsy and fungal culture of a tissue sample using Sabouraud's dextrose agar [17].

Sporotrichosis

Sporothrix schenckii is a saprophyte present in soil and organic debris. Infection is uncommon in cats and usually occurs via wound contamination, which may take place after inoculation of the organisms by contaminated claws or teeth from another cat. Lesions are common on the head and other extremities. Lesions initially present as abscesses, draining tracts, and cellulitis. Lesions ulcerate, drain a purulent exudate, and form crusted nodules. Large areas of necrosis may develop, and the organisms may spread to other areas of the body via normal grooming even after apparent clinical cure. Immunosuppressive doses of glucocorticoids have been reported to cause recurrence of disease [18].

Diagnosis via cytology may show pleomorphic round, oval, or cigar-shaped yeast that is often easily identified in exudate from cats but may be difficult to find in some cases. A biopsy of lesions shows a nodular to diffuse suppurative to granulomatous dermatitis with numerous fungal elements, especially in cats. Culture of tissue and fluid may also be diagnostic. This organism poses a zoonotic threat, and feline disease may result in human transmission [19].

Dermatophytosis

This is a common fungal infection in cats. Various dermatophytes cause lesions. The most commonly infectious agent is *Microsporum canis*; others are rare [20]. The incidence of disease may vary with housing practices and humidity [21]. Lesions may present as one or more areas of irregular or annular areas of alopecia, erythema, or crusts; however, there is a wide variety of clinical signs, and pruritus is also variable. Feline dermatophytosis may clinically mimic other dermatoses; for example, recurring chin folliculitis (chin acne) can be caused by *M canis*. Transmission may occur with direct contact or via fomites; hairs in the environment may remain infective for years. Infection seems to become established by mechanical disruption of the stratum corneum and invasion of keratin. Diagnosis is most commonly made by culture, which is the most reliable diagnostic test and the only method to identify the specific dermatophytes. Multiple cultures may be required for diagnosis. A Woods lamp examination is only positive for certain strains of *M canis*, and false-positive reactions can occur. Direct visualization of affected hair may reveal hyphae and arthrospores. Demonstration of organisms on a biopsy is definitive proof of infection; however, this method is not as sensitive as culture and should not be relied on for diagnosis [22].

Malassezia Dermatitis

Malassezia pachydermatis dermatitis most commonly affects the face of cats. Infection has also been associated with otitis, which may actually be more common in cats than the veterinary literature suggests. Clinical signs include pruritus, erythema, self-excoriation, and, less commonly, lichenification [23]. Malassezia may also be involved in feline chin acne [24].

Algae

Prototheca wickerhamii is a saprophytic algal organism found in salt and fresh water, soil, tree sap, and human and animal feces. Solitary to multiple firm papular to nodular masses or fluctuant subcutaneous growths have been described in cats, forming on the nose and surface of the ear. Diagnosis is via a biopsy and/or histopathologic examination as well as by culture [25].

BACTERIAL

Staphylococcal Folliculitis

This is rarely diagnosed in cats. When seen (Fig. 1), it is often noted as follicular papules and pustules on the face and head. Cats may present with a crusted papular eruption (miliary dermatitis) that is clinically indistinguishable from other causes of crusted papular lesions of cats. Diagnosis is made by cytology and bacterial culture, and a skin biopsy may be needed [26].

Dermatophilosis

Dermatophilus congolensis is rarely diagnosed in cats. It has been isolated from soft tissue fistulae and granulomatous lesions of the mouth [27].

Cat Bite Abscess

Aggressive behavior among cats resulting in bites during altercations may produce infections that present as well-circumscribed, fluctuant, painful swellings filled with purulent exudate. These cat bite abscesses may localize to the face in dominant cats. Bite marks are sometimes visible. Bacteria involved are representative of oral flora of cats, including *Pasteurella multocida*, *Fusobacterium* spp, *Clostridium* spp, *Peptostreptococcus* spp, *Bacteroides* spp, and others. Anaerobic bacteria are more frequently isolated than aerobic bacteria; however, they are more difficult to culture [28].

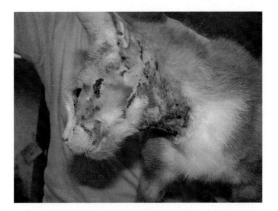

Fig. 1. Deep pyoderma and folliculitis in a cat with atopic dermatitis. Excoriations and pruritus are secondary to the *Staphylococcus* intermedius dermatitis, because the atopic dermatitis is well controlled.

Tuberculosis (mycobacterial infection)

This is a rare disease in cats. There is a higher incidence of infection with *Mycobacterium bovis* than with *Mycobacterium tuberculosis* in cats. An unnamed variant with cultural characteristics between *M bovis* and *M tuberculosis* has also been reported [29]. Diagnosis is made by observing acid-fast organisms via biopsy and histopathologic examination. Culture requires special conditions, such as enriched media, and usually requires 4 to 6 weeks to establish colonies. Cats may become inadvertently infected while living in the same household with tuberculous owners [30].

Cutaneous lesions are most commonly seen on the head, neck, and limbs and appear as nodules, ulcers, abscesses, and plaques that may discharge thick yellow to green pus with an unpleasant odor. Patients are often sick, exhibiting anorexia, weight loss, fever, lymphadenopathy, and involvement of the intestines and other organs. Clinical signs may be insidious, and serologic test results are unreliable. Skin testing with bacillus Calmette Guerin is not helpful in cats [31].

Feline Multisystemic Granulomatous Mycobacteriosis

Alopecia and nodules with thickened subcutaneous tissue involving the head, neck, and other areas of the body are caused by a newly described mycobacterium, *Mycobacterium visibilis*, identified in cats from North America. Lesions may be pruritic. Histopathologic examination from lesions revealed large numbers of thin filamentous organisms that were visible on hematoxylin-eosin–stained formalin-fixed tissue and also visible with acid-fast staining. Culture and gene sequence analysis suggests that this is a novel *Mycobacterium* species with a distinct genetic sequence from that of other mycobacteria [32].

Feline Leprosy

Feline leprosy [33] presents as single or multiple nonpainful, soft, fleshy nodules that may develop into nonhealing abscesses or fistulae and are confined to the skin or subcutis. Nodules may or may not be ulcerated. Lesions are common on the head, including nasal, buccal, and lingual mucosa, and the extremities. Regional lymphadenopathy is common. The organisms have a long incubation period and cannot be cultured. *Mycobacterium lepraemurium* is determined to be the causative agent based on transmission with fresh tissues from affected cats into rats and mice. These organisms are assumed to be contracted when hunting. Occurrence is most common in seaport cities of the western United States, New Zealand, Great Britain, Australia, and Netherlands, with a greater occurrence during the winter months [34].

Diagnosis is based on finding large numbers of acid-fast bacilli on direct smears and biopsies of lesions. A biopsy reveals two possible reaction patterns: a tuberculoid response—caseous necrosis and relatively few organisms (may be seen in zones of necrosis), or lepromatous leprosy—granuloma composed of solid sheets of large foamy macrophages with large numbers of acid-fast bacilli. Multinucleate histiocytic giant cells may contain bacilli. PCR amplification of the 16S rRNA gene sequence has been used as a diagnostic aid [35].

Actinomycosis

A rare pyogranulomatous or suppurative disease is caused by *Actinomyces* organisms. These are gram-positive, non–acid-fast, catalase-positive filamentous anaerobic rods that are opportunistic commensal inhabitants of the oral cavity. Infection is believed to arise from wound contamination. A 1-year-old domestic long-haired cat was presented to the author's clinic with a 5-month history of subcutaneous swelling of the chin area and moderate pruritus directed at the swelling and ear (Fig. 2). A fistulous tract dissecting to the left ear canal resulted in a purulent otitis. *Actinomyces* spp was isolated from the lesions, and the lesions were antibiotic responsive.

Yersinia pestis

Cats are highly susceptible to this bacterium, and rodent fleas are primary vectors. Sick rodents may become easy prey for cats, and fleas from rodents seek a new host. A localized abscess forms near the site of infection (often, the head and neck). The incubation period is 1 to 3 days if organisms are ingested or inhaled and 2 to 6 days if they are transmitted via flea bite. Infections are most common in endemic areas of the world. Diagnosis is by culture of the bipolar coccobacillus, which is a facultative anaerobic, nonmotile, non–spore-forming organism. These bacteria cannot penetrate unbroken skin but can invade mucous membranes [36].

PARASITIC

Chiggers and/or Trombiculosis

The adult form of *Trombicula autommalis* is a scavenger living on decaying vegetable material. The adult lifespan is approximately 10 months; eggs are laid in

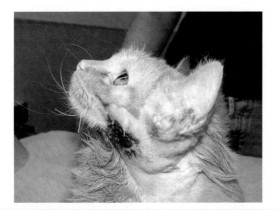

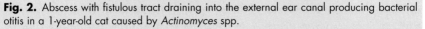

Fig. 2. Abscess with fistulous tract draining into the external ear canal producing bacterial otitis in a 1-year-old cat caused by *Actinomyces* spp.

moist ground and hatch to six-legged red larvae that are parasitic and feed on animals. These drop to the ground, become nymphs, and then become adults. Bites produce severe irritation and an intensely pruritic papulocrustous eruption. Bites may also cause nonpruritic papules, pustules, and crusts; secondary scaling and alopecia may result. Mites may be found in and around the ears of cats (distinguished from *Otodectes* by their intense orange-red color and their tight adherence to the skin). This is a seasonal disease that usually occurs in the summer and fall months. Diagnosis is based on visualization of the mite, history of environmental contact with woods and fields, and a skin biopsy demonstrating superficial perivascular dermatitis (spongiotic or hyperplastic) with many eosinophils [37].

Notoedres cati (notoedric mange)

Lesions attributed to *Notoedres cati* first appear at the medial proximal edge of the pinnae and then spread rapidly to the upper ear, face, eyelids, and neck. Female mites burrow into the horny layer of the epidermis, damaging keratinocytes, which leads to cytokine release (especially interleukin [IL]-1), causing cutaneous inflammation and clinical signs. The burrows appear on the skin surface in the center of minute papules; the skin then becomes thickened, wrinkled, and folded and later covered with dense, tightly adhering, yellow to gray crusts. Partial alopecia occurs in affected areas, intense pruritus develops, excoriations become secondarily infected, and peripheral lymphadenopathy usually results [38]. Diagnosis is confirmed via visualization of the mites from a skin scraping; however, distribution of lesions and intensity of pruritus are highly suggestive.

Sarcoptes scabiei

Although this mite more commonly produces disease in dogs, it is transferable to other species. Infestation in cats is rare and variable and may include pruritic pinnae and facial papules or generalized crusts, scales, and pruritus. Affected cats are often immunosuppressed before infestation [39,40].

Otodectes Infestation

Otodectes cynotis lives on the surface of the skin, feeding on epidermal debris and tissue fluid from the superficial epidermis. Hosts are exposed to and may become hypersensitized to mite antigens. Clinical symptoms are variable, especially in cats; some cats may have massive amounts of discharge but show no clinical signs, whereas other cats have intense otic pruritus with minimal discharge. Lesions may be restricted to the external ear canal, but mites are commonly found on other areas of the body (eg, neck, rump, and tail) [41].

Lice and Pediculosis

Biting lice (*Mallophaga*) move quickly and may be difficult to find and capture. *Felicola subrostratuas* is rarely found on cats. Movement of this louse may produce irritation and pruritus. The face and pinnae are most commonly affected. Scaling, crusts, and the presence of eggs adherent to hair shafts are the most common clinical findings. This mite is species-specific and is spread by direct contact or contaminated brushes, combs, and bedding [41].

Demodicosis

Demodex cati is a rare disease that usually affects the eyelids, periocular area, head, neck, and ear canal. Lesions are variably pruritic and consist of patchy erythema, scaling, crusting, and alopecia. It may also occur as a ceruminous otitis externa [42]. Generalized demodicosis caused by *D cati* is usually associated with underlying systemic disease.

Demodex gatoi is a short mite with a broad blunt abdomen; it is superficially located, inhabiting only the stratum corneum. In nonpruritic cats, skin scrapings reveal many mites and ova. In pruritic cats, however, especially if they lick their skin, mites may be difficult to find. Pruritus may be intense. Lesions include alopecia, scaling, excoriations, and crusts often concentrated on the head, neck, and elbows, whereas other cases have multifocal erythema and hyperpigmentation with broken stubby hairs. Histologically, minimal inflammation is observed; the epidermis may be acanthotic and hyperkeratotic with mites in the stratum corneum. *D gatoi* is contagious to other cats, and all cats in the home should be treated weekly with lime sulfur dips for 4 to 6 weeks [43].

Cuterebra

Eggs of *Cuterebra* spp are deposited on stones or vegetation around the burrows of small mammals. Animals pick up eggs or larvae as they come into mechanical contact with them. Cats are abnormal hosts, so larvae undergo aberrant migrations. Typical cases involving the skin are usually localized to the regions of the head, neck, or trunk. During the late summer or fall months, larvae enlarge and produce a swelling of 1 cm in diameter that develops into a fistula. Grubs should be mechanically removed without crushing, because retained parts may result in allergic or irritant reactions [41].

Leishmaniasis

This is a rare infection in cats but may be seen in areas in which the disease is endemic. Nodular lesions on the muzzle and ears have been observed in cats in Venezuela [44] and Texas. In one report, a cat infected with *L mexicana* relapsed 2 years after a radical pinnectomy, with lesions developing at the surgical site and also on the nasal mucosa and muzzle. The nasal planum developed hyperkeratosis and hypopigmentation [45].

Miscellaneous Helminthic Infections

Multiple cutaneous nodules were reported on the dorsal midline of the head and nuchal crest of a cat. These nodules had been present for more than 1 year with no change, and skin biopsies showed that the lesions contained male and female filarial nematode parasites morphologically compatible with *Dirofilaria immitis*. The results of serum antigen and antibody testing for *D immitis* were positive [46].

ALLERGIC
Food Allergy

The primary presenting complaint is a nonseasonal persistent pruritus. The lesions most commonly found on physical examination include erythema, alopecia, and miliary dermatitis type papules and crusts. Lesions consistent with eosinophilic granuloma complex may also be seen. Pruritus may be disproportionately severe in the head, neck, and otic region, although other body regions may be affected. This pruritus may or may not be glucocorticoid responsive. To diagnose food allergy, home-cooked diet trials are recommended for a minimum of 9 to 12 weeks. Some cats have been shown to be nonresponsive to commercially available restrictive diets (including baby foods and clam juice) [47].

Atopy

Diagnosis of atopic dermatitis is based on seasonally exacerbated pruritus and dermatitis and by ruling out other dermatoses that produce similar clinical signs. Cats show a more variable distribution of skin lesions than human beings and dogs. Pruritus may be present in the face, chin, and general head/neck along with other regions of the body. Indolent ulcers may be seen. Limited work on the pathogenesis in cats is available; however, the mechanisms seem similar to those of canine atopy-based on patch test studies and histologic examinations [48].

EOSINOPHILIC GRANULOMA COMPLEX

The clinical entities that comprise the eosinophilic granuloma complex are not a specific disease but are reaction pattern that most often results from an allergic etiology. Atopy, food allergy, and flea allergy have been implicated in inducing these lesions.

Feline Indolent Ulcer

Mucocutaneous and oral lesions may be present. Most commonly, a unilateral ulcer is present on the upper lip. These lesions are well-circumscribed red-brown alopecic lesions that are ulcerated and have a slightly raised border. Lesions are rarely pruritic or painful. They have been shown to develop in flea-allergic cats after exposure to only fleas (no other allergens) [49].

Eosinophilic Collagenolytic Granuloma
These well-circumscribed, raised, yellow-pink plaques may be found on the face, in the oral cavity, or in other body locations. The ulcerated surfaces may be covered with pinpoint white foci of collagen degeneration. Pruritus is usually mild.

Eosinophilic Plaque
This is a common feline cutaneous reaction pattern that may occur anywhere on the body. These well-demarcated erythematous lesions may appear ulcerated and exudative and may be seen on the preauricular skin of the head and in many other sites (Fig. 3). These lesions are usually highly pruritic [50].

Mosquito Bite Hypersensitivity
Lesions occur as a local reaction to mosquito bites. Lesions are present on the bridge of the nose and preauricular skin, because mosquitoes are most likely to feed on these areas of sparsely haired skin. Early lesions consist of erythematous papules or plaques that may be erosive or ulcerated as well as necrotic or crusted. More chronic lesions include nodules, pigment changes (melanoderma or leukoderma), alopecia, and scaling [51]. They are seasonal, appearing during warmer months. Lesions resolve with removal from mosquitoes but recur with re-exposure.

AUTOIMMUNE
Pemphigus Foliaceus
The most common initially affected area is the head, including the pinnae, face and/or head, nose, chin, or periocular skin. Other areas of the body may also

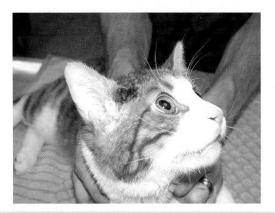

Fig. 3. Pruritic eosinophilic plaque in a young cat secondary to atopic dermatitis.

be affected, where the disease presents as pustules, crusts, erosions, scales, and alopecia. Mild to severe pruritus may be common (seen in 80% of cats in one report). The lesions are usually bilaterally symmetric. Intact pustules are rarely observed; the predominant lesions are serous or hemorrhagic crusts with associated scaling and alopecia. It is unclear if a history of previous skin disease plays any role in the development of pemphigus foliaceus in cats [52]. Drug-induced pemphigus foliaceus can occur in cats [53,54].

Pemphigus Erythematosus
This disease is uncommon in cats but has been reported. Primary lesions are transient. Cats typically present with crusts, scaling, alopecia, and erosions. Pruritus and pain are variable. The disease is often limited to the facial and/or nasal region. The lesions or disease may be photoaggrevated [55].

Discoid Lupus Erythematosus
This is a rare disease in cats; no age, breed, or sex predilection is reported. Lesions are most common on the pinnae and face. Erythema, scaling, crusting, and alopecia with variable pruritus have been described. Nasal dermatitis and depigmentation are less common. Lesions may be more severe when exposure to sunlight is increased. Diagnosis is based on correlating clinical signs and confirmatory biopsy findings. Affected cats are otherwise healthy [56,57].

Systemic Lupus Erythematosus
Systemic lupus erythematosus is rare in cats, with no apparent sex predilection. Affected cats range from 1 to 12 years of age. Siamese, Persian, and Himalayan cats may be predisposed. Associated syndromes reportedly include hematologic abnormalities, neurologic or behavioral abnormalities, fever, lymphadenopathy, polyarthritis, myopathy, oral ulceration, conjunctivitis, renal failure, and subclinical pulmonary disease. Cutaneous lesions are present in 20% of affected cats. Dermatologic abnormalities include seborrheic skin disease, exfoliative erythroderma, erythematous scaling and crusting, and alopecic scarring dermatitis most commonly involving the face, pinnae, and paws [58–60].

NEOPLASTIC/PRENEOPLASTIC
Solar Keratosis/Actinic Dermatitis
This well-known common syndrome usually affects white or orange-colored cats. Lesions often progress to squamous cell carcinoma. Lesions tend to develop in areas of sparsely haired skin, such as the nose and/or dorsal muzzle and pinnae. A higher incidence of disease is noted in sunny climates and locations. Lesions manifest early as scaling and hyperkeratosis with partial alopecia. Lesions can progress to hyperkeratotic plaques, papulated hyperplastic lesions, or focal crusts and/or erosions. Diagnosis is made by histopathologic findings on skin biopsies [61].

Squamous Cell Carcinoma
Exposure to ultraviolet radiation contributes strongly to the development of squamous cell carcinoma in cats. Cats living in geographic regions with

increased levels of sunlight and those spending time sunbathing in windows or outside have increased risk of developing squamous cell carcinoma. White-haired cats have a 13.4 times greater risk of developing squamous cell carcinoma than cats with pigmented skin. Although more common in older cats, tumors have been reported in cats as young as 1 year of age. More than 80% of lesions are found on the head, most commonly on the nasal planum, pinnae, and eyelids, most likely because of the sparse hair coverage in these areas and the sunlight's ability to penetrate the erect hair in these areas. Initial lesions may be subtle, as seen in actinic dermatitis, and may wax and wane, being mistaken for trauma or benign lesions. The tumors are usually locally aggressive, progressing to develop ulceration and destruction of surrounding tissue [62].

Multicentric Squamous Cell Carcinoma In Situ: Bowen's Disease

Lesions usually present in older cats and often involve the head and neck but may also affect other body regions. In contrast to actinic keratoses, these lesions are not related to sun exposure. Initially, lesions are often well-circumscribed, melanotic, hyperkeratotic macules and plaques that may progress to become verrucous in appearance. Cutaneous horns may develop on the surface of some lesions. Later lesions may appear as thick, crusted, ulcerated plaques that bleed easily. Lesions may progress to become invasive squamous cell carcinoma [63]. Approximately 45% of these lesions in cats have been found to have papillomavirus antigens present [64].

Cutaneous Lymphoma

Cutaneous T-cell lymphoma is rare in cats. These diseases can be subdivided into epitheliotropic and nonepitheliotropic lymphoma. Epitheliotropic T-cell lymphoma has been described to affect cats, in which lesions often affect the haired skin and, in some cases, the mucosa and nasal planum. Lesions vary from alopecia, scaling, and erythema to mucocutaneous and/or mucosal erythema, infiltration, depigmentation, and ulceration or may present as cutaneous plaques or nodules [65]. Sezary syndrome has been described in one cat in which lesions were especially prominent on the head, ears, trunk, and limbs. These lesions presented as diffuse generalized erythroderma, hyperhidrosis, exfoliation and secondary excoriations, patchy alopecia, and exudative crusts. In addition to skin lesions, this variant of epitheliotropic lymphoma has atypical lymphoid cell leukemia and peripheral lymphadenopathy composed of the same atypical lymphoid cells [66]. Nonepitheliotropic lymphoma may also present with ulceration, nodule formation, and erythema notable on the face and other body regions [67].

Cutaneous Lymphocytosis (pseudolymphoma)

This is a relatively uncommon disease that usually affects older cats. This description lacks specificity because it does not imply a specific disease or causation but simply a process of accumulation of lymphocytes in the skin. Some cats may present with lesions that have been described as ranging from alopecia, erythema, scaling, and crusting to miliary papules and nodules on the ear

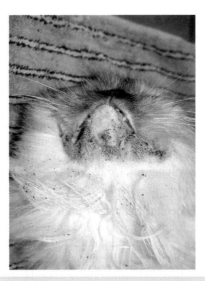

Fig. 4. Chin acne in a Himalayan cat secondary to atopic skin disease. Lesions resolve when allergic dermatitis is controlled and relapse when atopic dermatitis relapses.

this develops into a moderate to severe form that may be nonresponsive to antipruritic therapy. Some cats may improve when treated with corticosteroids or cyclosporine. Secondary infections with bacteria and *Malassezia* need to be treated if they occur. The cause of this disorder is unknown, although a genetic basis is suspected [79–81].

Intertrigo
Skin fold dermatitis can occur when face folds create an environment in which there is poor air circulation from skin apposition. Moisture, sebum, glandular secretions, and tear excretion provide an environment that favors skin maceration and bacterial or *Malassezia* yeast overgrowth [82].

Periocular Leukotrichia
This condition has been described in Siamese cats. There is no age predilection, but it is more commonly seen in female cats. A halo-like patchy or complete lightening of the hairs of the mask may occur after a precipitating factor, such as pregnancy, dietary deficiency, or systemic illness. The condition is transient and usually resolves within two hair cycles [83].

Preauricular Alopecia
The hair at the temporal region between the eye and ear is more sparse than on other parts of the head. This is a normal physiologic condition. In cats with a short hair coat, this area may appear alopecic [84].

Urticaria Pigmentosa
This has been described in several breeds, including Sphinx, Himalayan, Devon Rex, and Siamese cats. Lesions consist of a multifocal, partially

coalescing, variably hyperpigmented macular and crusted papular rash on the head, neck, pinnae, perioral skin, and chin. Lesions are variably pruritic. A familial history may be present. Diagnosis is by a biopsy and histopathologic examination. A moderate to severe perivascular to diffuse dermal and subcutaneous infiltrate of well-differentiated mast cells with small numbers of eosinophils and mast cells is seen on a biopsy. Treatment is symptomatic, and lesions may spontaneously regress [85,86].

Apocrine Nevus
This is described in a 14-month-old cat with pale to dark blue papules and nodules in several body locations, including the face and submaxillary region, that were present at birth. A biopsy revealed benign proliferation of apocrine glands consistent with a diagnosis of apocrine nevus [87].

Follicular Mucinosis
Lesions present as generalized alopecia with scaling or crusting that is more pronounced over the head, neck, and shoulders. The face and muzzle of affected cats were unusually thickened. Histologically, there is severe mixed inflammation of the wall of the follicular isthmus, accompanied by some follicular destruction in some cats. Sebaceous glands are not affected. All reported cases in cats had variable but often striking follicular mucin deposition as well as epidermal hyperkeratosis and crusting. The cause of the severe mural folliculitis has not been identified, and affected cats responded poorly to immunomodulating therapy. Follicular mucinosis may be a nonspecific finding, likely reflective of the follicular lymphocytic milieu, and does not always herald follicular lymphoma, although this has been reported in some cats [88].

Lentigo Simplex
Asymptomatic macular melanosis may begin in cats less than 1 year of age and typically affects the lips, gums, eyelids, and nose. Orange-colored cats are most commonly affected. Affected cats seem not to be at any increased risk for developing melanoma or any other diseases [89].

Lymphocytic Mural Folliculitis
Clinically, these nonpruritic lesions may vary from alopecia to crusting and scaling, with underlying erosions affecting the head, dorsal neck, and trunk. A diet-related disorder has been implicated in two cases [90].

Acquired Pinnal Folding
This is a sudden bilateral or lateral folding of the distal one third of pinnae; the folded portion is cool, thin, and palpably devoid of cartilage. All affected cats have received long-term (8 months to 2 years) daily applications of glucocorticoids containing otic preparations. Corticotropin stimulation tests show depressed serum cortisol, suggesting the presence of iatrogenic secondary adrenocortical insufficiency and iatrogenic Cushing's syndrome. Stopping glucocorticoid therapy may or may not resolve the fold [91–93].

Junctional Epidermolysis Bullosa

In cats, this congenital disorder presents as varying degrees of crusting and ulceration on the pinnae and lip margins, stomatitis, or claw and footpad lesions. Oral lesions may affect the gingival, pharynx, tongue, and hard palate. Defects in laminin-5 production are the cause of this disorder. The described cases have been heterogeneous. The disease has been severe enough to warrant euthanasia in one case, whereas other cats have continued to thrive into adulthood with only occasional ulcerations that heal with topical therapy [94].

Metastatic Calcinosis

This is a nodular focus of calcified tissue, typically described as a well-circumscribed, irregular, firm lesion with pale foci. Lesions have been described on the chin, and the ventral interdigital spaces of all feet may also be affected. Microscopic examination of exudate reveals refractile material that fails to take up stain. Calcification of tissue may develop secondary to renal disease. Metastatic calcification can be seen with any disease that produces a solubility product (SP) (Ca $\times$ P) greater than 7 g/L. One case reported a SP (Ca $\times$ P) of 14.83 g/L [95].

Feline Auricular Chondritis

This is a rare condition in which the pinnae become edematous and swell as well as becoming erythematous and painful, eventually appearing curled dorsally or medially and becoming deformed. The condition may be unilateral or bilateral. Pinnal cartilage necroses, with an associated lymphoplasmacytic inflammation and occasional neutrophilic infiltrates [96].

Erythema Multiforme

Reported cases are likely to occur secondary to a drug reaction; however, because provocative testing was not performed, this remains anecdotal. Lesions may present as well-demarcated patches of ulceration, superficial necrosis, and crusting present on the pinnae or as ulceration of mucocutaneous junctions. Lesions may also occur on nonfacial areas [97].

Table 2
Ear lesions categorized by problems

Structural/cartilage	
Acquired pinnal folding	Feline auricular chondritis
Crusting and scaling	
Pemphigus foliaceus	Pemphigus erythematosus
Feline leukemia virus (underlying erosions)	
Ulcerations	
Junctional epidermolysis bullosa	Erythema multiforme[a]
Otitis	
Malassezia	Otodectes cyanotis

[a]Diseases that fall into more than one problem category.

Table 3
Pruritic dermatoses[a]

Disorder	Degree of pruritus
Feline cow pox	Variable from case to case
FeLV dermatitis	Moderate to severe
Dermatophytosis	Variable from case to case
Malassezia	Often moderate to severe
Staphylococcal folliculitis	
Feline multisystemic granulomatous mycobacteriosis	Variable from case to case
Chiggers/trombiculosis	Intense pruritus
Notoedres	Intense pruritus
Otodectes	Variable, usually intense pruritus
Pediculosis	Variable, usually moderate to highly pruritic
Demodicosis	Variable
Food allergy	Variable, usually intense
Atopy	Variable, usually intense
Eosinophilic collagenolytic granuloma	Mild
Eosinophilic plaque	Highly pruritic
Pemphigus foliaceus	Variable, mild to intense
Pemphigus erythematosus	Variable
Xanthoma	Variable
Chin acne	Variable
Methimazole drug reaction	Intense
Idiopathic facial dermatitis of Persian cats	Initially none, then progresses to moderate/intense
Urticaria pigmentosa	Variable[b]

Abbreviations: FeLV, feline leukemia virus.
[a]Pruritus may be difficult to assess in cats because of their secretive nature and the difficulty in differentiating pruritus from normal grooming behavior.
[b]May or may not be present, with varying degrees of pruritus when present.

Foreign Body Reactions

Nodular ulcerative reactions on the chin have been described secondary to foreign body reactions from cacti (*Mammillaria* spp). The lesions consist of an eosinophilic collagenolytic foreign body reaction around foreign vegetative material [98].

Vasculitis

This is described as causing an ulcerative dermatitis with overlying crusts on the nose and pinnal margins and histologically showing severe epidermal necrosis with marked acute vasculitis and concurrent systemic panleukopenia [99].

Idiopathic Nasal Scaling in Bengal Cats

This syndrome is based on two reports from northern Europe of nasal planum scaling that progressed to thick crusts and then to exfoliation and erosive lesions. The age of onset is variable (between 4 months and 1 year of age). Resolution in some cats was spontaneous, whereas others responded to various treatments, including oral prednisolone and topical tacrolimus ointment. Occurrence of lesions in one breed suggests a heritable cause [100,101].

SUMMARY

Facial dermatitis is a common problem in cats. The skin of the face, head, and ears can be affected by a wide variety of diseases. A systematic consideration of the possible etiologies is required for accurate diagnosis and effective treatment of these disorders. Tables 1 through 3 provide summaries of differential diagnoses to consider when presented with a cat with facial dermatitis.

References

[1] Jazic E, Coyner KS, Loeffler DG, et al. An evaluation of the clinical, cytological, infectious, and histopathological features of feline acne. In: 20th Proceedings of North American Veterinary Forum. Sarasota (FL); 2005. p. 162.

[2] Sundberg JP, Van Ranst M, Montali R, et al. Feline papillomas and papillomaviruses. Vet Pathol 2000;37:1–10.

[3] Hargis AM, Ginn PE, Mansell JEKL, et al. Ulcerative facial and nasal dermatitis and stomatitis in cats associated with feline herpesvirus 1. Vet Dermatol 1999;10:267–74.

[4] Bennett M. Feline cowpox virus infection. J Small Anim Pract 1990;31:167.

[5] Gross TL. Giant cell dermatosis in FeLV-positive cats. Vet Dermatol 1993;4:117.

[6] Jacobs GJ, Medleau L. Cryptococcosis. In: Greene CE, editor. Infectious diseases of the dog and cat. Philadelphia: WB Saunders; 1998. p. 383.

[7] Gerdes-Grogan S, Dayrell-Hurt B. Feline cryptococcosis: a retrospective evaluation. J Am Anim Hosp Assoc 1997;33:118.

[8] Medleau L, Marks MA, Brown J, et al. Clinical evaluation of a cryptococcal antigen latex agglutination test for diagnosis of cryptococcosis in cats. J Am Vet Med Assoc 1990;196: 1470–3.

[9] Hodges RD, Legendre AM, Adams LG, et al. Itraconazole for the treatment of histoplasmosis in cats. J Intern Med 1994;8:409–13.

[10] Wolf AM. Histoplasmosis. In: Greene CE, editor. Infectious diseases of the dog and cat. Philadelphia: WB Saunders; 1998. p. 378–83.

[11] Rosser EJ. Cutaneous paecilomycosis in a cat. In: Proceedings of the 15th Annual Meeting of the American Association of Veterinary Dermatology and American College of Veterinary Dermatology, Concurrent Session. 1999; p. 37.

[12] Greene CE, Miller DM, Blue JL. Trichosporon infection in a cat. J Am Vet Med Assoc 1985;187:946–8.

[13] Greene CE, Chandler FW. Trichosporonosis. In: Greene CE, editor. Infectious diseases of the dog and cat. Philadelphia: WB Saunders; 1998. p. 418–9.

[14] Bostock DE, Coloe PJ. Phaeohyphomycosis caused by Exophiala Jeanselmei in a domestic cat. J Comp Pathol 1982;92:479.

[15] Kettlewell P, McGinnis MR, Wilkinson GT. Phaeohyphomycosis caused by Exophiala spinifera in two cats. J Med Vet Mycol 1989;27:257.

[16] Dhein CR, Leathers CW, Padhye AA, et al. Phaeohyphomycosis caused by Alternaria alternata in a cat. J Am Vet Med Assoc 1988;193(9):1101–2.

[17] Fondati A, Grazia-Gallo M, Romano E, et al. A case of feline Phaeohyphomycosis due to Fonsecaea pedrosoi. Vet Dermatol 2001;12(5):297.

[18] Rosser EJ. Sporotrichosis. In: Griffin CE, et al, editors. Current veterinary dermatology: the science and art of therapy. St. Louis (MO): Mosby–Year Book; 1993. p. 49–53.

[19] Rosser EJ, Dunstan RW. Sporotrichosis. In: Greene CE, editor. Infectious diseases of the dog and cat. Philadelphia: WB Saunders; 1998. p. 399–402.

[20] Moriello KA, DeBoer DJ. Feline dermatophytosis: recent advances and recommendations for therapy. Vet Clin North Am Small Anim Pract 1995;25:901–21.

[21] Simpanya MF, Baxter M. Isolation of fungi from the pelage of cats and dogs using the hair-brush technique. Mycopathologia 1996;134:129.

[22] Foil CS. Dermatophytosis. In: Griffin CE, et al, editors. Current veterinary dermatology: the science and art of therapy. St. Louis (MO): Mosby–Year Book; 1993. p. 22–33.

[23] Morris DO. *Malassezia* dermatitis and otitis. Vet Clin North Am Small Anim Pract 1999;29:1303–10.

[24] Mason KV. *Malassezia pachydermatis*–associated dermatitis. In: August JR, editor. Consultations in feline internal medicine 3. Philadelphia: WB Saunders; 1997. p. 221–3.

[25] Dillberger JE, Homer B, Daubert D, et al. Protothecosis in two cats. J Am Vet Med Assoc 1988;192(11):1557.

[26] Scott DW, Miller WH, Griffin CE. Bacterial skin diseases. In: Muller and Kirk's small animal dermatology. 6th edition. Philadelphia: WB Saunders; 2001. p. 300.

[27] Baker GJ, Breeze RG, Dawson CO. Oral dermatophilosis in a cat: a case report. J Small Anim Pract 1972;13:649–53.

[28] Greene CE. Feline abscesses. In: Greene CE, editor. Infectious diseases of the dog and cat. Philadelphia: WB Saunders; 1998. p. 328–30.

[29] Blunden AS, Smith KC. A pathological study of a mycobacterial infection in a cat caused by a variant with cultural characteristics between *Mycobacterium tuberculosis* and M. *bovis*. Vet Rec 1996;138:87–8.

[30] Greene CE, Gunn-Moore DA. Tuberculous mycobacterial infections. In: Greene CE, editor. Infectious diseases of the dog and cat. Philadelphia: WB Saunders; 1998. p. 316–9.

[31] Lemarie SL. Mycobacterial dermatitis. Vet Clin North Am Small Anim Pract 1999;29:1299.

[32] Appleyard GD. Histologic and genotypic characterization of a novel *Mycobacterium* species found in three cats. J Clin Microbiol 2002;40(7):2425–30.

[33] Lawrence WE. Cat leprosy: infection by a bacillus resembling *Mycobacterium lepraemurium*. Aust Vet J 1963;39:390–3.

[34] Lewis DT, Kunkle GA. Feline leprosy. In: Greene CE, editor. Infectious diseases of the dog and cat. Philadelphia: WB Saunders; 1998. p. 321.

[35] Hughs MS, Ball NW, Beck LA, et al. Determination of the etiology of presumptive feline leprosy by 16S rRNA gene analysis. J Clin Microbiol 1997;35(10):2464.

[36] Macy DW. Plague. In: Greene CE, editor. Infectious diseases of the dog and cat. Philadelphia: WB Saunders; 1998. p. 295–300.

[37] Sosna CB, Medleau L. The clinical signs and diagnosis of external parasite infestation. Vet Med 1992;564.

[38] Wall R, Shearer D. Veterinary ectoparasites. 2nd edition. Blackwell Science; 2001. p. 33–4.

[39] Patterson S. Skin diseases of the cat. Blackwell Science; 2000. p. 77–8.

[40] Bonrstein S, Gidlund K, Karlstam E, et al. Vet Dermatol 2004;15(Suppl 1):34.

[41] Scott DW, Miller WH, Griffin CE. Parasitic skin diseases. In: Muller and Kirk's small animal dermatology. 6th edition. Philadelphia: WB Saunders; 2001. p. 451.

[42] Kontos V, Sotiraki S, Himonas C. Two rare disorders in the cat: demodectic otitis externa and sarcoptic mange. Feline Pract 1998;26(6):18.

[43] Morris DO, Beale KM. Feline demodicosis—a retrospective of 15 cases. In: Proceedings of the Annual Meeting of the American Association of Veterinary Dermatology and American College of Veterinary Dermatology. 1997. p. 13127.

[44] Bonfante-Garrido R, Urdaneta I, Urdaneta R, et al. Natural infection of cats with leishmania in Barquisimeto, Venezuela. Trans R Soc Trop Med Hyg 1991;85:53.

[45] Barnes JC, Stanley O, Craig TM. Diffuse cutaneous leishmaniasis in a cat. J Am Vet Med Assoc 1993;202:416.

[46] Hill JR. Nodular cutaneous dirofilariasis in a cat. Vet Dermatol 2000;11(Suppl 1):63.

[47] Rosser E. Food allergy in the cat: a prospective study of 13 cats. In: Ihrke PJ, Mason IS, White SD, editors. Advances in veterinary dermatology, vol. II. New York: Pergamon Press; 1993. p. 33.

[48] Roosje PJ, Thepen TH, Rutten VP, et al. Feline atopic dermatitis: a review. Vet Dermatol 2000;11(Suppl):12.

[49] Colombini S, Hodgin EC, Foil CS, et al. Induction of feline flea allergy dermatitis and the incidence and histopathological characteristics of concurrent indolent lip ulcers. Vet Dermatol 2001;12:155.

[50] Patterson S. Skin diseases of the cat. Oxford (UK): Blackwell Science; 2000. p. 231–8.

[51] Mason KV, Evans AG. Mosquito bite-caused eosinophilic dermatitis in cats. J Am Vet Med Assoc 1991;198(12):2086–8.

[52] Preziosi DE, Goldschmidt MH, Greek JS, et al. Feline Pemphigus foliaceus: a retrospective analysis of 57 cases. Vet Dermatol 2003;14:313.

[53] McEwan NA, McNeil PE, Kirkham D. Drug eruption in a cat resembling Pemphigus foliaceus. J Small Anim Pract 1987;28:713.

[54] Mason KV, Day MJ. A Pemphigus foliaceous-like eruption associated with the use of ampicillin in a cat. Aust Vet J 1987;64:223.

[55] Scott DW, Miller WH, Griffin CE. Immune-mediated disorders. In: Muller and Kirk's small animal dermatology. 6th edition. Philadelphia: WB Saunders; 2001. p. 690.

[56] Kalaher S. Discoid lupus erythematosus in a cat. Feline Pract 1991;19:7.

[57] Willemse T, et al. Discoid lupus erythematosus in cats. Vet Dermatol 1989;1:19.

[58] Scott DW, et al. Immune mediated dermatoses in domestic animals: ten years after. Part II. Compend Contin Educ Small Anim Pract 1987;9:539.

[59] Pedersen NC. Systemic lupus erythematosus in the cat. Feline Pract 1991;19:5.

[60] Vitale CB, et al. Systemic lupus erythematosus in a cat: fulfillment of the American Rheumatism Association criteria with supportive skin histopathology. Vet Dermatol 1997;8:133.

[61] Foil CS. Facial, pedal, and other regional dermatoses. Vet Clin North Am Small Anim Pract 1995;25(4):923–44.

[62] Ruslander D, Kaser-Hotz B, Sardinas JC. Cutaneous squamous cell carcinoma in cats. Compend Contin Educ Pract Vet 1997;19(10):1119.

[63] Baer KE, Helton K. Multicentric squamous cell carcinoma in situ resembling Bowen's disease in cats. Vet Pathol 1993;30:535–42.

[64] Clark EG, et al. Primary viral skin disease in three cats caused by three different viruses and confirmed by immunohistochemical and/or electron microscopic techniques on formalin-fixed tissue. In: Proceedings of the Annual Meeting of the American Association of Veterinary Dermatology and American College of Veterinary Dermatology. 1993. p. 56.

[65] Scott DW, Miller WH, Griffin CE. Neoplastic and nonneoplastic tumors. In: Muller and Kirk's small animal dermatology. 6th edition. Philadelphia: WB Saunders; 2001. p. 1333.

[66] Schick RO, Murphy GF, Goldschmidt MH. Cutaneous lymphosarcoma and leukemia in a cat. J Am Vet Med Assoc 1993;203(8):1155–8.

[67] Komori S, Nakamura S, Takahashi K, et al. Use of lomustine to treat cutaneous nonepitheliotropic lymphoma in a cat. J Am Vet Med Assoc 2005;226(2):237–9.

[68] Gilbert S, Affolter VK, Gross TL, et al. Clinical, morphological and immunohistochemical characterization of cutaneous lymphocytosis in 23 cats. Vet Dermatol 2004;15:3.

[69] Teifke JP, Kidney BA, Lohr CV, et al. Detection of apapillomavirus-DNA in mesenchymal tumour cells and not in the hyperplastic epithelium of feline sarcoids. Vet Dermatol 2003;14:47.

[70] Vogelnest LJ. Cutaneous xanthomas with concurrent demodicosis and dermatophytosis in a cat. Aust Vet J 2001;79(7):470–5.

[71] Bagnasco GB, Properzi R, Porto R, et al. Feline cutaneous neuroendocrine carcinoma (Merkel cell tumor): clinical and pathological findings. Vet Dermatol 2003;14:111.

[72] Goldschmidt M, Liu S, Shofer F. Feline dermal melanoma: a retrospective study. In: Ihrke P, Mason I, White I, editors. Advances in veterinary dermatology. New York: Pergamon Press; 1992. p. 285.

[73] Diters RW, Walsh KM. Feline basal cell tumors: a review of 124 cases. Vet Pathol 1984;21:51–6.

[74] Day DG, Couto CG, Weisbrode SE, et al. Basal cell carcinoma in two cats. J Am Anim Hosp Assoc 1991;27:339–47.

[75] Buerger RG, Scott D. Cutaneous mast cell neoplasia in cats: 14 cases (1975–1985). J Am Vet Med Assoc 1987;190(11):1440–4.

[76] Luther P, et al. The dilated pore of Winer—an overlooked cutaneous lesion of cats. J Comp Pathol 1989;101:375.

[77] Jazic E, Coyner KS, Loeffler DG, et al. An evaluation of the clinical, cytological, infectious and histopathological features of feline acne. In: 20th Proceedings of the North American Veterinary Dermatology Forum. Sarasota (FL); 2005. p. 162.

[78] Kunkle G. Adverse cutaneous reactions in cats given methimazole. Derm Dialog 1993;Spring/Summer:4.

[79] Bond R, Curtis CF, Ferguson EA, et al. An idiopathic facial dermatitis of Persian cats. Vet Dermatol 2000;11:35.

[80] Power HT. Newly recognized feline skin diseases. In: Proceedings of the American Association of Veterinary Dermatology and American College of Veterinary Dermatology, Concurrent Session Notes. San Antonio (TX); 1998. p. 30.

[81] Bond R, Curtis C, Mason I, et al. An idiopathic facial dermatitis of thirteen Persian cats. In: Thoday K, Foil C, Bond R, editors. Advances in veterinary dermatology, vol. 4. Oxford (UK): Blackwell Publishing; 2002. p. 307.

[82] Small animal dermatology. 6th edition. p. 1105.

[83] Scott D. Feline dermatology 1983–1985: the secret sits. J Am Anim Hosp Assoc 1987;23:255.

[84] Scott DW, Miller WH, Griffin CE. Acquired alopecias. In: Muller and Kirk's small animal dermatology. 6th edition. Philadelphia: WB Saunders; 2001. p. 900.

[85] Vitale C, Ihrke P, Olivry T, et al. Case report feline urticaria pigmentosa in three related Sphinx cats. Vet Dermatol 1996;7:227.

[86] Noli C, Scarampella F. Feline urticaria pigmentosa-like disease in two unrelated Devon Rex cats. In: Proceedings of the Meeting of the American Association of Veterinary Dermatology and American College of Veterinary Dermatology. Maui (HI); 1999. p. 65.

[87] Shibata K, Nagata M, Ito M, et al. Apocrine nevus in a cat. Vet Dermatol 2003;14:226.

[88] Gross TL, Olivry T, Vitale C, et al. Degenerative, mucinotic mural folliculitis in cats. Vet Dermatol 2001;12(5):279.

[89] Scott D. Lentigo simplex in orange cats. Comp Anim Pract 1987;1:23–5.

[90] Declercq J. A case of diet-related lymphocytic mural folliculitis in a cat. Vet Dermatol 2000;11:75.

[91] Rest JR. Floppy pinnae in Siamese cats. Vet Rec 1998;143(20):568.

[92] Weaver M. Floppy pinnae in Siamese cats. Vet Rec 1998;143(25):700.

[93] Scott DW. Feline dermatology 1986–1988: looking to the 1990s through the eyes of many counselors. J Am Anim Hosp Assoc 1990;26:515.

[94] Alhaidari Z, Olivry T, Spadafora A, et al. Junctional epidermolysis bullosa in two domestic shorthair kittens. Vet Dermatol 2005;17:69–73.

[95] Declercq J, Bhatti S. Calcinosis involving multiple paws in a cat with chronic renal failure and in a cat with hyperthyroidism. Vet Dermatol 2005;16:74–8.

[96] Bunge MM, Foil CS, Taylor HW. Relapsing polychondritis in a cat. J Am Anim Hosp Assoc 1992;28:203.

[97] Scott CW, Miller WH. Erythema multiforme in dogs and cats: literature review and case material from the Cornell University College of Veterinary Medicine (1988–96). Vet Dermatol 1999;10:297–309.

[98] Cornegliana L, Vercelli A. Collagenolytic granuloma in three domestic shorthaired (DSH) cats following foreign body penetration. Vet Dermatol 2000;11(Suppl 1):30.

[99] Berrocal A. A case of autoimmune vasculitis affecting ears and nose in a cat with panleu-kopenia enteritis. Vet Dermatol 2000;11(Suppl 1):62.

[100] Bergvall K. A novel ulcerative nasal dermatitis of Bengal cats. Vet Dermatol 2004; 15(Suppl 1):28.

[101] Auxilia S, Abramo F, Ficker C, et al. Juvenile idiopathic nasal crusting in three Bengal cats. Vet Dermatol 2004;15(Suppl 1):52.

Canine and Feline Eosinophilic Skin Diseases

Paul B. Bloom, DVM[a,b,]*

[a]Allergy and Dermatology Clinic for Animals, 31205 Five Mile Road, Livonia, MI 48158, USA
[b]Department of Small Animal Clinical Sciences, Department of Dermatology,
Michigan State University, East Lansing, MI, USA

EOSINOPHILIC DERMATOSIS

Eosinophilic dermatosis (ED) is a histologic diagnosis rather than a clinical diagnosis. It includes a heterogeneous group of diseases that are secondary to underlying antigenic stimulation (hypersensitivity reaction) in most cases. EDs all have one thing in common—the eosinophil. Eosinophils are phagocytic cells in the granulocyte lineage, as are neutrophils and basophils, that are produced in the bone marrow. Phagocytic cells contain granules that may or may not stain with dyes. Those cells with granules that take up acidic dyes, such as eosin, are called eosinophils. Eosinophils are involved in the inflammatory response to foreign material, especially parasites. They are one of the major sources of inflammatory mediators associated with type I hypersensitivity reactions. An eosinophil-derived cytokine, transforming growth factor-β_1 (TGFβ_1) may also contribute to chronic inflammation.

A variety of molecules are involved in the activation and attraction of eosinophils [1–3], including the following:

1. Chemokines
    a. Regulated on activation normal T-cell expressed and secreted (RANTES)
    b. Monocyte chemoattractant protein (MCP)
    c. Macrophage inflammatory protein-1 (MIP-1)
    d. Eotaxin
2. Cytokines
    a. Interleukin (IL) 1-β, IL-3, IL-4, and IL-5
    b. Granulocyte macrophage colony-stimulating factor (GM-CSF)
    c. Tumor necrosis factor-α (TNFα)
    d. TGFβ_1
3. Lipid mediators
    a. Eicosanoids
        i. Leukotriene (LT) B_4, LTC_4, LTD_4, and LTE_4

*Allergy and Dermatology Clinic for Animals, 31205 Five Mile Road, Livonia, MI 48158.
E-mail address: dermdoc@cvm.msu.edu

0195-5616/06/$ – see front matter
doi:10.1016/j.cvsm.2005.09.015

ii. Prostaglandin D_2 (PGD$_2$)
iii. Thromboxanes
   b. Platelet-activating factor
4. Complement fragments (C3a and C5a)
5. Adhesion molecules (expressed on eosinophil or vascular endothelium)
   a. Selectins
       i. L selectin/GlyCAM-1
       ii. PSGL-1/P selectin
       iii. ESL-1/E selectin
   b. Integrins
       i. LFA-1/ICAM-1
       ii. Mac-1/ICAM-1
       iii. VLA-4/VCAM-1
6. Mast cell degranulation products
   a. Histamine and its metabolite, imidiazoleactic acid
   b. Eosinophilic chemoattractant factor A
7. Immunoglobulins
   a. IgG
   b. IgA
8. Helminth-associated molecules

Little of an eosinophil's lifespan is spent in circulation; rather, it is primarily spent in the tissues. Once an eosinophil has arrived at its final destination, it begins the work of destroying the insult that attracted it to that site, such as a parasite, by phagocytosis or by releasing toxic compounds. Eosinophils can phagocytize small antigens; however, to kill large parasites, they extrude cellular contents via degranulation. Four major granules—secondary granules, small granules, lipid bodies, and primary granules—are found in the cytoplasm of eosinophils. These granules contain a wide variety of proteins, many with enzymatic activity. Major basic protein, eosinophilic cationic protein, eosinophilic peroxidase, and eosinophilic-derived neurotoxin reside within the secondary granule along with a number of cytokines, enzymes, and other proteins. Small granules contain a variety of enzymes, including arylsulfatase and acid phosphatase, whereas lipid bodies are responsible for eicosanoid formation. The function of the primary granule that contains Charcot-Leyden crystals is unknown at this time [1,2]. Taken together, these compounds are responsible for tissue destruction and inflammation. They have profound vasoactive and neurogenic properties that manifest clinically as erythema, wheals, and pruritus. Further details about the content and function of these cytoplasmic granules are beyond the scope of this article.

As mentioned previously, there are a variety of stimuli that can activate eosinophils, whereupon they can phagocytize foreign material or degranulate and release the contents of their granules. As previously mentioned, they can also synthesize the cytokines, including TNFα, IL-1, IL-3, IL-4, IL-5, IL-8, and GM-CSF, that are involved in an inflammatory response (type I hypersensitivity reaction) [2]. The degranulation of the eosinophils along with the production of cytokines evokes a profound inflammatory reaction in the tissue in which the parasite resides. The parasite is then killed by this immunologic response. Unfortunately, this same immunologic response, whether uncontrolled or misdirected, can also respond inappropriately to other antigens, producing a hypersensitivity reaction.

There are a number of EDs that affect cats and dogs. In some of these diseases, the eosinophil is a major "player," whereas in others, it is just part of the mixed inflammatory response. Causes of eosinophilic skin disorders in cats and dogs include hypersensitivity reactions (environmental allergens, insects [fleas and mosquitoes], food, intestinal parasites, and drugs), endogenous (free keratin and hair shafts) or exogenous (imbedded insect parts), infectious (bacterial or fungal infection [dermatophytosis]), viral (feline herpesvirus [FHV]-1 and retroviruses [feline leukemia virus [FeLV], feline immunodeficiency virus]), parasitic (*Cheyletiella, Otodectes, Sarcoptes, Notoedres*, and pediculosis), and idiopathic (unknown). In cats, ED should not be thought of as a disease but rather as a cutaneous reaction pattern to a variety of different stimuli. Regardless of the trigger, a number of different causes can cause similar immunologic, histologic, and clinical findings.

EDs described in cats or dogs include miliary dermatitis, "eosinophilic granuloma complex" (EGC, which includes feline indolent ulcer [IU], eosinophilic plaque [EP], and eosinophilic granuloma [EG]), feline mosquito bite hypersensitivity (MBH), canine eosinophilic folliculitis and furunculosis, and canine eosinophilic dermatitis and edema (Wells'-like syndrome).

EOSINOPHILIC GRANULOMA COMPLEX
Background
In cats, the most common EDs are feline miliary dermatitis (FMD) and EGC. Regardless of which form of ED is present, the underlying cause is essentially the same. The most commonly identified underlying cause is a hypersensitivity reaction to insects (fleas and mosquitoes), environmental allergens (atopic dermatitis [AD]), or foods. Before condemning the cat to lifelong drug therapy, all attempts should be made to identify and, if possible, eliminate the underlying trigger(s).

In human beings, AD is a chronic inflammatory skin disease caused by cutaneous hyperreactivity to environmental triggers and is characterized by elevated serum IgE levels [4]. There are also human patients with severe AD who generate IgE antibodies directed against human proteins (self-antigens). The autoallergens identified to date have been intracellular proteins, perhaps released as the result of self-trauma from scratching. This suggests that although the IgE immune responses are initiated by environmental allergens, chronic allergic skin disease can be maintained by the release of human proteins derived from damaged skin [4]. A recent article [5] suggests that *Felis domesticus* allergen I (Feld I) could be an autoallergen responsible for chronic inflammatory reactions in cats with EGC.

EGC consists of the EP, EG, and IU. Clinically, these are distinct entities, but making a diagnosis based on histopathologic findings is potentially confusing, because even though each of these clinical presentations has "typical" histologic changes, all forms can be observed on the same cat at the same time [6]. In fact, some lesions may have histologic features consistent with more than one of the reaction patterns [7]. It is best to think of the histopathologic changes associated with EGC as a reaction pattern rather than as a specific diagnosis.

Because EP, EG, and IU are most commonly a manifestation of a hypersensitivity reaction [7,8], differentiating among these, clinically or histologically, is not essential in establishing the underlying cause, nor is it helpful in choosing a treatment plan. Using histopathologic examination to rule in or rule out other similar-appearing diseases (eg, neoplasia, infection) is critical, because treatment and prognosis for these other diseases would be drastically different. Histopathologic examination should be performed in cases that clinically appear atypical or for those cases that fail to respond to prescribed treatment.

Because the diseases in the EGC have overlapping histopathologic findings, they are discussed as a group rather than individually. Histologic findings consistent with EGC are a variation on a theme. Findings vary depending on the stage (early versus late) and location of the lesion. Histologic findings may include epidermal hyperplasia with variable degrees of spongiosis and eosinophilic exocytosis, erosions, ulcerations, or epidermal coagulation necrosis. A luminal eosinophilic folliculitis and furunculosis may be present. There is a superficial to deep perivascular to interstitial to diffuse predominantly eosinophilic dermal infiltrate. A variable number of histiocytes, mast cells, and lymphocytes are present in the dermis. Mineralization of flame figures, which are distinct dermal deposits of collagen coated with amorphous to granular eosinophilic debris, may be present. A palisading granulomatous reaction containing epithelioid and multinucleated giant cells may form around flame figures as a result of proteins being released from degranulated eosinophils. In the past, these flame figures were described as collagenolysis or collagen degeneration. Subsequent studies have revealed that the collagen is normal (normal staining with Masson-Trichrome) and that the appearance of the collagen is attributable to its coating with substances from degranulated eosinophils [9].

EP may be singular, or there may be multiple lesions (Fig. 1). They are grossly alopecic and erosive to ulcerative erythematous patches or plaques most typically involving the ventral abdomen, perianal, and medial thigh regions. These highly pruritic lesions may also appear in the axillary regions, dorsal trunk, or flexor surface of the elbows. Although tissue and blood eosinophilia is a common finding, peripheral lymphadenopathy is only occasionally present. Direct impression smear cytology may show large numbers of eosinophils. As mentioned previously, it is important to identify and treat any underlying hypersensitivity. This is discussed further in the section on diagnosis and treatment.

FMD is closely related to EP. These two diseases are histologically similar but clinically distinct. FMD consists of pruritic, multifocal, erythematous papulocrusts that are frequently found on the trunk, neck, and face. Histologically,

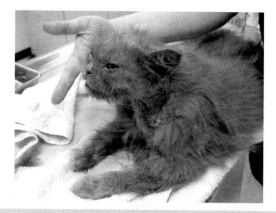

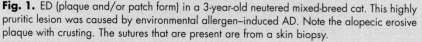

Fig. 1. ED (plaque and/or patch form) in a 3-year-old neutered mixed-breed cat. This highly pruritic lesion was caused by environmental allergen–induced AD. Note the alopecic erosive plaque with crusting. The sutures that are present are from a skin biopsy.

FMD is characterized by multifocal spongiosis, eosinophilic and neutrophilic exocytosis with serocellular crusting, and areas of epidermal coagulation necrosis. There is superficial and middermal perivascular to interstitial dermatitis with eosinophils and mast cells, intraepidermal eosinophilic pustules, and sometimes eosinophilic folliculitis [10]. There is a group of cats with FMD that the owners report as not being pruritic. It is unclear whether these cats are "closet" itchers or whether the papulocrusts are truly a primary lesion of the disease and not a result of self-trauma. In this subgroup of cats, the lesions on the haired skin are discovered by the owners incidentally as they are petting their cat. The lesions also may be found during the physical examination as the hair coat and skin are palpated or when a fine-toothed comb is passed through the hair coat. It is easiest to think of EP as a coalescence of miliary dermatitis lesions. Diagnosis and treatment are discussed elsewhere in this article.

An IU appears as an erosive to ulcerative lesion with slightly raised edges occurring most commonly on the midline of the upper lip or adjacent to the upper canine tooth. It may also involve the hard palate [6]. It is a reddish-brown to yellow lesion that is not painful or pruritic. Regional lymphadenopathy may be present [6,8]. An IU may be a precancerous lesion that progresses to SCC [8]. Blood eosinophilia and tissue eosinophilia are uncommon. A recent article expands our rule-out list for causes of IU [11]. In that article, it was reported that infection with *Microsporum canis* may be responsible for lip ulcers. This serves as additional proof on how a wide variety of antigens can stimulate a nonspecific reaction (ED) in cats. Diagnosis and treatment are discussed elsewhere in this article.

EG (linear granuloma or collagenolytic granuloma) is nonpruritic and appears as a mildly erythematous, alopecic, eroded, or ulcerated nodule or plaque. It is an off-white to yellow to pink lesion that may occasionally have white granules in the middle of the nodule. The nodular form is most commonly found in the oral cavity (tongue, hard palate, or glossopharyngeal arches) or on the chin. It is speculated that the oral cavity lesion may be a local reaction to imbedded insect parts in some cats [8]. When EG involves the chin ("chin edema"), affected cats have a "pouty" appearance because of the swelling of the area. EG may also involve the footpad or the conjunctiva [8]. Lesions also frequently appear on the caudal thigh as a linear plaque that is nonpruritic. The linear plaque is frequently detected only by "accident" when the owner is petting the cat or during a physical examination. Peripheral eosinophilia may be present. Diagnosis and treatment are discussed elsewhere in this article.

EG and IU are unique in that there is a subset of cats with these lesions that have no detectable underlying cause. This was discovered in a study involving a closed breeding colony of interrelated specific pathogen-free cats that had a high incidence of EG and IU. Intradermal tests (IDTs) and food trials failed to identify an underlying hypersensitivity reaction. This led to the theory that there is a genetic heritable eosinophil dysregulation predisposing to the development of these lesions [7,8,12]. In this study, however, it was also reported that the lesions would wax and wane, with spring and summer exacerbations, suggesting the presence of an unidentified environmental trigger. By 2 to 3 years of age, these cats became asymptomatic. Thus, if EG or IU occurs in a young cat, there is a possibility (perhaps small) of a heritable basis and that the cat may "outgrow" the disease over time. Because there is no way to predict which cats are going to become asymptomatic and which are going to continue to have symptoms, it is best to approach each case as though the disease is going to continue to be a problem and there is an identifiable and treatable underlying hypersensitivity.

A new approach (and possibly less confusing) to EGC would be to group the diseases based on a clinical description of the lesions. These descriptions would replace EP, IU, and EG. Only two forms, the papular and/or plaque form and the ulcerative form, would need to be identified. The former would encompass the EP and EG lesions and would be firm flat-topped papules that may coalesce into plaques with alopecia or erythema and would have a variable amount of pruritus. These lesions may involve the ventral abdomen, inguinal regions, and inner thighs. The linear plaque that involves the caudal thighs would also be included in this form. The ulcerative form would replace the IU. It would appear as a nonpruritic painless ulceration on the midline of the upper lip or adjacent to the upper canine teeth. The ulcerative form may also involve the oral cavity.

Eosinophilic Granuloma Complex or Feline Miliary Dermatitis Diagnosis and Treatment

As is the case with most dermatologic diseases, a diagnosis is made by using a combination of signalment, history (including response to therapy), clinical findings, laboratory testing, and response to therapy.

Because ED lesions are fairly distinctive, it is tempting to forget that other diseases can appear similar to ED lesions. For IU, the differential diagnosis would include SCC and infectious ulcers (herpes, calicivirus, FeLV infection, and *Cryptococcus*). For EP or EG rule outs, the differential diagnosis would include cutaneous epitheliotropic T-cell lymphoma, infectious granulomas (demodicosis, bacterial [including *Mycobacterium*], or fungal), mast cell tumor, and SCC [6,8].

The minimum database (MDB) for a cat presented with clinical signs consistent with ED depends on which form of ED is present but usually includes the following:

1. Skin scrapings (superficial and deep, because cats have superficial and deep forms of *Demodex* mites). Clear acetate tape preparations should be performed, as should combing the hair coat thoroughly with a fine-toothed comb to rule out other ectoparasites (eg, *Cheyletiella*, fleas).
2. Wood's lamp examination and dermatophyte culture. Because feline dermatophytosis is known as the "great imitator," all cats with skin disease should have a fungal culture performed. The use of the Wood's lamp examination alone is discouraged, because only 30% to 80% of the strains of *M canis* (the most common feline dermatophyte) fluoresce. Also, there are a variety of other causes of fluorescence, including scales, medication, and bacteria (eg, *Pseudomonas*) [13]. It is best to use the Wood's lamp as an aid in selecting which hairs to submit for fungal culture.
3. If the lesions appear atypical or do not respond to therapy, skin biopsy and histopathologic examination of the sample are appropriate. Other diagnostics that may be of value on an individual basis include macerated tissue cultures for bacteria or fungi. In the author's experience, complete blood cell counts (CBCs) and cytologic examination of lesions have been of little value.

Because EGC and FMD are most commonly associated with a hypersensitivity reaction, diagnostics for an allergic disease should be performed. In addition to the testing mentioned previously, all cats deserve an aggressive therapeutic trial for ectoparasites (especially directed toward fleas). This would include the administration of fipronil, imidacloprid, or selamectin biweekly for 30 days and then monthly for 2 more months (note that the administration of these products biweekly is an off-label use). The limitation of imidacloprid, which is an excellent insecticide, is that it is not an ascaricide; thus, it is not effective against mites. Depending on the region of the country, this factor may or may not be important.

In addition to the affected cat, all four-legged haired pets are treated with one of these products monthly for 3 months. Lufenuron may be administered orally to all these pets for 3 months. Environmental treatment should include aggressive vacuuming and "spot" treating the areas where the pets spend most of their time. A spray containing a combination of a pyrethrin and an insect growth regulator should be used for the spot treatment. Initially, while awaiting the response to this insecticidal treatment, a 21-day course using a tapering dose of oral prednisolone may be used for symptomatic relief.

If there is a response to therapy, it may be that flea allergy is the trigger; alternately, it may be the case that the cat has seasonal environmental allergen–induced disease and the seasons have changed or the problematic aeroallergens are no longer present. This may or may not present a diagnostic challenge depending on the historical information obtained. If the cat has a history of the lesions being present year round, it could be concluded that the seasonal change was not responsible for the improvement. If the lesions have not been present (or recurrent) for at least a year, the underlying disease may not be clarified until longer follow-up on the case occurs. During this time, continuation of the flea treatment should be maintained. (Please note that if a long-acting injectable glucocorticoid [GC], such as methylprednisone acetate, is administered simultaneously with flea control treatment, assessment of response is not possible until at least 4 months after the injection).

If the diagnostics performed were negative and the treatment for ectoparasites is unsuccessful in managing the skin disease, the next step depends on the severity of the disease and the frequency of its occurrence. If the symptoms occur once or twice a year, are fairly mild, and respond to a short course of oral prednisolone or an injection of a long-acting GC, symptomatic therapy is appropriate. If, conversely, the lesions are getting progressively more severe, more frequent, or require more than once- or twice-yearly GC therapy, investigation and treatment for cutaneous adverse food reactions (CAFRs) or environmental allergen–induced AD should occur.

It is critical to understand that environmental allergen–induced AD is a diagnosis of exclusion. Blood testing, or even an IDT, does not diagnose environmental allergen–induced AD. These tests are used to select antigen for allergen-specific immunotherapy (ASIT) once the diagnosis has been made. The diagnosis of environmental allergen–induced AD may be made historically (seasonal symptoms despite appropriate ectoparasite control) or may not be established until therapeutic trials and laboratory testing (as mentioned previously) have been performed.

When all the previously mentioned diagnostics and therapies have failed to diagnose and "cure" the problem and the symptoms are nonseasonal, a food trial should be performed. It is beyond the scope of this article to discuss the diagnosis of CAFRs in detail, but the author believes that the commercially available diets may rule in CAFR but cannot rule it out. The author is a firm believer that the only proper way to rule out a CAFR is by a home-prepared diet containing a novel protein and, in the case of dogs, a novel carbohydrate. Blood testing or an IDT is worthless. There are commercial diets that are novel protein based or contain hydrolyzed proteins. The limitation of these products is that a certain unknown percentage (it has not been established what percentage based on double-blind placebo-controlled trials) of dogs and cats respond to the novel protein or hydrolyzed diets. Thus, failure to respond to these diets does not rule out a CAFR.

Regardless of which method is used for the elimination diet trial, the new food should be fed for a minimum of 8 weeks in dogs and 12 weeks in cats. One possible explanation for the need for such a prolonged trial is because of the presence of histamine-releasing factors. Histamine-releasing factors are a heterogeneous group of cytokines generated by chronic antigenic exposure and may cause histamine release in the absence of antigen. This release may continue for weeks after antigen is removed [14].

If the cat's symptoms recur in spite of the ectoparasiticidal and food trials, the next step is to perform an IDT or serum "allergy" test to select an allergen for ASIT. The author prefers IDT over a blood test. The reader is encouraged to read elsewhere about the "pros and cons" of these testing methods.

If the owner declines ASIT, symptomatic treatment is needed while awaiting the response to a food trial or ASIT, the cat has failed to respond to ASIT, or the symptoms are infrequent, options for symptomatic relief include (please note that these therapies may be used concurrently with ASIT) the following:

1. Systemic antibiotics, such as amoxicillin–clavulanic acid (22 mg/kg administered every 12 hours), cefpodoxime proxetil (5 mg/kg administered every 24 hours; not approved for cats), cephalexin (22–30 mg/kg administered every 12 hours), cefadroxil (10–20 mg/kg administered every 12 hours), clindamycin (5–10 mg/kg administered every 12 hours; watch for esophageal irritation leading to esophageal stricture in cats). These may be useful in cats with mild IUs. Treatment should be for 4 to 6 weeks.
2. Systemic GCs, prednisolone (1–2 mg/kg every 12 hours and then tapering to every other day) rather than prednisone. Cats have unpredictable absorption or metabolism (to the active form) of prednisone; thus, only prednisolone should be used. As an alternative, methylprednisolone acetate (5 mg/kg) can be administered subcutaneously. For severe lesions, methylprednisolone acetate can be given two to three times 2 weeks apart. This is not a long-term therapy, nor should it be a standard therapy. Side effects associated with GCs in cats include diabetes mellitus, congestive heart failure, weight gain, demodicosis, dermatophytosis, and feline cutaneous fragility syndrome. Other oral steroids that may be useful in cases that fail to respond or become resistant to the effect of the previously mentioned GCs include oral triamcinolone (0.1–0.2 mg/kg administered every 24 hours) or dexamethasone (0.1–0.2 mg/kg administered every 24 hours). If these two GCs are used long term, it is best to administer them only every 3 days so that there is less suppression of the adrenal-pituitary axis. Intralesional triamcinolone may be useful for a severe refractory IU or oral EG.
3. Antihistamines and ω-3 or ω-3/6 fatty acid combinations can be administered. The antihistamine is used concurrently with an ω-fatty acid supplement. The author has been underwhelmed with the response to these therapies in cats with EGC.
   a. Hydroxyzine: 1.0–2.0 mg/kg administered two to three times daily for 14 days.
   b. Chlorpheniramine: 0.4–0.5 mg/kg administered twice daily for 14 days. This pill is extremely bitter tasting.
   c. Diphenhydramine: 1.0–2.0 mg/kg administered two to three times daily for 14 days. The liquid form has an alcohol base that cats strongly dislike.
   d. Clemastine: 0.05–0.10 mg/kg administered twice daily for 14 days
   e. Amitriptyline: 1.0–2.0 mg/kg administered once to twice daily for 21 days.

  f. Cyproheptadine: 0.5 to 1.0 mg/kg administered every 8 hours for 14 days. Warn owners about possible polyphagia. The author has also seen some anxiousness at the higher dose. This can be avoided by slowly increasing the dose over 5 to 7 days.

  g. Fatty acids: if a ω-3/6 combination product is used, prescribe double the bottle dose. If the product contains only ω-3, use it so that the cat receives eicosapentaenoic acid at a dose of 40 mg/kg daily.

4. Chlorambucil is a nitrogen mustard derivative, cell cycle–nonspecific, alkylating antineoplastic and/or immunosuppressive agent. Its cytotoxic activity stems from cross-linking with cellular DNA. The reader should become familiar with this drug if he or she is going to use it for EGC. It should only be used in severe steroid-refractory cases of EGC. It is used in combination with GCs. The initial dose is 0.1–0.2 mg/kg administered every 24 hours (usually one half of the 2-mg tablet or 1 mg daily). Once the disease is in remission, tapering of the GC is begun, eventually going to an every other day dose of the GC. Chlorambucil effectiveness has a lag effect and may not be fully appreciated until 4 to 8 weeks on therapy. Once the cat is off the GC, or the minimum dose of the GC has been determined based on relapses, treatment every 48 hours with chlorambucil is attempted. If the disease flairs at any point, go back two to three dosage steps (doses of GC and chlorambucil used two to three steps previously) and then begin to taper again, stopping before the ineffective dose. Side effects associated with chlorambucil therapy are myelosuppression (anemia, leukopenia, and thrombocytopenia), gastrointestinal (anorexia, vomiting, and diarrhea), and, rarely, hepatotoxicity. CBCs, including platelet counts, in addition to measuring liver enzymes, should be performed every other week for the first 3 months, monthly for 3 months, and then every 3 months for as long as the cat is on the chlorambucil. In addition, urinalysis and urine cultures should be done every 6 months to evaluate for asymptomatic bacteriuria.

5. Cyclosporine (CSA), which is a calcineurin inhibitor, may be used in cases of EGC. By inhibiting calcineurin, an important enzyme responsible for T-cell activation, CSA prevents the transcription of proinflammatory genes. CSA also inhibits the activation of mast cells, eosinophils, lymphocytes, Langerhans cells, and keratinocytes. The dose the author uses in cats is 5–7 mg/kg of the microemulsified form (mCSA) administered every 24 hours. There have mixed results with this drug [15,16]. The author has been pleased with the response to this drug and believes that it controls the disease adequately in 60% to 75% of the cats with EGC. Side effects in cats are limited and are primarily gastrointestinal, especially vomiting. Other side effects reported include cutaneous papillomatosis, hyperplastic gingivitis, hirsutism, papillomatosis, and activation of latent *Toxoplasma* infection. To minimize the most limiting factor of CSA (vomiting), the following protocol is used for a 10-lb cat: 10 mg of mCSA is administered once daily for 4 days, 20 mg administered once daily for 4 days, and then 30 mg administered once daily for 45 days. For the first 10 days, metoclopramide 2.5–5.0 mg is administered 30 minutes before mCSA. For the first 14 days, the mCSA is administered with a meal. After that, it is administered 2 hours before a meal. The product is available in a capsule form as well as in a liquid form. The liquid allows more flexible dosing but is extremely bitter tasting.

6. Comicronized palmidrol is an analogue of palmitoyl-ethanolamide. Palmitoyl-ethanolamide is produced in the area of mast cell degranulation by the surrounding tissue. It is an anti-inflammatory molecule that exerts it action by binding cannabinoid receptors (CB2) on mast cells. These receptors downregulate mast cell degranulation. In a preliminary study administering 10 mg/kg twice daily for 30 days to 15 cats with EG or EP, 10 (67%) of 15 cats showed clinical improvement of clinical signs and lesions [17].

7. Other treatment options, depending on the form of EGC, that have been reported to be effective include the following: doxycycline (25 mg administered every 12 hours; the medication must be followed with food or water to help prevent esophagitis and subsequent esophageal stricture), oral gold (auranofin, 0.1 mg/kg daily), surgical excision, cryotherapy, laser excision or ablation, α-interferon (3000 IU daily), and megestrol acetate (which should only be used as an absolute last resort because of serious side effects associated with its use, including adrenocortical suppression, transient diabetes mellitus, personality changes, increased weight, stump pyometra, mammary hypertrophy, neoplasias, and hepatotoxicity) at a dosage of 2.5 to 5.0 mg administered every 24 hours for 5 days and then at 2.5 to 5.0 mg administered semiweekly to weekly [18].

MOSQUITO BITE HYPERSENSITIVITY
Background

MBH is an uncommon ED of cats that was first described in 1988 [19]. Some authors consider it to be a member of the EGC, whereas others believe that it is a separate entity. Either way, it seems to be a hypersensitivity reaction to mosquito bites. There is significant geographic variability of this disease in the United States, correlating to the density of mosquitoes in a particular region. Also, because of the insect etiology, the disease is seasonal, correlating to the mosquito season in a particular area.

MBH only affects cats that are exposed to mosquitoes; therefore, the disease primarily affects indoor and outdoor or exclusively outdoor cats. There is no age, breed, or sex predilection. Affected areas include the poorly haired areas on the dorsal muzzle, the pinnae, preaural regions, periorbitally, skin around the nipples, and the footpads. Lesions progress from an erythematous papule or plaque to an erosion or ulcer that develops a crust. Alopecia and depigmentation of these areas may be present. Edema may develop on the muzzle or the footpads. Peripheral lymphadenopathy, fever, and eosinophilia are frequently present [6,20]. Histopathologic examination reveals a superficial and deep nodular to diffuse predominantly eosinophilic dermatitis, with eosinophilic luminal folliculitis and furunculosis and an occasional flame figure [10,21].

The differential diagnosis depends on the specific areas affected but could include pemphigus foliaceus or erythematosus, environmental allergen–induced AD, CAFR, flea bite hypersensitivity, dermatophytosis, demodicosis, neoplasia (eg, SCC, mast cell tumor), discoid lupus erythematosus, actinic dermatitis, *Cryptococcus* infection, and idiopathic EGC.

Mosquito Bite Hypersensitivity Diagnosis

As mentioned previously, the diagnosis of dermatologic disease is dependent on the combination of signalment, history, clinical findings, and response to therapy. In MBH, the history, symptoms occurring during mosquito season with known exposure to mosquitoes, clinical findings as described previously, and rapid and complete response to treatment consisting of avoidance of mosquito exposure or treatment with steroids support the diagnosis.

The MDB for a cat presented with signs consistent with MBH should include skin scrapings (superficial and deep), Wood's lamp examination, and fungal cultures to rule out demodicosis and dermatophytosis, respectively. Because of the seriousness of the rule-out diseases, it is advisable to biopsy the lesions and have histopathologic evaluation of tissue samples before instituting therapy. Remember that many of the differentials may be steroid-responsive diseases but that the long-term prognosis for control may be different than for MBH.

Mosquito Bite Hypersensitivity Treatment

Many cases need symptomatic treatment with systemic GCs (oral prednisolone or injectable methylprednisolone acetate using doses as previously discussed) in addition to minimizing or avoiding mosquito bites. Avoiding mosquito bites by restricting the cat to indoors (especially during and after dusk) is an effective treatment if the cat cooperates. An additional option includes applying insect repellents to the affected areas (use cautiously, because many are toxic in cats).

FELINE HERPESVIRUS DERMATITIS AND STOMATITIS

FHV is best known for its contribution to the upper respiratory syndrome (rhinotracheitis) of cats. Cats with this syndrome may present with oral or corneal ulcers along with sneezing and ocular and nasal discharge. The ulcers occur because herpesvirus is an epitheliotropic DNA virus capable of causing epithelial necrosis. A less common presentation is a syndrome of facial, truncal, oral cavity (stomatitis), or footpad ulceration associated with FHV infection. The face, especially the nasal planum, tends to have the most severe involvement.

Historically, affected cats have chronic ocular or respiratory disease or had an upper respiratory infection as a kitten. Eighty percent of all previously infected cats go on to become infected for life even though they may not be symptomatic (carrier state) [22]. Persistent infection with periodic or continuous shedding is common. Whenever a carrier cat undergoes stress or administration of GCs or another immunosuppressive therapy, there is a risk of a recrudescence of the virus, most commonly presenting with upper respiratory tract signs. Some cats develop a dermatitis or stomatitis in addition to or instead of the respiratory signs. The author has also seen the nasal planum affected in cats given intranasal vaccines containing FHV. In these cases, the disease is self-limiting and treatment is not necessary.

Clinical findings include vesicles, erosions, ulcers, and crusts that may involve the face (especially the nasal planum), footpads, trunk, or gums (stomatitis). Signs of an upper respiratory infection (fever, anorexia, conjunctivitis, corneal or oral ulcers, nasal and ocular discharge, or sneezing) may be present. The differential diagnosis includes FeLV-associated dermatitis, cutaneous drug reaction, erythema multiforme, MBH, EGC, pemphigus vulgaris, and systemic lupus erythematosus [23–25].

Feline Herpesvirus Diagnosis

Historical clues would include a poor response or exacerbation of clinical signs when GCs are administered, a history of upper respiratory infection, the presence of concurrent immunosuppressive diseases (eg, FeLV, FIV) or neoplasia, or a history of refractory gingivitis and/or stomatitis. Diagnosis is confirmed by histopathologic examination in which there are intranuclear inclusion bodies present. Polymerase chain reaction (PCR) from conjunctival smears, fluorescent antibody from conjunctival smears, serology, and immunohistochemistry (IHC) for FHV antigen may help to support a diagnosis of FHV infection; however, because of the high incidence of FHV infection in the "normal" cat population, overinterpretation of a positive result is a concern. Recently, the IHC test was reported to be an accurate test for FHV infections [24].

Histopathologic examination reveals necrotic, ulcerative, and crusting dermatitis with a primarily eosinophilic infiltrate and intranuclear viral inclusion bodies in the surface keratinocytes and follicular outer root sheath epithelial cells [10]. The nuclei of these cells exhibit margination of chromatin, and the cytoplasm has a foamy appearance. When viral inclusion bodies are present, the diagnosis is straightforward. Unfortunately, the viral inclusions are not always readily seen, and in those cases, differentiating FHV dermatitis from MBH or EGC is difficult.

No specific treatment is available. Symptomatic treatment for the upper respiratory signs should be administered. This may include ophthalmic medications and/or oral antibiotics for secondary infections and supportive care (eg, removing discharge from the eyes and nose, hand feeding if anorexic). Additional treatments that have not been evaluated with evidence-based medicine but have been anecdotally reported to be of value include the following:

1. α-Interferon, a cytokine with antiviral, antineoplastic, and immunomodulating properties, has been used to treat cats with FHV infections. Dose recommendations range from 1.5 to 2 million U/m^2 body surface area (BSA) administered subcutaneously three times a week (this is the dose used in human patients for herpes virus infections) to as low as 1000 IU/d administered orally. Side effects are uncommon, but malaise may be seen using the subcutaneous protocol. The author prefers to use the oral form at 3000 IU/d administered orally.

2. Concurrent lysine therapy at a dose of 250 to 500 mg administered twice daily. If a nonveterinary product is used, be certain that it does not contain propylene glycol, which is toxic in cats. Herpesvirus depends on exogenous arginine for replication. Lysine suppresses the incorporation of arginine into viral proteins; therefore, it has a virostatic effect. In a recent in vitro study [26], high concentrations of lysine did reduce the replication of FHV but

pace than those treated with GCs. Yet, in those cases treated with antibiotics versus GCs, clinical findings were identical on days 21 through 30.

CANINE EOSINOPHILIC DERMATITIS WITH EDEMA (WELLS' SYNDROME)

Wells' Syndrome Background in Human Beings

Wells' syndrome is an eosinophilic cellulitic disease of human beings. Clinically, people with Wells' syndrome present with a history of sudden onset of annular erythematous or edematous patches that rapidly evolve into plaques. These plaques may be single or multiple and may occur anywhere on the body. The patient may report mild pruritus, and there may be pain associated with the lesions. Papules, vesicles, bullae, erosions, ulcerations, or nodules may also be present. The disease may be recurrent [29,30].

The cause is unknown, but cases have been associated with an arthropod bite or sting, cutaneous viral infections, cutaneous parasitic infestations (eg, toxocariasis, ascariasis, onchocerciasis), leukemia, myeloproliferative disorders, AD, fungal infections, and cutaneous drug reactions [31–34]. Because of the many causes of this disease, it is best to think of Wells' syndrome as a reaction pattern rather than as a specific diagnosis.

The pathogenesis is unclear; however, there has been a study in which an increase in the IL-5 level was identified [29]. In this study, the increase in the circulating IL-5 level was associated with a relative increase in circulating CD3+CD4+ T cells. This increase in IL-5 could explain the increase in blood and tissue eosinophilia that is present in this disease. Degranulation of the eosinophils then occurs, leading to the clinical signs of edema and inflammation.

Wells' Syndrome Diagnosis

Diagnosis is made by histologic examination of a skin biopsy. Histopathologic findings on biopsies include a dermal infiltrate of eosinophils and histiocytes. In older lesions, the dermal infiltrate changes from eosinophilic to histiocytic with giant cells that surround some of the collagen fibers (flame figures). Flame figures represent eosinophilic debris coating collagen bundles [35–37].

Wells' Syndrome Treatment

Treatment for Wells' syndrome depends on the triggering event. This may include antifungal therapy, antihistamines, topical or systemic GCs, CSA, and dapsone [29].

Canine Well's-Like Syndrome

ED with edema (Wells'-like syndrome) is a rarely reported disease in dogs. A case report of a dog that had urticaria with ED was not identified as Wells'-like syndrome, but it may have been this disease [38]. In that report, the authors believed that the disease was triggered by a heartworm preventative, diethylcarbamazine. The first report of dogs with Wells'-like syndrome was published in 1999 [39]. In that study of nine dogs with this disease, all dogs presented with "target" lesions, erythematous patches with a central pallor, on the pinnae and ventrum. In some areas, these lesions progressed to erythematous serpiginous plaques. In four of nine dogs, there was also involvement on the extremities. Some of these lesions were purpuric and failed to blanch with diascopy, which is most consistent with hemorrhage from damaged and/or dysfunctional blood vessels. Edema, ranging from facial to generalized, was present in six of nine dogs. Fever (six of nine dogs) and lymphadenopathy (four of nine dogs) were also reported in this study. Urinalysis, tick titers for Rocky Mountain spotted fever, *Ehrlichia canis*, *Borrelia burgdorferi*, and antinuclear antibody (ANA) were all within normal limits or negative. CBCs revealed mild stress leukograms (neutrophilia with lymphopenia). Hypoalbuminemia was also reported. Histopathologic abnormalities reported from skin biopsies included superficial to deep perivascular to interstitial eosinophilic dermatitis with dermal edema and vascular dilatation. Four of nine dogs had flame figures, although, surprisingly, dermal hemorrhage, as suggested by the clinical findings, was not present.

Seven of the dogs were treated with anti-inflammatory doses of GCs for up to 4 weeks. Five of these seven dogs had the disease resolve within 4 weeks. In the other two dogs, the disease waxed and waned. The final two dogs were treated with antihistamines or received no therapy. Both of these dogs had resolution of their disease. The authors speculated that cutaneous drug reactions were the cause in seven of nine dogs and that an arthropod bite was causative in one case. Historically, five of the nine dogs had a history of allergic skin disease, perhaps suggesting that they were "prone" to hypersensitivity reactions. The other possibility is that because most cases were seen in the late summer or early fall months, environmental allergens may have triggered the disease. This author has seen a case in a 6-year-old intact female Labrador Retriever with

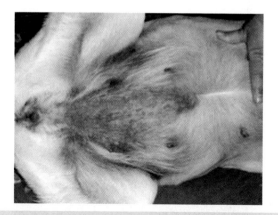

Fig. 4. This 6-year-old intact female Labrador Retriever was presented for fever, lethargy, and these extensive lesions on the ventral abdomen that occurred within a week of receiving vaccination and a long-acting heartworm injection (moxidectin). Over the next year, these symptoms and lesions recurred two more times without any known precipitating trigger. Note the erythematous patches involving the ventral abdomen

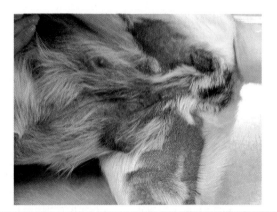

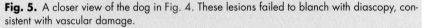

Fig. 5. A closer view of the dog in Fig. 4. These lesions failed to blanch with diascopy, consistent with vascular damage.

a history of seasonal atopy that was diagnosed with ED with edema (Figs. 4–6). The disease began shortly after administration of a long-lasting injectable form of heartworm preventative. The disease continued to wax and wane, regardless of the therapy (including immunosuppressive doses of GCs).

SUMMARY

EDs include a heterogeneous group of diseases that are secondary to underlying antigenic stimulation (hypersensitivity reactions) in most cases. Treatment options may include GCs, antifungal agents, antibiotics, food trials, ASIT, or

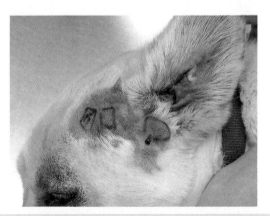

Fig. 6. The dog in Fig. 4 also had extensive involvement of the pinnae and temporal regions. Like many of the dogs reported with Wells'-like syndrome, this dog had a history of allergic skin disease but had never before had any involvement of the these areas.

CSA. To avoid the indiscriminate administration of chronic GCs or random therapeutic trials, a systematic approach to the diagnosis of these diseases should be performed.

References

[1] Zucker Franklin D. Eosinophil structure and maturation. In: Mahmoud AAF, Austen KF, editors. The eosinophil in health and disease. New York: Grune & Stratton; 1980. p. 43–60.

[2] Giembycz MA, Lindsay MA. Pharmacology of the eosinophil. Pharmacol Rev 1999;51: 213–340.

[3] Simon D, Braathen LR, Simon HU. Eosinophils and atopic dermatitis. Allergy 2004;59(6): 561–70.

[4] Leung DYM, Boguniewicz M, Howell M, et al. New insights into atopic dermatitis. Clin Invest 2004;113:651–7.

[5] Wisselink MA, van Ree R, Willemse T. Evaluation of *Felis domesticus* allergen I as a possible autoallergen in cats with eosinophilic granuloma complex. Am J Vet Res 2002;63:338–41.

[6] Mason K, Burton G. Eosinophilic granuloma complex. In: Guaguere E, Prelaud P, editors. A practical guide to feline dermatology. Paris: Merial Limited; 2000. p. 12.1–9.

[7] Rosenkrantz WS. Feline eosinophilic granuloma complex. In: Griffin CE, Kwochka KW, MacDonald JM, editors. Current veterinary dermatology. The science and art of therapy. St. Louis (MO): Mosby–Year Book; 1993. p. 319–24.

[8] Scott DW, Miller WH, Griffin CE. Muller and Kirk's small animal dermatology. 6th edition. Philadelphia: WB Saunders; 2001. p. 1148–53.

[9] Fernandez CJ, Scott DW, Erb HN. Staining abnormalities of dermal collagen in eosinophil or neutrophil-rich inflammatory dermatoses of horses and cats as demonstrated with Masson's trichrome stain. Vet Dermatol 2000;11(1):43–8.

[10] Affolter VK. Eosinophilic skin disease. In: 16th Proceedings of the Annual Meeting of the American Academy of Veterinary Dermatology and American College of Veterinary Dermatology. Norfolk (VA); 1996.

[11] Moriello KA. Important factors in the pathogenesis of feline dermatophytosis. Veterinary Medicine 2003;98:845–58.

[12] Power HT, Ihrke PJ. Selected feline eosinophilic skin diseases. Vet Clin North Am Small Anim Pract 1995;25:833–49.

[13] Scott DW, Miller WH, Griffin CE. Muller and Kirk's small animal dermatology. 6th edition. Philadelphia: WB Saunders; 2001. p. 119.

[14] Scott DW, Miller WH, Griffin CE. Muller and Kirk's small animal dermatology. 6th edition. Philadelphia: WB Saunders; 2001. p. 617.

[15] Guaguère E, Prélaud P. Efficacy of cyclosporin in the treatment of 12 cases of eosinophilic granuloma complex [abstract]. Vet Dermatol 2000;11(1):31.

[16] Noli C, Scarampella F. A prospective pilot study on the use of cyclosporin on feline allergic disease. Vet Dermatol 2004;15(1):33.

[17] Scarampella F, Abramo F, Noli C. Clinical and histological evaluation of an analogue of palmitoylethanolamide, PLR 120 (comicronized palmidrol INN) in cats with eosinophilic granuloma and eosinophilic plaque: a pilot study. Vet Dermatol 2001;12(1):29–39.

[18] Plumb DC. Megestrol acetate. In: The veterinary drug handbook. Ames (IA): PharmaVet Publishing; 2002.

[19] Mason KV, Evans AG. Mosquito bite caused eosinophilic dermatitis in cats. J Am Vet Med Assoc 1991;198:2086–8.

[20] Foster AP. New feline skin diseases—frustrating feline eosinophilic skin diseases. In: Clinical Programme Proceedings of the Fifth World Congress.

[21] Scott DW, Miller WH, Griffin CE. Muller and Kirk's small animal dermatology. 6th edition. Philadelphia: WB Saunders; 2001. p. 636.

[22] Lagerwerf W. Feline upper respiratory viruses part one: rhinotracheitis. Winn Foundation Handout. Manasquan (NJ): Winn Feline Foundation; 2002.

[23] Heiman M, Fontaine J. Feline idiopathic ulcerative dermatosis [abstract]. Vet Dermatol 2000;11(Suppl 1):31.

[24] Hargis AM, Ginn PE, Mansell JEKL, et al. Ulcerative facial and nasal dermatitis and stomatitis in cats associated with feline herpesvirus 1. Vet Dermatol 1999;10:267–74.

[25] Scott DW, Miller WH, Griffin CE. Muller and Kirk's small animal dermatology. 6th edition. Philadelphia: WB Saunders; 2001. p. 524.

[26] Maggs DJ, Collins BK, Thorne JG, et al. Effects of L-lysine and L-arginine on in vitro replication of feline herpesvirus type-1. Am J Vet Res 2000;61(12):1474–8.

[27] Gross TL. Canine eosinophilic furunculosis of the face. In: Ihrke PJ, Mason IS, White SD, editors, Advances in veterinary dermatology, vol. 2. New York: Pergamon Press; 1993. p. 239–46.

[28] Scott DW, Miller WH, Griffin CE. Muller and Kirk's small animal dermatology. 6th edition. Philadelphia: WB Saunders; 2001. p. 641–2.

[29] Brown J, Schwartz RA. Wells syndrome (eosinophilic cellulitis). Omahal (NE): eMedicine. com; 2003.

[30] Spigel GT, Winkelmann RK. Wells' syndrome. Recurrent granulomatous dermatitis with eosinophilia. Arch Dermatol 1979;115(5):611–3.

[31] Tsuda S, Tanaka K, Miyasato M, et al. Eosinophilic cellulitis (Wells' syndrome) associated with ascariasis. Acta Derm Venereol 1994;74(4):292–4.

[32] Hurni MA, Gerbig AW, Braathen LR, et al. Toxocariasis and Wells' syndrome: a causal relationship? Dermatology 1997;195(4):325–8.

[33] Kaufmann D, Pichler W, Beer JH. Severe episode of high fever with rash, lymphadenopathy, neutropenia, and eosinophilia after minocycline therapy for acne. Arch Intern Med 1994;154(17):1983–4.

[34] van den Hoogenband HM. Eosinophilic cellulitis as a result of onchocerciasis. Clin Exp Dermatol 1983;8(4):405–8.

[35] Newton JA, Greaves MW. Eosinophilic cellulitis (Wells' syndrome) with florid histological changes. Clin Exp Dermatol 1988;13(5):318–20.

[36] Stern JB, Sobel HJ, Rotchford JP. Wells' syndrome: is there collagen damage in the flame figures? J Cutan Pathol 1984;11(6):501–5.

[37] Moossavi M, Mehregan DR. Wells' syndrome: a clinical and histopathologic review of seven cases. Int J Dermatol 2003;42(1):62–7.

[38] Vitale CB, Ihrke PJ, Gross TL. Putative diethylcarbamazine-induced urticaria with eosinophilic dermatitis in a dog. Vet Dermatol 1994;5(4):197–202.

[39] Holm KS, Morris DO, Gomez SM, et al. Eosinophilic dermatitis with edema in nine dogs, compared with eosinophilic cellulitis in humans. J Am Vet Med Assoc 1999;215(5):649–53.

Atopy: New Targets and New Therapies

Rosanna Marsella, DVM

Blanche Saunders Dermatology Laboratory, Department of Small Animal Clinical Sciences, College of Veterinary Medicine, University of Florida, PO Box 100126, Gainesville, FL 32610–0126, USA

In the past decade in human medicine, atopy and atopic dermatitis (AD) have been the foci of great research effort because of their increased incidence, lifelong and complex nature, and therapeutic challenges. In veterinary medicine, canine AD has represented a similar challenge for clinicians and researchers. A special Task Force of the American College of Veterinary Dermatology was charged with the mission of reviewing the existing literature and providing clinicians with guidelines for diagnostic criteria and treatment options. From that work, it became evident that there are more questions than answers and that we are just now beginning to unfold the complex, variable, and dynamic nature of this disease. It became obvious that previously accepted definitions and dogmas are insufficient to explain clinical observations and that a more comprehensive approach is necessary to understand and manage our patients successfully [1].

IgE, TYPE I HYPERSENSITIVITY, AND ITS MODULATION

Atopy was traditionally defined as type I hypersensitivity to inhaled allergens. It is now evident that although IgE-mediated reactions play an important role in the capture of the allergens and in the effector phase [2], additional abnormalities are necessary to explain atopy and AD fully [3]. This is supported by several observations. Clinically, antihistamines have limited efficacy, although it could be argued that the limited response may be caused, at least in part, by an inappropriate extrapolation of doses [4,5]. Little information is available regarding the pharmacokinetics of these drugs in small animals; therefore, most of the doses have been extrapolated from human medicine. It is interesting to note that the limited response to antihistamine therapy is not limited to the first-generation antihistamines but has also been reported with the second-generation drugs, such as cetirizine. In one recent study, cetirizine satisfactorily reduced pruritus in only 18% of AD patients when used at a daily

E-mail address: marsellar@mail.vetmed.ufl.edu

0195-5616/06/$ – see front matter
doi:10.1016/j.cvsm.2005.09.004

dose of 1 mg/kg [6]. Similarly, partial success has been reported with other treatments that have focused on type I hypersensitivity, such as leukotriene inhibitors [7] and essential fatty acids [8].

To question the absolute role of IgE in canine AD further, past attempts to establish a model using high-IgE dogs had limited success [9] and allergy testing focused on the detection of IgE is not able to differentiate between normal and affected individuals [10]. Although some of these findings could be explained by the complex nature of IgE [11,12] and speculation that different isoforms of IgE might have different pathogenetic potential, it is also reasonable to consider that additional mechanisms may play a decisive role in the pathogenesis of AD. A subtype of AD, called "intrinsic" or "nonallergic" AD, has been recently identified in which an IgE response is not detectable [13]. Affected individuals have all the other clinical features of AD.

Despite these controversies, modulation or abolition of the IgE component of the disease is still an appealing strategy to control, at least in part, symptoms associated with AD. Great effort has been placed on testing anti-IgE therapies in people [14,15]. Recently, omalizumab, a humanized IgG1 monoclonal antibody against IgE, has been shown to be effective in the treatment of allergic asthma and allergic rhinitis [16]. Omalizumab recognizes and masks an epitope in the CH3 region of IgE responsible for binding to the high-affinity FcϵR on mast cells and basophils. Omalizumab markedly reduces serum levels of free IgE and downregulates IgE receptors on circulating dendritic cells. These findings suggest that blocking IgE may also inhibit more chronic aspects of allergic inflammation involving T-cell activation. Although most of the research has focused on respiratory diseases [17], anti-IgE therapy may also have a role in AD, especially in those individuals in which an IgE response is detectable. Anti-IgE therapy is currently being explored in dogs, and vaccination with an anti-IgE peptide was demonstrated to decrease total IgE [18].

LYMPHOCYATES, CYTOKINE AND CHEMOKINE IMBALANCES, AND THEIR MODULATION

Current research is now focusing on the role of cytokines involved in the determination of the type of lymphocytic response and the chemokines responsible for the recruitment of inflammatory cells at the site of allergen challenge [19]. Numerous similarities exist between canine AD and the human counterpart [20], and it seems that in dogs and people, cytokine imbalances geared toward a predominant T helper (Th) 2 response play an important role [21]. More specifically, in canine AD, there is overexpression of interleukin (IL)-4 mRNA and reduced transcription of transforming growth factor (TGF)-β compared with normal dogs [22]. In the same study, higher levels of γ-interferon (IFN), TNFα, and IL-2 mRNA were found in lesional compared with nonlesional and healthy skin, whereas there were no significant differences in IL-10, IL-6, or IL-12 transcription. There is also evidence that chemokines, such as thymus and activation regulated chemokine (TARC), play an important role in the recruitment of Th2 lymphocytes in lesional skin in dogs with AD

[23,24]. Finally, in a recent study evaluating atopy patch test reactions, it was demonstrated that early phases of the reactions are characterized by a predominant Th2 response, whereas later reactions are dominated by a Th1 cytokine profile [25]. All these findings support the consideration of treatment options focused on the modulation of the lymphocytic response, such as calcineurin inhibitors [26].

Calcineurin Inhibitors: Cyclosporine, Tacrolimus, and Pimecrolimus

Calcineurin inhibitors have the ability to block most of the allergic reaction by inhibiting cytokine production and modulating T-cell proliferation and activation and antigen presentation [27–29]. Cyclosporine also inhibits eosinophil function and survival [30,31], decreases the number of Langerhans cells in the epidermis, and inhibits the lymphocyte-activating functions of these antigen-presenting cells [32,33]. Cyclosporine is successfully used in human medicine for recalcitrant AD; however, the severity of the adverse effects has limited its use to severe cases that fail more conventional therapies [34].

Several studies have been published in veterinary medicine evaluating the efficacy and safety of cyclosporine in dogs [35]. Oral cyclosporine at a dose of 5 mg/kg was found to have similar efficacy to prednisolone at a dose of 0.5 mg/kg in a 6-week study [36]. The efficacy of cyclosporine therapy is dose dependent [37,38], but monitoring of blood levels has not been found to be of benefit in predicting and monitoring the clinical response of dogs with AD [39].

In a recent retrospective study that evaluated the response of atopic dogs treated with cyclosporine for a minimum of 6 months, it was found that 55% of dogs needed ongoing cyclosporine to control clinical signs of AD, although daily administration was not necessary [40]. In the same study, laboratory abnormalities were detected in 25% of dogs and therapy was discontinued in 45% because of a limited response (22%) or after achieving a clinical response (24%). Adverse effects of cyclosporine at the dose used for AD have been found to be mostly gastrointestinal disorders (eg, vomiting), development of oral growths, and hirsutism, although concerns have been raised regarding the potential of cyclosporine to induce or precipitate the development of lymphoma [41]. It is important to report that a recent retrospective study evaluating the incidence of lymphoma in 32 dogs receiving cyclosporine for a variety of conditions failed to demonstrate development of lymphoma [42]. Dogs received cyclosporine for a period that varied from 2 weeks to 2 years, with an average of 4 months.

Topical calcineurin inhibitors, such as tacrolimus, may be a suitable alternative to cyclosporin, especially in dogs with localized AD. Tacrolimus ointment has been demonstrated to be safe and effective for short- and long-term treatment of AD in pediatric and adult patients [43,44], although studies on rodents have recently raised concerns about the potential for carcinogenicity and prompted warnings about long-term use [45].

Few studies in veterinary medicine have evaluated tacrolimus' efficacy in dogs with AD. In a 4-week, double-blind, placebo-controlled, crossover study, tacrolimus ointment at 0.1% significantly decreased the severity of symptoms when evaluated by owners and investigators [46]. Dogs with localized disease responded better than dogs with generalized disease. Minimal absorption was observed with topical application, and tacrolimus was detected in the blood of animals receiving the active ingredient. Levels were below the level of toxicity, and no adverse effects were reported. No changes in complete blood cell count and chemistry parameters were detected.

In another single-blind study using dogs with localized AD, after 6 weeks of therapy, the percentage reduction from baseline scores was higher for tacrolimus-treated sites than for placebo-treated sites [47]. In the tacrolimus-treated dogs, lesions decreased by 50% or greater in 75% of dogs. Adverse drug events consisted of minor irritation in some lesional areas treated with tacrolimus. The irritation could possibly be linked to the ability of tacrolimus to activate nociceptive C-fibers [48].

In human medicine, it is reported that pimecrolimus has a similar mechanism of action and safety profile as tacrolimus but less efficacy [49]. Pimecrolimus permeates less through the skin than tacrolimus and has a lower potential for transcutaneous resorption after topical administration, resulting in a lower risk of systemic effects. Pimecrolimus has high anti-inflammatory activity in animal models of skin inflammation, including a model reflecting neurogenic inflammation, but a more favorable balance of anti-inflammatory versus immunosuppressive activity than tacrolimus [50]. To date, no published studies have been conducted to evaluate the efficacy of pimecrolimus in the treatment of canine AD.

Alternative Modalities of Allergen-Specific Immunotherapy

Multiple open studies and clinical observations suggest that allergen-specific immunotherapy (ASIT) is effective in decreasing clinical signs of AD in dogs [51]. ASIT requires repeated subcutaneous injections, and it may take months before clinical improvement can be observed. The success rate of conventional ASIT in dogs has been reported to vary from 50% to 70% [52].

To abbreviate the induction period, rush ASIT protocols have been explored in veterinary medicine [53]. In one study, the safety of a rush protocol was evaluated in 30 dogs with AD [54]. In this study, allergen extracts were administered in increasing concentrations every 30 minutes for 6 hours to a maintenance concentration of 20,000 protein nitrogen U/mL. In 22 (73%) dogs, rush ASIT safely replaced the prolonged induction period (15 weeks) of weekly injections, which consists of increasing concentrations of allergen extract. In 7 (23%) dogs, the induction period was abbreviated to 4 weeks. Of the 8 dogs that developed problems during rush ASIT, increased pruritus necessitated premature cessation of rush ASIT in 7 and 1 developed generalized wheals. The authors concluded that rush ASIT performed at a veterinary hospital is a safe method for treatment of dogs with AD.

Although the exact mechanisms of ASIT in dogs have not been completely elucidated, it has been shown that ASIT causes a shift toward a Th1 bias by enhancing γ-IFN expression [55]. More specifically, it was found that the ratio of γ-IFN/IL-4 was low in atopic dogs compared with normal controls before the beginning of ASIT. The level of γ-IFN after ASIT increased significantly, whereas that of IL-4 mRNA was not changed.

An alternate method of suppressing Th2 responses is to take advantage of the innate immune response mounted against bacterial DNA. Oligodeoxynucleotides (ODNs) containing sequence motifs centered on unmethylated CG dinucleotides (CpG ODNs) resemble bacterial DNA and, like bacterial DNA, are immunostimulatory [56]. For this reason, these agents may represent a novel therapeutic approach that restores immune tolerance and suppresses Th2 reactions in atopic individuals [57]. Promising results have been reported with the incorporation of CpG adjuvants in ASIT in human medicine [58]. Similarly, complexes of liposomes and noncoding plasmid DNA may be used to increase Th1 responses, in place of CpG oligonucleotides, because they also stimulate the release of γ-IFN [59].

In a recent open study, seven dogs with refractory AD were treated with liposome–nucleic acid complexes mixed with the ASIT [60]. In this pilot study, the dogs underwent a series of six intradermal injections (weeks 0, 2, 4, 6, 10, and 14). The dose of allergen extract used was decreased by 90% from the dose used in conventional ASIT, based on the known prior potency of the liposome-DNA complex vaccines. Owners assessed pruritus using a visual analog scale, and lesion scores were determined using the Canine Atopic Dermatitis Extent and Severity Index. Circulating levels of γ-IFN, IL-4, TNFα, and IL-10 were measured at the beginning and end of the study. Injections were well tolerated in all dogs, and owners reported a significant improvement in pruritus. A significant decrease in IL-4 production was also reported, although the production of other cytokines did not change significantly with treatment. It is important to note that this study was not blind or controlled; therefore, although these results are encouraging, further investigations with larger numbers of dogs in a controlled and blind study are necessary.

Another alternative approach for ASIT is nonspecific immunotherapy, such as that using MS-antigen. MS-antigen is a peptide extracted from the urine of human allergic patients and is marketed in Japan for nonspecific immunotherapy. In one report, this peptide was successfully used in two dogs that had failed conventional ASIT [61]. Increasing doses of MS-antigen were given every 3 to 4 days initially. Frequency was increased to once weekly to once monthly based on the response. Although various mechanisms of action have been postulated for this compound, the exact mechanism is not known. Various immunomodulatory properties have been reported, including decrease of histamine release, increase of cyclic adenosine monophosphate, and suppression of leukotriene D4. Other antiallergic compounds that have been used in human medicine for nonspecific immunotherapy include histaglobin and neutropin. Histaglobin has been reported to downregulate the release of IL-1β, TNFα, IL-6, and IL-10 in human peripheral blood mononuclear cell cultures [62] and to decrease or resolve symptoms of AD and rhinitis [63,64]. So far, no studies have been conducted in dogs to evaluate the efficacy of this therapy.

NEUROPEPTIDES AND THEIR MODULATION

Evidence is building on the relation between the nervous system and the immune system and the potential role for stress and neuropeptides, such as substance P (SP), in the pathogenesis of atopy and AD [65,66]. This is confirmed by the increased plasma concentration of SP and the increased expression of SP in lesional skin of patients with AD [67,68]. In a study evaluating the ability of neuropeptides to affect the T-cell cytokine profile, it was found that the effect is not cytokine specific [69].

Only one study has been reported in veterinary medicine investigating SP concentrations in the skin of normal dogs and dogs with AD. This evaluation was combined with an investigation of the clinical efficacy of 0.025% capsaicin lotion as therapy for canine AD in a double-blind crossover study [70]. In this study, SP concentrations in the skin did not correlate with the severity of the pruritus and did not change significantly over time and with treatments. At the end of the study, significant improvement was reported by owners, suggesting that this treatment could be considered as an adjunctive therapy for canine AD. Initial worsening was noted in some dogs in the first 7 to 10 days of therapy, possibly attributable to increased release of SP.

BARRIER FUNCTION, ITS NORMALIZATION, AND REDUCTION OF ALLERGEN EXPOSURE

In human medicine, AD is characterized by dry skin and increased transepidermal water loss. It is hypothesized that a defective extrusion of lipid-containing organelles, the lamellar bodies, results in changes in the chemical composition of the epidermal lipid barrier and increased transepidermal water loss [71,72]. Extensive research has been done on topical and oral fatty acid supplementation that might help to restore a normal barrier function in patients with AD [73].

At this time, it is not known if a defective lipid barrier is also present in atopic dogs. Studies in veterinary medicine have yielded controversial results. In one study, water absorption/desorption values of dogs with AD did not differ from those of normal dogs [74]. In another study, normal and atopic canine skin was evaluated using transmission electron microscopy to determine structural differences within stratum corneum lipids [75]. The deposition of stratum corneum lipid lamellae in atopic canine skin appeared markedly heterogeneous compared with that seen in normal canine skin. When present, the lamellae often exhibited an abnormal structure. The continuity and thickness of the intercellular lipid lamellae were significantly less in nonlesional atopic canine skin than in normal canine skin, suggesting that the epidermal lipid barrier may be defective in atopic canine skin. Additional studies are clearly needed to characterize the biochemical defect and possibly to correct it with nutritional or pharmacologic intervention. If transepidermal water loss is increased in atopic dogs, oral supplementation with essential fatty acids and topical application of oils may lead to a normalization of the barrier [76–78].

The other consequence of an abnormal skin barrier is increased penetration of allergens. It is now known that epicutaneous exposure of allergens plays a significant role in canine AD patients [79]. Decrease of allergen exposure can therefore be accomplished by frequent bathing. Unfortunately, epicutaneous exposure is not the only clinically relevant route of exposure. A recent study demonstrated that ingestion of the allergen as well as inhalation and epicutaneous exposure is able to trigger allergic reactions [80]. The approach to affected patients should therefore be multifaceted, with topical therapy being one of the multiple strategies adopted to reduce allergen exposure and decrease clinical signs.

For animals with hypersensitivity to house dust mites, in addition to frequent bathing, it may be useful to use products like benzyl benzoate, an acaricide utilized for the control of house dust mites. In a recently published study, the use of benzyl benzoate led to resolution of lesions and pruritus in 48% of cases of canine AD. In addition, 36% of dogs had moderate improvement, with a decrease of pruritus and minimal skin lesions, but still required some medication [81].

NEW STRATEGIES FOR THE FUTURE
Probiotics
Great interest exists in human medicine regarding early prevention and treatment of AD using microbial probiotics. Probiotics can beneficially boost Th1 immune responses and decrease the likelihood of development of AD [82,83]. Cultures of beneficial live microorganisms characteristic of commensal microflora are administered with probiotic functional foods to provide a microbial challenge for the maturation of gut-associated lymphoid tissue of infants. The probiotic effects are attributed to the normalization of the increased intestinal permeability, the balance of gut microecology, the improvement of the immunologic defense barrier (IgA), the downregulation of proinflammatory cytokines characteristic of allergic inflammation, and the increase of Th1 cytokines (eg, γ-IFN) [84,85].

Most probiotic studies have been conducted using *Lactobacillus rhamnosus* (*Lactobacillus* GG), a specific strain safe to use at an early age, which is effective in promoting local antigen and immune responses and able to survive passage through and transiently colonize the gastrointestinal tract.

To date, there are no studies evaluating this therapy in dogs, although it may be a safe and promising adjunctive treatment for young dogs belonging to breeds with high risk of AD.

Cytokine and Anticytokine Therapy
Therapy with cytokines, such as γ-IFN and IL-4 receptor, have been evaluated in rodents and human beings [86,87]. Because of the potential interference with other immunologic functions of the host, this type of therapy has been replaced

with anticytokines. Anticytokines belong to a new family of biologic response modifiers, which interfere with the biologic functions of cytokines [88]. Anticytokines, such as soluble TNF receptors and IL-1ra inhibitors, have been used to control septic shock and autoimmune diseases and represent promising strategies for the control allergic diseases.

Peptide Immunotherapy

Peptide therapy targets T cells directly with short peptides containing multiple T-cell receptor epitopes [89]. Short allergen peptides, native sequences or altered peptide ligands, are attractive for immunotherapy because they are unlikely to contain epitopes for IgE binding or to induce anaphylaxis. Peptide therapy induces a significant dose-dependent decrease in peptide-stimulated IL-4 production consistent with a shift in T-cell phenotype or peptide-specific T-cell tolerance and may represent an attractive future option of alternative immunotherapy in our patients.

Antisense Oligonucleotides

Antisense oligonucleotides (ASOs) are short single-stranded DNA fragments that are targeted against a specific mRNA. The use of ASOs targeted to the transcripts encoding biologically active proteins in the immunology system provides a novel and highly selective therapeutic strategy to obtain the selective blockage of a specific gene [90]. The advantages of ASOs are high specificity and less adverse drug events than typical immunosuppressive drugs. ASO specific for IL-10 has been demonstrated to resolve AD lesions in a mouse model after topical application [91].

Blockade of Recruitment of Cells

E-selectin on dermal postcapillary venules and homing receptors on lymphocytes play critical roles in the migration of effector T cells into inflamed skin. Cutaneous lymphocyte antigen-1 (CLA-1) is particularly important for homing of T cells in the skin. Modifiers of CLA have been tested in mice and successfully prevented migration of lymphocytes to inflamed skin [92,93]. Additionally, inhibitors of chemokines, such as RANTES and TARC, are being developed to block recruitment of leukocytes at the site of allergen challenge [94].

Targeted Therapy Based on Genetic Testing

It is becoming increasingly evident that AD is a polygenetic disease, with multiple genes being considered as candidates. It is hypothesized that different mutations may be present in different patients and that AD encompasses a variety of genetic alterations, although, clinically, they all lead to similar manifestations. DNA microarray studies are presently allowing the simultaneous comparison of thousands of mRNAs that may help to identify the disease-specific pattern of tissue inflammatory responses [95]. In the future, we may be able to identify the mutations responsible for canine AD in the various breeds of dogs, predict the likelihood of development of disease of young animals, recognize the specific mutations of the affected individual, and prescribe more targeted therapy.

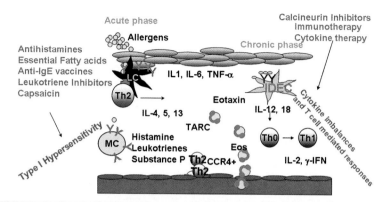

Fig. 1. Proposed pathogenesis for canine AD. Currently, it is accepted that type I hypersensitivity reactions are mixed with T-cell–mediated reactions. Eosinophils are attracted by eotaxin, whereas Th2 cells are attracted by TARC. IDEC, inflammatory dendritic cells; LC, Langerhans cell; MC, mast cell; Th, T helper.

SUMMARY

Because of the multifactorial nature of AD (Fig. 1), the best therapeutic approach is to use combinations of multiple modalities individualized for each patient. Recent research has emphasized the complexity of this disease, indicating how type I hypersensitivity is intermingled with T-cell imbalances and, possibly, abnormalities of the barrier function. New strategies for patient management include modulation of the lymphocytic response through the use of calcineurin inhibitors, potential inhibition of the IgE response through the use of anti-IgE vaccines, and alternative modalities for immunotherapy. Decrease of allergen exposure by frequent bathing, adjunctive antihistamine therapy, and neuropeptide modulation may help in controlling clinical signs. Future strategies may include the use of probiotics, inhibitors of cytokines and chemokines, and a targeted approach based on the genetic mutations of the individual patient.

References

[1] Olivry T, DeBoer DJ, Griffin CE, et al. The ACVD task force on canine atopic dermatitis: forewords and lexicon. Vet Immunol Immunopathol 2001;81(3–4):143–6.

[2] Olivry T, Moore PF, Affolter VK, et al. Langerhans cell hyperplasia and IgE expression in canine atopic dermatitis. Arch Dermatol Res 1996;288(10):579–85.

[3] Halliwell RE, DeBoer DJ. The ACVD task force on canine atopic dermatitis (III): the role of antibodies in canine atopic dermatitis. Vet Immunol Immunopathol 2001;81(3–4):159–67.

[4] DeBoer DJ, Griffin CE. The ACVD task force on canine atopic dermatitis (XXI): antihistamine pharmacotherapy. Vet Immunol Immunopathol 2001;81(3–4):323–9.

[5] Olivry T, Mueller RS, and the International Task Force on Canine Atopic Dermatitis. Evidence-based veterinary dermatology: a systematic review of the pharmacotherapy of canine atopic dermatitis. Vet Dermatol 2003;14(3):121–46.

[6] Cook CP, Scott DW, Miller WH Jr, et al. Treatment of canine atopic dermatitis with cetirizine, a second generation antihistamine: a single-blinded, placebo-controlled study. Can Vet J 2004;45(5):414–7.

[7] Crow DW, Marsella R, Nicklin CF. Double-blinded, placebo-controlled, cross-over pilot study on the efficacy of zileuton for canine atopic dermatitis. Vet Dermatol 2001;12(4): 189–95.

[8] Olivry T, Marsella R, Hillier A. The ACVD Task Force on Canine Atopic Dermatitis (XXIII): are essential fatty acids effective? Vet Immunol Immunopathol 2001;81(3–4):347–62.

[9] Egli KS, Schiessl B, Roosje PJ, et al. Evaluation of the usefulness of sensitization to aeroallergens as a model for canine atopic dermatitis in genetically predisposed Beagles. Am J Vet Res 2002;63(9):1329–36.

[10] DeBoer DJ, Hillier A. The ACVD task force on canine atopic dermatitis (XVI): laboratory evaluation of dogs with atopic dermatitis with serum-based "allergy" tests. Vet Immunol Immunopathol 2001;81(3–4):277–87.

[11] Zhang K, Max EE, Cheah HK, et al. Complex alternative RNA splicing of epsilon-immunoglobulin transcripts produces mRNAs encoding four potential secreted protein isoforms. J Biol Chem 1994;269:456–62.

[12] Peng Z, Arthur G, Rector ES, et al. Heterogeneity of polyclonal IgE characterized by differential charge, affinity to protein A, and antigenicity. J Allergy Clin Immunol 1997;100: 87–95.

[13] Wuthrich B, Schmid-Grendelmeier P. The atopic eczema/dermatitis syndrome. Epidemiology, natural course, and immunology of the IgE-associated ("extrinsic") and the nonallergic ("intrinsic") AEDS. J Investig Allergol Clin Immunol 2003;13(1):1–5.

[14] Milgrom H. Attainments in atopy: special aspects of allergy and IgE. Adv Pediatr 2002;49: 273–97.

[15] MacGlashan D Jr. Anti-IgE antibody therapy. Clin Allergy Immunol 2002;16:519–32.

[16] Holgate ST, Djukanovic R, Casale T, et al. Anti-immunoglobulin E treatment with omalizumab in allergic diseases: an update on anti-inflammatory activity and clinical efficacy. Clin Exp Allergy 2005;35(4):408–16.

[17] D'Amato G, Liccardi G, Noschese P, et al. Anti-IgE monoclonal antibody (omalizumab) in the treatment of atopic asthma and allergic respiratory diseases. Curr Drug Targets Inflamm Allergy 2004;3(3):227–9.

[18] Wang CY, Walfield AM, Fang X, et al. Synthetic IgE peptide vaccine for immunotherapy of allergy. Vaccine 2003;21:1580–90.

[19] Nuttall T, Knight PA, McAleese SM, et al. Expression of Th1, Th2 and immunosuppressive cytokine gene transcripts in canine atopic dermatitis. Clin Exp Allergy 2002;32:789–95.

[20] Marsella R, Olivry T. Animal models of atopic dermatitis. Clin Dermatol 2003;21(2): 122–33.

[21] Olivry T, Dean GA, Tompkins MB, et al. Toward a canine model of atopic dermatitis: amplification of cytokine-gene transcripts in the skin of atopic dogs. Exp Dermatol 1999;8(3): 204–11.

[22] Nuttall TJ, Knight PA, McAleese SM, et al. T-helper 1, T-helper 2 and immunosuppressive cytokines in canine atopic dermatitis. Vet Immunol Immunopathol 2002;87(3–4):379–84.

[23] Maeda S, Fujiwara S, Omori K, et al. Lesional expression of thymus and activation-regulated chemokine in canine atopic dermatitis. Vet Immunol Immunopathol 2002; 88(1–2):79–87.

[24] Maeda S, Okayama T, Omori K, et al. Expression of CC chemokine receptor 4 (CCR4) mRNA in canine atopic skin lesion. Vet Immunol Immunopathol 2002;90(3–4):145–54.

[25] Marsella R, Olivry T, Maeda S. Investigation on the pathogenesis of canine atopic dermatitis using epicutaneous allergen challenge (atopy patch test) in IgE hyper-responsive beagles: cellular and cytokine kinetics [abstract]. Vet Dermatol 2005;16: 203.

[26] Marsella R. Calcineurin inhibitors: a novel approach to canine atopic dermatitis. J Am Anim Hosp Assoc 2005;41(2):92–7.

[27] Schreiber SL, Crabtree GR. The mechanism of action of cyclosporine A and FK-506. Immunol Today 1992;12:136–42.

[28] Hess AD. Mechanisms of action of cyclosporine: considerations for the treatment of autoimmune diseases. Clin Immunol Immunopathol 1993;68:220–8.

[29] Rostaing L, Puyoo O, Tkaczuk J, et al. Differences in Type 1 and Type 2 intracytoplasmic cytokines, detected by flow cytometry, according to immunosuppression (cyclosporine A vs. tacrolimus) in stable renal allograft recipients. Clin Transplant 1999;13(5):400–9.

[30] Caproni M, Dagata A, Cappelli G, et al. Modulation of serum eosinophil cationic protein levels by cyclosporin in severe atopic dermatitis. Br J Dermatol 1996;135:336–7.

[31] Meng Q, Ying S, Corrigan CJ, et al. Effects of rapamycin, cyclosporin A, and dexamethasone on interleukin 5-induced eosinophil degranulation and prolonged survival. Allergy 1997;52:1095–101.

[32] Teunissen MB, De Jager MH, Kapsenberg ML, et al. Inhibitory effect of cyclosporin A on antigen and alloantigen presenting capacity of human epidermal Langerhans cells. Br J Dermatol 1991;125:309–16.

[33] Thomson AW. The effects of cyclosporin A on non-T cell components of the immune system. J Autoimmun 1992;5(Suppl A):167–76.

[34] Lee SS, Tan AW, Giam YC. Cyclosporin in the treatment of severe atopic dermatitis: a retrospective study. Ann Acad Med Singapore 2004;33(3):311–3.

[35] Steffan J, Horn J, Gruet P, et al. Remission of the clinical signs of atopic dermatitis in dogs after cessation of treatment with cyclosporin A or methylprednisolone. Vet Rec 2004;154(22):681–4.

[36] Olivry T, Rivierre C, Jackson HA, et al. Cyclosporine decreases skin lesions and pruritus in dogs with atopic dermatitis: a blinded randomized prednisolone-controlled trial. Vet Dermatol 2002;13(2):77–87.

[37] Steffan J, Alexander D, Brovedani F, et al. Comparison of cyclosporine A with methylprednisolone for treatment of canine atopic dermatitis: a parallel, blinded, randomized controlled trial. Vet Dermatol 2003;14(1):11–22.

[38] Olivry T, Steffan J, Fisch RD, et al and the European Veterinary Dermatology Cyclosporine Group. Randomized controlled trial of the efficacy of cyclosporine in the treatment of atopic dermatitis in dogs. J Am Vet Med Assoc 2002;221:370–7.

[39] Steffan J, Strehlau G, Maurer M, et al. Cyclosporin A pharmacokinetics and efficacy in the treatment of atopic dermatitis in dogs. J Vet Pharmacol Ther 2004;27(4):231–8.

[40] Radowicz SN, Power HT. Long-term use of cyclosporine in the treatment of canine atopic dermatitis. Vet Dermatol 2005;16(2):81–6.

[41] Blackwood L, German AJ, Stell AJ, et al. Multicentric lymphoma in a dog after cyclosporine therapy. J Small Anim Pract 2004;45(5):259–62.

[42] Santoro D, Marsella R. Investigation of a possible correlation between atopic dermatitis, the use of cyclosporine A and development of lymphomas in dogs [abstract]. Vet Dermatol 2005;16:203.

[43] Pascual JC, Fleisher AB. Tacrolimus ointment (Protopic) for atopic dermatitis. Skin Therapy Lett 2004;9(9):1–5.

[44] Breuer K, Werfel T, Kapp A. Safety and efficacy of topical calcineurin inhibitors in the treatment of childhood atopic dermatitis. Am J Clin Dermatol 2005;6(2):65–77.

[45] Niwa Y, Terashima T, Sumi H. Topical application of the immunosuppressant tacrolimus accelerates carcinogenesis in mouse skin. Br J Dermatol 2003;149(5):960–7.

[46] Marsella R, Nicklin CF, Saglio S, et al. Investigation on the clinical efficacy and safety of 0.1% tacrolimus ointment (Protopic) in canine atopic dermatitis: a randomized, double-blinded, placebo-controlled, cross-over study. Vet Dermatol 2004;15(5):294–303.

[47] Bensignor E, Olivry T. Treatment of localized lesions of canine atopic dermatitis with tacrolimus ointment: a blinded randomized controlled trial. Vet Dermatol 2005;16(1):52–60.

[48] Senba E, Katanosaka K, Yajima H, et al. The immunosuppressant FK506 activates capsaicin- and bradykinin-sensitive DRG neurons and cutaneous C-fibers. Neurosci Res 2004;50(3):257–62.

[49] Paller AS, Lebwohl M, Fleischer AB Jr, and the US/Canada Tacrolimus Ointment Study Group. Tacrolimus ointment is more effective than pimecrolimus cream with a similar safety profile in the treatment of atopic dermatitis: results from 3 randomized, comparative studies. J Am Acad Dermatol 2005;52(5):810–22.

[50] Grassberger M, Steinhoff M, Schneider D, et al. Pimecrolimus—an anti-inflammatory drug targeting the skin. Exp Dermatol 2004;13(12):721–30.

[51] Griffin CE, Hillier A. The ACVD task force on canine atopic dermatitis (XXIV): allergen-specific immunotherapy. Vet Immunol Immunopathol 2001;81(3–4):363–83.

[52] Mueller RS, Bettenay SV. Long-term immunotherapy of 146 dogs with atopic dermatitis—a retrospective study. Aust Vet Pract 1996;26:128–32.

[53] Patterson R, Harris KE. Rush immunotherapy in a dog with severe ragweed and grass pollen allergy. Ann Allergy Asthma Immunol 1999;83(3):213–6.

[54] Mueller RS, Bettenay SV. Evaluation of the safety of an abbreviated course of injections of allergen extracts (rush immunotherapy) for the treatment of dogs with atopic dermatitis. Am J Vet Res 2001;62(3):307–10.

[55] Shida M, Kadoya M, Park SJ, et al. Allergen-specific immunotherapy induces Th1 shift in dogs with atopic dermatitis. Vet Immunol Immunopathol 2004;102(1–2):19–31.

[56] Tokunaga M, Hazemoto N, Yotsuyanagi T. Effects of oligopeptides on gene expression: comparison of DNA/peptide and DNA/peptide/liposome complexes. Int J Pharm 2004;269:71–80.

[57] Hussain I, Kline JN. CpG oligodeoxynucleotides: a novel therapeutic approach for atopic disorders. Curr Drug Targets Inflamm Allergy 2003;2(3):199–205.

[58] Marshall JD, Abtahi S, Eiden JJ, et al. Immunostimulatory sequence DNA linked to the Amb a 1 allergen promotes T(H)1 cytokine expression while down regulating T(H)2 cytokine expression in PBMCs from human patients with ragweed allergy. J Allergy Clin Immunol 2001;108(2):191–7.

[59] Raz E, Tighe H, Sato Y, et al. Preferential induction of a Th1 immune response and inhibition of specific IgE antibody formation by plasmid DNA immunization. Proc Natl Acad Sci USA 1996;93:5141–5.

[60] Mueller RS, Veir J, Fieseler KV, et al. Use of immunostimulatory liposome-nucleic acid complexes in allergen-specific immunotherapy of dogs with refractory atopic dermatitis—a pilot study. Vet Dermatol 2005;16(1):61–8.

[61] Park SJ, Yoshida N, Nishifuji K, et al. Successful treatment of two dogs with allergic dermatitis by anti-allergic peptides (MS-antigen). J Vet Med Sci 2002;64(1):63–5.

[62] Ayoub M, Mittenbuhler K, Sutterlin BW, et al. The anti-allergic drug histaglobin inhibits NF-kappaB nuclear translocation and down-regulates proinflammatory cytokines. Int J Immunopharmacol 2000;22(10):755–63.

[63] Paci A, Taddeucci-Brunelli G, Barachini P, et al. Therapy of atopic dermatitis in children. Study on the use of a desensitizing preparation. Pediatr Med Chir 1986;8(6):839–44.

[64] Gushchin IS, Luss LV, Il'ina NI, et al. Therapeutic effectiveness of histaglobin preparations in patients with allergic rhinitis and chronic urticaria. Ter Arkh 1999;71(3):57–62.

[65] Wright RJ, Cohen RT, Cohen S. The impact of stress on the development and expression of atopy. Curr Opin Allergy Clin Immunol 2005;5(1):23–9.

[66] Ohmura T, Hayashi T, Satoh Y, et al. Involvement of substance P in scratching behaviour in an atopic dermatitis model. Eur J Pharmacol 2004;491(2–3):191–4.

[67] Jarvikallio A, Harvima IT, Naukkarinen A. Mast cells, nerves and neuropeptides in atopic dermatitis and nummular eczema. Arch Dermatol Res 2003;295(1):2–7.

[68] Toyoda M, Nakamura M, Makino T, et al. Nerve growth factor and substance P are useful plasma markers of disease activity in atopic dermatitis. Br J Dermatol 2002;147(1):71–9.

[69] Gordon DJ, Ostlere LS, Holden CA. Neuropeptide modulation of Th1 and Th2 cytokines in peripheral blood mononuclear leucocytes in atopic dermatitis and non-atopic controls. Br J Dermatol 1997;137(6):921–7.

[70] Marsella R, Nicklin CF, Melloy C. Double blinded-placebo controlled, cross-over study to evaluate the clinical efficacy of 0.025% capsaicin lotion for the management of atopic dermatitis and cutaneous Substance P concentrations. Vet Dermatol 2002;13:131–9.

[71] Leung DY, Boguniewicz M, Howell MD, et al. New insights into atopic dermatitis. J Clin Invest 2004;113(5):651–7.

[72] Linde YW. Dry skin in atopic dermatitis. Acta Derm Venereol 1992;177(Suppl):9–13.

[73] Chamlin SL, Kao J, Frieden IJ, et al. Ceramide-dominant barrier repair lipids alleviate childhood atopic dermatitis: changes in barrier function provide a sensitive indicator of disease activity. J Am Acad Dermatol 2002;47:198–208.

[74] Chesney CJ. Measurement of skin hydration in normal dogs and in dogs with atopy or a scaling dermatosis. J Small Anim Pract 1995;36:305–9.

[75] Inman AO, Olivry T, Dunston SM, et al. Electron microscopic observations of stratum corneum intercellular lipids in normal and atopic dogs. Vet Pathol 2001;38:720–3.

[76] Marsh KA, Ruedisueli FL, Coe SL, et al. Effects of zinc and linoleic acid supplementation on the skin and coat quality of dogs receiving a complete and balanced diet. Vet Dermatol 2000;11(4):277–84.

[77] Campbell KL, Kirkwood AR. Effect of topical oils on transepidermal water loss in dogs with seborrhea sicca. In: Ihrke PJ, Mason K, White SD, editors. Advances in veterinary dermatology. New York: Pergamon Press; 1993. p. 157–62.

[78] DeBoer DJ. Canine atopic dermatitis: new targets, new therapies. J Nutr 2004;134 (8 Suppl):2056S–61S.

[79] Olivry T, Buckler KE, Dunston SM, et al. Positive 'atopy patch tests' reactions in IgE-hyperresponsive beagle dogs are dependent upon elevated allergen-specific IgE serum levels and are associated with IgE-expressing dendritic cells. Vet Dermatol 2002;13:219.

[80] Marsella R, Nicklin C, Lopez J. Studies on the role of the various routes of allergen exposure in atopic dermatitis using a colony of high IgE producing Beagle dogs sensitized to house dust mites [abstract]. Vet Dermatol 2005;16:204.

[81] Swinnen C, Vroom M. The clinical effect of environmental control of house dust mites in 60 house dust mite-sensitive dogs. Vet Dermatol 2004;15(1):31–6.

[82] Kalliomaki M, Salminen S, Arvilommi H, et al. Probiotics in primary prevention of atopic disease: a randomized placebo-controlled trial. Lancet 2001;357:1076–9.

[83] Kalliomaki M, Salminen S, Poussa T, et al. Probiotics and prevention of atopic disease: 4-year follow-up of a randomised placebo-controlled trial. Lancet 2003;361:1869–71.

[84] Pohjavuori E, Viljanen M, Korpela R, et al. Lactobacillus GG effect in increasing IFN-gamma production in infants with cow's milk allergy. J Allergy Clin Immunol 2004;114:131–6.

[85] Ogden NS, Bielory L. Probiotics: a complementary approach in the treatment and prevention of pediatric atopic disease. Curr Opin Allergy Clin Immunol 2005;5(2): 179–84.

[86] Grassegger A, Hopfl R. Significance of the cytokine interferon gamma in clinical dermatology. Clin Exp Dermatol 2004;29(6):584–8.

[87] Nasert S, Millner M, Herz U, et al. Therapeutic interference with interferon-gamma (IFN-gamma) and soluble IL-4 receptor (sIL-4R) in allergic diseases. Behring Inst Mitt 1995;96: 118–30.

[88] Tartour E, Lee RS, Fridman WH. Anti-cytokines: promising tools for diagnosis and immunotherapy. Biomed Pharmacother 1994;48(10):417–24.

[89] Marcotte GV, Braun CM, Norman PS, et al. Effects of peptide therapy on ex vivo T-cell responses. J Allergy Clin Immunol 1998;101(4 Pt 1):506–13.

[90] Varga LV, Toth S, Novak I, et al. Anti-sense strategies: functions and applications in immunology. Immunol Lett 1999;69(2):217–24.

[91] Sakamoto T, Miyazaki E, Aramaki Y, et al. Improvement of dermatitis by iontophoretically delivered antisense oligonucleotides for interleukin-10 in NC/Nga mice. Gene Ther 2004;11(3):317–24.

[92] Dimitroff CJ, Kupper TS, Sackstein R. Prevention of leukocyte migration to inflamed skin with a novel fluorosugar modifier of cutaneous lymphocyte-associated antigen. J Clin Invest 2003;112:1008–18.

[93] Bochner BS. Adhesion molecules as therapeutic targets. Immunol Allergy Clin North Am 2004;24(4):615–30.

[94] Grzela K, Lazarczyk M, Dziunycz P, et al. Molecular therapy versus standard treatment in allergy. Int J Mol Med 2004;14(1):3–22.

[95] Nomura I, Gao B, Boguniewicz M, et al. Distinct patterns of gene expression in the skin lesions of atopic dermatitis and psoriasis: a gene microarray analysis. J Allergy Clin Immunol 2003;112(6):1195–202.

Food Allergies: Update of Pathogenesis, Diagnoses, and Management

Robert A. Kennis, DVM, MS

Department of Clinical Sciences, College of Veterinary Medicine, Auburn University, Auburn, AL 36849, USA

Food allergies have been defined in human beings. Possible reactions include type I, type III, and type IV hypersensitivities. An oral allergy syndrome has also been described. Oral allergy syndrome is a form of contact allergy affecting the oropharynx that is associated with local IgE-mediated activation of mast cells. The term *food allergy* describes an immune-mediated process that may include any or all of the aforementioned reactions. Nonimmunologic adverse food reactions may also occur, such as food intolerance, which is an abnormal physiologic response to an ingested food item or food additive. Also, toxic reactions may occur because of the ingestion of bacterial or fungal toxins. Food intolerances probably account for most human adverse food reactions (eg, "jitters" from too much caffeine) [1].

Dogs may present with cutaneous clinical signs of food allergy. These may be attributable to immunologic or nonimmunologic causes. Because it is sometimes difficult to define the true pathogenesis, the term *cutaneous adverse food reactions* should be used [2]. The term *food allergy* is used when immune-mediated disease is discussed, regardless of the type of hypersensitivity reaction.

PATHOGENESIS

The major food allergens have been identified as water-soluble glycoproteins ranging from 10,000 to 60,000 d [3]. They are generally stable to treatment with heat, acid, and proteases. The most common food allergens include beef, chicken, corn, wheat, cow's milk, soy, eggs, and fish, but virtually any ingested food item may induce a cutaneous adverse food reaction [4]. Type I (immediate hypersensitivity) and type IV (delayed hypersensitivity) reactions have been reported in dogs. Mixed IgE-mediated, non–IgE-mediated, and late-phase IgE reactions may also be implicated [5]. The true pathogenesis of food allergies in dogs has not been defined.

E-mail address: kennira@vetmed.auburn.edu

0195-5616/06/$ – see front matter
doi:10.1016/j.cvsm.2005.09.012

The best protective mechanism for the development of tolerance is an intact intestinal mucosal barrier. Oral tolerance is a state of immunologic unresponsiveness to potential allergens. It has been shown that anergy and active suppression are the principal mechanisms of oral tolerance in mice under experimental circumstances [6]. Secretory IgA binds allergens and removes them in the mucus. Those antigens that pass through the intestinal barrier are bound by IgA and secreted through the liver into bile.

A type I reaction is characterized by the production of IgE antibodies and the activation of mast cells. Antigens may pass through a disrupted mucosal barrier or may enter circulation as antibody or antigen complexes. The allergens are processed by antigen-presenting cells and are subsequently presented to T cells. CD4+ T cells may be categorized into T helper (Th) 1 and Th2 subsets. The Th2 cells play a role in the activation of B cells, leading to the production of antibodies in which Th1 cells activate macrophages and a "cell-mediated" response. Most Th cells recognize processed antigen in association with major histocompatability complex (MHC) II molecules on the surface of antigen-presenting cells (eg, dendritic cells, macrophages) and bind to the T-cell receptor (TCR). This interaction leads to T-cell activation. Concurrently, antigen may bind directly to B cells via the B-cell receptor, which is, in fact, an IgD or IgM antibody, leading to B-cell activation. Activated T cells provide "help" to the activated B cells by cell-cell interactions and the production of cytokines. The secreted cytokines of an activated Th2 cell include interleukin (IL)-4, IL-5, IL-6, IL-10, and IL-13. These promote the class switching of B-cell antibodies to the formation of antigen-specific IgE. IgE antibodies bind to mast cells via the fixed complement ϵ high-affinity receptor (FcϵRI). When specific antigen "cross-links" IgE molecules on a mast cell, a signal is sent to release chemical mediators of inflammation, such as histamine and leukotrienes. The development of allergy is caused by a breakdown of oral tolerance.

The oral allergy syndrome has been described in a dog with Japanese cedar allergy. Cross-reactivity between Japanese cedar and tomato allergens was demonstrated by enzyme-linked immunosorbent assay (ELISA) inhibition. When the patient was fed fresh tomato, salivation, tightness, and swelling of the lips and quivering of the tongue occurred within 15 minutes after provocation. A similar finding was not observed when the same dog was challenged with tomato juice that was heated [7]. This study clearly demonstrated cross-reactivity between cedar and tomato antigens. To date, this is the only published report of the oral allergy syndrome in a dog. Similar oral allergy syndrome reactions could partially explain why some dogs with adverse food reactions exhibit pruritus of the muzzle region after eating, however. Numerous cross-reactions between environmental allergens and food allergens have been implicated in the oral allergy syndrome in human beings (Table 1) [8,9].

The role of type 1 hypersensitivity as a cause of canine food allergy has been investigated using an atopic dog model [10–12]. Dogs were selected based on their ability to produce higher than normal levels of IgE. Selected dogs were then purposefully bred [13]. Their puppies were sensitized to various food

Table 1
Pollens and foods causing oral allergy syndrome in human being

Pollen	Cross-reacting foods
Alder	Almonds, apples, celery, cherries, hazelnuts, parsley, pears, peaches
Birch	Almonds, apricots, apples, buckwheat, caraway, carrots, celery, cherries, coriander, dill, fennel, hazelnuts, honey, kiwi, lentils, nectarines, parsley, parsnips, peanuts, peppers, plums, potatoes, prunes, spinach, sunflower seeds, spinach, walnuts, wheat
Grasses	Melons, oranges, peanuts, swiss chard, tomatoes, watermelons, wheat
Mugwort	Apples, carrots, celery, coriander, fennel, kiwi, melons, parsley, peanuts, peppers, sunflower seeds, watermelons
Plane	Apples, chickpeas, green beans, hazelnuts, kiwi, lettuce, maize, melons, peanuts
Ragweed	Apples, bananas, cantaloupes, chamomile tea, cucumbers, honeydews, zucchini, watermelons

Data from Vieths S, Scheurer B, Ballmer-Weber B. Current understanding of cross-reactivity of food allergens and pollen. Ann NY Acad Sci 2002;964:47–68; Zarkadas M, Scott FW, Salminen J, et al. Common allergenic foods and their labeling in Canada—a review. Can J Allergy Clin Immunol 1999;4:118–41.

allergens via subcutaneous injections. Later in life, these dogs demonstrated cutaneous or gastrointestinal signs when challenged orally with the food items to which they had been sensitized. It was shown that these dogs had elevated IgE to the sensitized food items, had wheal and flare reactions with intradermal injections of the relevant food extracts, and had immediate and late-phase reactions when relevant food extracts were injected into gastric mucosa via an endoscope [14]. These findings suggested that sensitized dogs producing high IgE could be useful as a model of canine food allergy. Additional studies with this model helped to elucidate the hypothesis of genetic predispositions for the development of high levels of IgE [10,11,13].

This canine model producing high IgE has been used in additional investigations. One finding is that these dogs have a statistically significant difference in IgE levels detected by ELISA for individual food items compared with control dogs. These differences were not altered when sensitized allergens were given as food items in the diet or when an elimination test diet was used [14]. Further, only the sensitized dogs exhibited wheal and flare when whole-food allergen extracts were injected subcutaneously. None of the atopic food allergen–sensitized dogs exhibited cutaneous or gastrointestinal signs when challenged with soy- or corn-based diets, however, even though they had been sensitized to these items via subcutaneous injections. These results differed from the data obtained from previous studies [11,13].

A spontaneous dog model of IgE-mediated food hypersensitivity has also been investigated. These test dogs exhibited cutaneous and/or gastrointestinal signs when challenged with cow's milk or dairy products, and their symptoms resolved when fed an elimination test diet. Relative concentrations of serum IgE detected by ELISA to wheat, corn, and cow's milk were elevated in test dogs compared with control dogs. These dogs also had an increase in IgE to corn when a corn-based diet was fed. A concurrent increase in the severity of clinical signs was seen during the feeding of the corn-based diet [15]. From an investigative standpoint, the spontaneous food-allergic dog model may prove to be better than the atopic dog, food allergen–sensitized model for the study of type I hypersensitivity reactions as a parallel to dogs with cutaneous adverse food reactions.

Investigations support the hypothesis that dogs with concurrent gastrointestinal disease may also have associated elevations in serum IgE to food items. In one study, atopic dogs had more food allergen–specific IgE than control dogs. Also, dogs with gastrointestinal disease had more food allergen–specific IgG compared with atopic and control dogs. It was summarized that increased antigen exposure follows increased mucosal permeability [16]. In another study, it was shown that normalization of intestinal permeability followed by an elimination test diet helped to define dietary hypersensitivity, whereas those dogs with persistent abnormalities in gastrointestinal permeability are more likely to have underlying intestinal disease and food intolerance [17]. Together, all these studies help to define that true IgE-mediated adverse food reactions are dependent on genetic predisposition and an abnormality in gastrointestinal function.

Although the IgE hypersensitivity reaction is assumed to be the most common cause of cutaneous adverse food reactions in dogs and people, there is some recent evidence to support the finding that elevated levels of serum IgE may not always be present. In one study, it was shown that people diagnosed with food hypersensitivity based on a double-blind, placebo-based, controlled food challenge (DBPCFC) exhibited localized IgE responses when symptomatic without statistically significant differences in serum IgE compared with control patients [18]. This finding may help to explain why serum testing and intradermal skin testing with food allergens in dogs have been inaccurate–the IgE-mediated response may be occurring at the intestinal level and may not be reflected in serum or cutaneous mast cell reactivity.

DIAGNOSIS

There is no evidence that there is any sex predilection for cutaneous adverse food reactions. The age of onset is variable, and clinical signs maybe seen in dogs less than 6 months of age and greater than 11 years of age [4]. There is some evidence to support the finding that certain breeds have an increased risk for the development of food allergy [19,20]. In dogs, the most common signs associated with cutaneous adverse food reactions include nonseasonal pruritus of the face, feet, ears, axillae, forelegs, or perianal regions. Any or all of these regions may be affected, or the dog may have generalized skin disease [4,21,22]. Additionally, dogs may present with chronic or recurrent otitis or pyoderma [4,21,22].

The "gold standard" for diagnosis of food allergy in human beings is the DBPCFC. During the challenge, capsules of food items are ingested and the patient is evaluated. The oral allergy syndrome causes a burning or tingling sensation of the oral cavity and sometimes tinnitus [1]. Clearly, these subtleties could not be evaluated in canine patients. The oral allergy syndrome may partially explain facial pruritus in the dog, however. Skin prick testing using whole-food items has demonstrated a negative predictive value in human beings. Serum allergy testing for IgE antibodies is sometimes used but may only be helpful in evaluating type I hypersensitivity reactions.

The only accurate diagnosis of canine food allergy is based on an elimination test diet leading to the resolution of clinical signs, followed by a provocative food challenge. Clinical signs may recur in minutes to hours or up to 2 weeks after the challenge item is fed [23]. The duration required to perform an elimination test diet is not clearly defined. The length of time recommended for the elimination diet is variable, and a period ranging from 3 to 10 weeks has been suggested [19–21]. It has been demonstrated that an 8-week food trial is adequate in most situations [19]. Some authors contend that there is usually some evidence of improvement of clinical signs within the first month, although all the signs may not have completely resolved. Also, there have been other reports of food-allergic dogs failing to show clinical improvement until the food trial was extended for 12 full weeks [19].

One of the most difficult challenges in achieving an accurate diagnosis of food allergy is owner compliance. In a recent study, suspected food-allergic dogs were to be fed a homemade diet elimination food trial for 6 to 8 weeks. Of the 28 dogs enrolled in the study, 10 did not complete the food trial as prescribed [24]. There are many reasons for noncompliance in general. These may include cost, time of preparation, intolerance or dislike of the selected food items, inability to limit exposure to other items (treats), exacerbation of clinical signs, poor doctor and client communication, or a client who does not believe that food is a cause of the clinical signs.

The selection of an appropriate elimination test diet is dependent on the dietary history. Most dogs have eaten commercial diets containing a variety of different ingredients from protein and carbohydrate sources. Selecting items that are unique to the diet can be challenging. Ideally, the test diet would be free of preservatives or additives, although documented adverse reactions to preservatives and food additives in canine patients are rare [25]. Studies have suggested that commercial diets are not as accurate in diagnosing food allergy as home-prepared diets [19,23,25]. Therefore, it is recommended that a home-cooked elimination diet should be considered the gold standard for diagnostic purposes.

There are profound limitations associated with a home-prepared diet using a unique or novel protein source. First, some protein sources may be expensive for the owner to purchase or may only be found in limited quantities. Second, home-cooked diets entail some work by the owner that he or she might find tedious. Finally, home-prepared diets are not usually complete and balanced [26]. For clinically healthy dogs, the short duration of the feeding trial should not lead to major nutritional deficiencies. Dogs with concurrent metabolic illness should be carefully evaluated before recommending a home-cooked diet, however. Most home-prepared diets are low in calcium [27]. Nondietary calcium, vitamins, and essential fatty acids should be added to the diet [4,26].

Many "novel" protein sources can be considered for an elimination test diet. A short list of fresh food items includes pinto beans, tofu, venison, duck, rabbit, fish (various species), squid, ostrich, alligator, and other wild game. Canned tuna in water or salmon is also an option. Care should be taken if selecting fish as a test diet. One study suggests that a home-cooked diet containing fish and potato was inadequate in diagnosing food allergy in four of eight cases and that there may be an emergence of fish allergies in canine food-allergic patients [24]. This may be attributable to the presence of fish and fish meal in many commercial diets. In another study, it was found that the two most common canine food allergens identified were beef and soy [23]. This would suggest that tofu might not be the best protein source for a dietary trial.

The selection of a carbohydrate source is also based on dietary history. Food elimination diets have been performed using rice or potato, but these ingredients have found their way into many commercial diets and may not be suitable as test ingredients. Sweet potato or brown rice should be considered as a novel carbohydrate source at this time. New commercial diets available through mail order may contain these items as well.

The test diet may be composed of a 50:50 protein-to-carbohydrate source by volume, although less protein may be used for financial reasons. This diet should be fed for a minimum of 10 to 13 weeks or until clinical signs abate [4,19]. A partial improvement in clinical signs may be seen in some cases because of resolution of concurrent problems such as atopy, flea allergy, or concurrent infection with bacteria or *Malassezia* yeast. Recurrence of clinical signs may occur in 3 to 7 days on dietary food challenge. Once a documented reaction is noted, the dog should be placed back on the test diet. It may only take a few days for the pruritus and lesions to improve. It is recommended to use individual food items for the identification of offending allergens. This should aid in the long-term management of the patient. In one study, it was found that the mean number of offending allergens per dog was 2.4, with 80% of dogs reacting to one or two items and 64% reacting to two or more tested proteins [23]. Once the offending allergens are identified, strict avoidance is essential. Sensitivity to commercial dietary products based on the same ingredients as those used in home-cooked diets has been noted [20,28].

Home-prepared test diets are not without potential adverse reactions. Some dogs may not tolerate a home-cooked diet and may exhibit vomiting or diarrhea. Some dogs may be reluctant to eat the chosen diet. Also, weight gain or weight loss should be carefully monitored during the dietary trial. Hungry dogs are likely to scrounge for food and may accidentally ingest items that negate the food trial.

During the food trial, it is imperative that nothing passes the dogs lips except for the selected diet and water. Flavored heartworm preventive should be changed to a nonflavored tablet or alternative product. By the same token, chewable flavored antibiotic or vitamin tablets must be avoided. All treats, including rawhide chews and pig's ears, are also off limits. Part of the difficulty in achieving an accurate food trial stems from the client's desire to offer the dog treats. Children within the household who do not understand the implications of an elimination test diet can also affect the outcome of the trial. Even treats that are labeled "hypoallergenic" should be avoided.

Several commercial diets have been formulated for the diagnosis and management of food-allergic dogs. Novel protein sources, such as rabbit, venison, duck, kangaroo, and others, are available from commercial producers. Potato and oats have been used in combination with the various protein sources. These diets seem to be a reasonable alternative to home cooking when cost or owner effort is the limiting factor. Commercial diets containing lamb were once considered effective as testing and management sources for canine food allergy. Because of the prevalence of lamb-based diets (including puppy formulations), however, this protein source has lost its "novel" status. There are also many commercial diets available that contain fish (eg, catfish, whitefish, salmon). Recent data suggest that fish is no longer considered to be a novel protein [24].

Within the past few years, new diets have emerged that extend beyond the novel protein concept. Diets containing hydrolyzed proteins are now commercially available. It had been demonstrated that modification of wheat proteins led to the mitigation of allergic responses in a colony of highly inbred and sensitized research dogs [29]. These findings helped to introduce the idea of formulating hypoallergenic diets for dogs. Hydrolyzed diets have been shown to be beneficial for human beings with known allergic reactions [30]. Enzymatic hydrolysis of proteins can lead to smaller protein peptide fragments that are more digestible and less allergenic. Small proteins may still be immunogenic, however.

Hydrolyzed diets have been investigated for dogs suspected of having food allergy. In one study, 34 of 36 dogs improved during the test period when fed a commercially prepared soy isolate hydrolysate and rice diet and relapsed when challenged with the original diet. Interestingly, 1 dog did not respond to the hydrolyzed soy diet but did improve when a home-prepared soy diet was fed [31]. These findings suggest that a commercially prepared hydrolyzed soy diet could be used as an elimination test diet for many dogs. The percentage of dogs with a favorable response was high, although this may reflect the selection process for inclusion in the study.

Hydrolyzed chicken-based diets are also commercially available. In one study using a hydrolyzed chicken and corn starch diet as a test diet for dogs suspected of having adverse food reactions, 9 of 46 dogs were diagnosed with an adverse food reaction as the sole cause of nonseasonal pruritus. Concurrent gastrointestinal signs were noted in 21 of these dogs, and they all improved during the test diet [32].

The colonoscopy allergen provocation test has recently been described to evaluate the type I hypersensitivity reaction in human beings [33]. Allergens are directly injected into the mucosa of the colon, and observations are made of wheal and flare reaction. This procedure has been evaluated using the atopic dog model and showed good reproducibility [34]. The preliminary results of this diagnostic test on dogs with adverse food reactions seem to be promising [34]. Colonoscopy allergen provocation testing demonstrated sensitivity and specificity of 75% and 73%, respectively, when evaluated in nine food-allergic dogs (atopic dog model). This novel approach to the diagnosis of adverse food reactions is only useful for detecting the type I reaction. Further data must be collected before conclusions can be drawn on the usefulness of this procedure. A similar procedure has been described for injecting food allergens into the gastric mucosa using an endoscope [35]. This procedure has limitations with reproducibility and sensitivity.

Skin prick testing using whole-food allergens is used to rule out IgE-mediated food hypersensitivity in human beings [1]. This test is associated with low sensitivity and high specificity (few false-positive reactions). It is sometimes used for infants and young children who may not be amenable to oral food challenge [36]. Skin prick testing is not commonly used in dogs. Intradermally injected food allergens have been investigated in dogs. This procedure showed low sensitivity and high specificity similar to skin prick testing in people [37].

MANAGEMENT

Long-term management of the food-allergic dog requires strict avoidance of the offending food items. Some dogs may exhibit new dietary sensitivities within 1 to 3 years [22]. Therefore, it might be best to limit the variety of items fed to the patient in case a new elimination test diet is needed. The owner should keep a journal of offending foods and note any adverse reactions, including pruritus, infections, or seizures.

FUTURE CONSIDERATIONS

We are a long way from understanding the complete pathogenesis of cutaneous adverse food reactions in dogs. Further investigations may lead to better and easier diagnostic tests.

It has been hypothesized that there is an immunologic window of opportunity for dogs to become sensitized to food allergens [20]. If it is shown that dogs become sensitized at a young age, it might be possible to limit sensitization to those food items that affected dogs are not likely to consume during the remainder of their lives. Feeding a novel protein antigen at a young age may lead to sensitization, but this protein could easily be avoided at an older age [12]. There might still be a chance of new sensitivities developing later in life, however [22]. Hydrolyzed protein diets could also be considered instead of novel proteins. Hydrolyzed diet formulas are given to atopy-prone people to reduce allergenic activity [38]. Also, reduced exposure of human infants to allergenic foods caused by food allergen avoidance on the part of the reactive mother has been shown to decrease food sensitization, primarily during the first year of life [38]. Additional studies are needed to investigate whether hydrolyzed diets or limited antigen exposure to proteins of the nursing bitch would be of benefit in reducing the risk of development of cutaneous adverse food reactions in dogs.

References

[1] Sampson HA. Food allergy. Part 1: immunopathogenesis and clinical disorders. J Allergy Clin Immunol 1999;103(5 Pt 1):717–28.

[2] Hillier A, Griffin CE. The ACVD task force on canine atopic dermatitis (X): is there a relationship between canine atopic dermatitis and cutaneous adverse food reactions? Vet Immunol Immunopathol 2001;81(3–4):227–31.

[3] Sampson HA, Burks AW. Mechanisms of food allergy. Annu Rev Nutr 1996;16:161–77.

[4] Griffin CE. Skin immune system and allergic diseases. In: Scott DW, Miller WH, Griffin CE, editors. Muller and Kirk's small animal dermatology. Philadelphia: WB Saunders; 2001. p. 543–666.

[5] Halliwell R. Dietary hypersensitivity in the dog: a monograph. Vernon (CA): Kal Kan Foods; 1992.

[6] Kaminogawa S. Food allergy, oral tolerance and immunomodulation—their molecular and cellular mechanisms. Biosci Biotechnol Biochem 1996;60(11):1749–56.

[7] Fujimura M, Ohmori K, Masuda K, et al. Oral allergy syndrome induced by tomato in a dog with Japanese cedar (Cryptomeria japonica) pollinosis. J Vet Med Sci 2002;64(11):1069–70.

[8] Vieths S, Scheurer S, Ballmer-Weber B. Current understanding of cross-reactivity of food allergens and pollen. Ann NY Acad Sci 2002;964:47–68.

[9] Zarkadas M, Scott FW, Salminen J, et al. Common allergenic foods and their labeling in Canada—a review. Can J Allergy Clin Immunol 1999;4:118–41.

[10] de Weck AL, Mayer P, Stumper B, et al. Dog allergy, a model for allergy genetics. Int Arch Allergy Immunol 1997;113(1–3):55–7.

[11] Ermel RW, Kock M, Griffey SM, et al. The atopic dog: a model for food allergy. Lab Anim Sci 1997;47(1):40–9.

[12] Kennis RA. Use of atopic dogs to investigate adverse reactions to food. J Am Vet Med Assoc 2002;221(5):638–40.

[13] Frick OL. Food allergy in atopic dogs. Adv Exp Med Biol 1996;409:1–7.

[14] Kennis RA, Hannah S, Ermel R, et al. Changes in IgE antibodies to soy in sensitized and control dogs after challenge using three diets in a cross over study [abstract]. Vet Dermatol 2002;13(4):218.

[15] Jackson HA, Jackson MW, Coblentz L, et al. Evaluation of the clinical and allergen specific serum immunoglobulin E responses to oral challenge with cornstarch, corn, soy and a soy hydrolysate diet in dogs with spontaneous food allergy. Vet Dermatol 2003;14(4):181–7.

[16] Foster AP, Knowles TG, Moore AH, et al. Serum IgE and IgG responses to food antigens in normal and atopic dogs, and dogs with gastrointestinal disease. Vet Immunol Immunopathol 2003;92(3–4):113–24.

[17] Rutgers HC, Batt RM, Hall EJ, et al. Intestinal permeability testing in dogs with diet-responsive intestinal disease. J Small Anim Pract 1995;36(7):295–301.

[18] Lin XP, Magnusson J, Ahlstedt S, et al. Local allergic reaction in food-hypersensitive adults despite a lack of systemic food-specific IgE. J Allergy Clin Immunol 2002;109(5):879–87.

[19] Rosser EJ Jr. Diagnosis of food allergy in dogs. J Am Vet Med Assoc 1993;203(2):259–62.

[20] White SD. Food hypersensitivity in 30 dogs. J Am Vet Med Assoc 1986;188(7):695–8.

[21] MacDonald JM. Food allergy. In: Griffin CE, Kwochka KW, MacDonald JM, editors. Current veterinary dermatology: the science and art of therapy. St. Louis (MO): Mosby–Year Book; 1993. p. 121–32.

[22] White SD. Food hypersensitivity. Vet Clin North Am Small Anim Pract 1988;18(5):1043–8.

[23] Jeffers JG, Meyer EK, Sosis EJ. Responses of dogs with food allergies to single-ingredient dietary provocation. J Am Vet Med Assoc 1996;209(3):608–11.

[24] Tapp T, Griffin C, Rosenkrantz W, et al. Comparison of a commercial limited-antigen diet versus home-prepared diets in the diagnosis of canine adverse food reaction. Vet Ther 2002;3(3):244–51.

[25] Reedy LM. Food hypersensitivity. In: Reedy LM, Miller WH, Willemse T, editors. Allergic skin diseases of dogs and cats. Philadelphia: W.B. Saunders Company; 1997. p. 173–88.

[26] Roudebush P, Crowell CS. Results of a hypoallergenic diet survey of veterinarians in North America with a nutritional evaluation of homemade diet prescriptions. Vet Dermatol 1992;3:23–8.

[27] Roudebush P. Hypoallergenic diets for dogs and cats. In: Bonagura JD, editor. Kirk's current veterinary therapy XIII. Philadelphia: WB Saunders Company; 2000. p. 530–5.

[28] Leistra MH, Markwell PJ, Willemse T. Evaluation of selected-protein-source diets for management of dogs with adverse reactions to foods. J Am Vet Med Assoc 2001;219(10):1411–4.

[29] Buchanan BB, Adamidi C, Lozano RM, et al. Thioredoxin-linked mitigation of allergic responses to wheat. Proc Natl Acad Sci USA 1997;94(10):5372–7.

[30] Terracciano L, Isoardi P, Arrigoni S, et al. Use of hydrolysates in the treatment of cow's milk allergy. Ann Allergy Asthma Immunol 2002;89(6 Suppl.1):86–90.

[31] Biourge VC, Fontaine J, Vroom MW. Diagnosis of adverse reactions to food in dogs: efficacy of a soy-isolate hydrolysate-based diet. The American Society for Nutritional Sciences 2004;134(2062s):1–8.

[32] Loeffler A, Lloyd DH, Bond R, et al. Dietary trials with a commercial chicken hydrolysate diet in 63 pruritic dogs. Vet Rec 2004;154(17):519–22.

[33] Bischoff SC, Mayer J, Wedemeyer J, et al. Colonoscopic allergen provocation (COLAP): a new diagnostic approach for gastrointestinal food allergy. Gut 1997;40(6):745–53.

[34] Allenspach K. Food allergy in dogs: new insights. In: Proceedings of the 2004 American College of Veterinary Internal Medicine Forum. Lakewood (CO): American College of Veterinary Internal Medicine; 2004. p. 1–3.

[35] Guilford WG, Strombeck DR, Rogers Q, et al. Development of gastroscopic food sensitivity testing in dogs. J Vet Intern Med 1994;8(6):414–22.

[36] Rance F, Juchet A, Bremont F, et al. Correlations between skin prick tests using commercial extracts and fresh foods, specific IgE, and food challenges. Allergy 1997;52(10):1031–5.

[37] Kunkle G, Horner S. Validity of skin testing for diagnosis of food allergy in dogs. J Am Vet Med Assoc 1992;200(5):677–80.

[38] Dahlgreen UI, Hanson LA, Telemo E. Maturation of immunocompetence in breast fed vs. formula fed infants. In: Woodward B, Draper HH, editors. Advances in nutritional research. New York: Kluwer Academic/Plenum Publishers; 2001. p. 311–25.

Bacterial Skin Diseases: Current Thoughts on Pathogenesis and Management

Elizabeth R. May, DVM

Department of Veterinary Clinical Sciences, Veterinary Teaching Hospital, Iowa State University, 1600 South 16th Street, Ames, IA 50011, USA

Historically, most cases of bacterial skin disease in the dog and cat have been associated with *Staphylococcus* species, specifically *Staphylococcus intermedius* and, less commonly, *Staphylococcus aureus*. Recently published information, however, suggests that newly reported *Staphylococcus* organisms should be considered in addition to *S intermedius* and *S aureus* in pyoderma cases. The question of zoonotic transfer and the concern surrounding methicillin-resistant *Staphylococcus* mandate a new or modified approach to bacterial skin diseases in small animals. This article focuses on the characteristics of the newly reported *Staphylococcus* species as well as on the importance of recognizing and treating emerging pathogens.

BACTERIAL FLORA OF THE SKIN: AN OVERVIEW
Resident, Transient, and Nomad Populations
Normal canine and feline skin is host to various species and strains of bacteria that are considered normal inhabitants [1]. In the dog, these organisms are acquired from the dam within the first 7 days after birth [2]; this information has not been documented in cats. Traditionally, these organisms have been divided into resident and transient organisms based on their ability to replicate on normal skin and hair. Although resident bacteria are, in fact, capable of multiplication on normal skin, transient organisms are acquired from the environment and are not capable of multiplying on the normal skin of most animals [1]. Thus, transient organisms are not considered pathogenic unless isolated from lesional skin. In addition, a nomadic population exists. Nomads are capable of brief adherence and colonization, and their isolation is thought to reflect environmental contamination [3]. Thus, the current classification scheme identifies residents as those organisms that are isolated more than 75% of the time the skin is cultured, nomads are isolated less than 75% but

E-mail address: ermay@iastate.edu

0195-5616/06/$ – see front matter
doi:10.1016/j.cvsm.2005.09.014

more than 25% of the time the skin is cultured, and transients can only be isolated less than 25% of the time the skin is cultured [3]. An alternative method of classification involves the number of colonies isolated. The method used by Cox and colleagues [4] defined resident organisms as those with 10 or more colonies isolated from a specimen and transient organisms as those with less than 10 colonies isolated per specimen. This method is more restrictive, however, in that species that are consistently isolated with high frequency from multiple sites, regardless of the colony count, should be considered to have colonized the individual [5–7]. By evaluating colony count only, less common but important species may not be considered relevant. Therefore, the frequency and persistence of isolation should be considered when differentiating normal inhabitants from those organisms causing secondary colonization or contamination rather than secondary infections. This differentiation is crucial in generating an effective therapeutic plan for the appropriate pathogenic organism based on culture and sensitivity data, especially when multiple organisms are reported.

Frequently, additional organisms may be cultured from the skin. On isolating one such organism from the skin of a patient with skin disease, the clinical picture may become confused. The significance of the isolation of a transient organism must be questioned unless it is involved in a pathologic process as a secondary invader. Therefore, although the isolate may not be the expected organism, when it is present in high numbers in a relatively pure culture, the clinician should evaluate the site of culture as well as the method of collection. A culture obtained from the surface of the skin in an area that is pruritic or painful to the patient, for example, would be expected to contain transient contaminant organisms from the oral cavity, because the animal licks or chews that site. If the lesion is a closed pustule or nodule, however, the isolate may be an important pathogen. It has been demonstrated recently that culturing an epidermal collarette (Fig. 1) is also a reliable method of identifying pathogens if performed correctly [8].

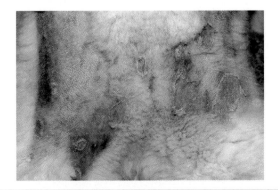

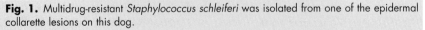

Fig. 1. Multidrug-resistant *Staphylococcus schleiferi* was isolated from one of the epidermal collarette lesions on this dog.

Colonization of the Skin

It is well documented that the oral, nasal, and anal mucocutaneous sites serve as a reservoir for *S intermedius* colonization in the dog [2,4,9,10]. In addition, the ear is another site from which *S intermedius* can frequently be isolated [11,12]. These locations seem to serve as carrier sites for seeding the rest of the skin and hair through normal grooming activity. It is not clear, however, why some dogs become resident carriers of *S intermedius* with higher numbers of bacteria than others. Offspring of dogs that had been classified as resident carriers also had significantly higher populations of *S intermedius*, and it seemed that a dominant strain was consistently isolated from the adult dogs and their puppies [13]. This continued transfer of strains of *S intermedius* between generations has been suggested as a potential reservoir for retention of genes for staphylococcal antibiotic resistance [14]. This concept needs to be investigated further, because exchange and acquisition of new strains occur between dogs with normal daily contact. Animals receiving antibiotic therapy may be especially at risk for acquisition of resistant organisms, because this situation may, in fact, encourage the transfer of organisms via antibiotic-induced reduction of the normal resident population of *Staphylococcus* [15].

Coagulase-Negative *Staphylococcus* Species

Coagulase-negative *Staphylococcus* species (CoNS) have long been considered resident organisms that are nonpathogenic in small animals and human beings [1,16]. Because of their relatively low virulence and ubiquitous nature, they typically have not been speciated by most human and veterinary laboratories but reported simply as CoNS. With the emergence of nosocomial infections linked to CoNS in Europe and now in the United States, however, the current recommendation is to identify clinically significant CoNS to the species level [17–19]. Although some CoNS isolates remain true contaminants, it is especially valid to speciate a CoNS, including an antibiotic susceptibility profile, when repeated cultures are obtained or no other isolate is identified in patients with clinical disease.

According to past reports, the most numerous CoNS isolated from dogs is *Staphylococcus epidermidis*, whereas *Staphylococcus simulans* is isolated from cats (Table 1). More recently, the coagulase-negative subspecies of *Staphylococcus schleiferi* and *Staphylococcus sciuri* have also been isolated from dogs.

EMERGING PATHOGENS

Coagulase-Negative *Staphylococcus* Species

CoNS caused 27% to 27.9% of nosocomial blood stream infections in hospitals participating in surveillance programs in the early 1990s [16]. In addition, based on data obtained during this assessment, CoNS are among the five most commonly reported pathogens isolated from hospitalized patients in these same hospitals. Why is this important? How does this relate to veterinary medicine? The answers are progressively more relevant as the rate of nosocomial and community-acquired infections with CoNS continues to increase in human

Table 1
Cutaneous microflora of the skin

Organism	Resident	Transient
Dog	Staphylococcus intermedius	Escherichia coli
	Micrococcus spp	Proteus mirabilis
	S epidermidis (CoNS)	Corynebacterium spp
	S xylosus (CoNS)	Bacillus spp
	S sciuri (CoNS)	S sciuri (CoNS)
	α-Hemolytic streptococci	Pseudomonas spp
	Clostridium spp	
	Propionibacterium acnes	
	Acinetobacter spp	
	Gram-negative aerobes	
Cat	S intermedius	Other Staphylococcus spp (CoPS)
	S aureus	S capitis (CoNS)
	S simulans (CoNS)	S epidermis (CoNS)
	Micrococcus spp	S haemolyticus (CoNS)
	α-Hemolytic streptococci	S hominis (CoNS)
	Acinetobacter spp	S sciuri (CoNS)
		S warneri (CoNS)
		β-Hemolytic streptococci
		E coli
		P mirabilis
		Pseudomonas spp
		Alcaligenes spp
		Bacillus spp

Abbreviations: CoNs, coagulase-negative Staphylococcus species; CoPS, coagulase-positive staphylococcus species.

and veterinary health care settings. In human hospitals, immunocompromised patients as well as hospitalized patients with implant devices, such as intravenous catheters or pacemakers, have been overrepresented because they are the population most susceptible to such infections. The significance of the problem in the veterinary field has also grown with the increase in numbers of immunocompromised patients as well as advances and demands for sophisticated veterinary health care. The increased incidence of CoNS infections coincides with the development of more invasive medical procedures and advances in medicine for human beings and animals, increasing the risks for opportunistic infection to occur.

In spite of this growing concern, little is known about the true incidence of infections caused by CoNS in veterinary patients. Historically, clinical microbiologists as well as clinicians discounted the presence of CoNS as contaminants in clinical specimens, because they are considered less virulent and because these organisms comprise a significant component of the resident microflora of people and animals. Differentiating pathogenic from contaminant strains thus has and still does pose a large problem. In the human health field, anything other than *S aureus*, which is coagulase-positive, was simply not reported or was reported as CoNS [16,17]. Unfortunately, this approach continues today and has been perpetuated in veterinary microbiology laboratories as well. Because of the lack of concern with the pathogenicity of CoNS in the human health field, the same trend has existed within the veterinary health field up to the time of the most recent changes that have occurred in regard to the pathogenesis of CoNS.

Staphylococcus schleiferi

In the early 1990s, *S schleiferi*, a coagulase-variable organism, was recognized as a human as well as veterinary pathogen. Two subspecies were initially identified and isolated from patients: a coagulase-negative subspecies, *S schleiferi schleiferi*, from human beings in 1988 [20] and a coagulase-positive subspecies, *S schleiferi coagulans*, from the external auditory meatus of dogs with otitis externa in 1990 [21]. In human medicine, both subspecies have been associated with wound infections [22,23], endocarditis [24,25], osteomyelitis [24,26], bacteremia [24], urinary tract infections [27], and meningitis [28]. In the veterinary literature, *S schleiferi coagulans* has been associated with pyoderma [29–31] as well as with otitis externa [21] in dogs. *S schleiferi schleiferi* and *S schleiferi coagulans* were both isolated from dogs with pyoderma in the most recent veterinary study [30]. This was the first report to associate *S schleiferi schleiferi* with canine pyoderma as well as demonstrating the presence of methicillin-resistant variants.

S schleiferi coagulans was first identified in 1988, but only recently has this subspecies been reported as a pathogen in human and veterinary medicine. Before that, the most recent reclassification of *Staphylococcus* species isolated from domestic animals occurred in 1976, when *S intermedius* was differentiated from *S aureus* [10]. Thus, it is likely that *S schleiferi coagulans* is underreported by automated staphylococcal identification systems because it is phenotypically similar to *S aureus* [23,24], and therefore is similar to *S intermedius*. In addition, the CoNS have historically been considered nonpathogenic [32], and all staphylococcal organisms other than *S aureus* were reported simply as CoNS in human medicine [17]. Based on this information, it is expected that the coagulase-negative subspecies *S schleiferi schleiferi* has also been underreported.

Virulence Factors

The virulence factors of *S aureus* have been well documented; however, less information is available related to the virulence factors of *S intermedius* specifically [10,33,34]. In vivo, many strains of staphylococci, including those associated with pyoderma, possess a capsule, or slime layer [34,35]. This polysaccharide layer inhibits chemotaxis and phagocytosis by leukocytes [34] and also facilitates adherence of CoNS, especially in regard to implant devices, such as intravenous catheters. The presence or absence of the slime layer is often used in the laboratory to differentiate clinically relevant isolates of CoNS from nonpathogenic strains [35]. Constituents of the cell wall of *S aureus* include peptidoglycans, teichoic acid, clumping factor, and protein A. The cell wall of *S intermedius* also consists of peptidoglycans, which provide stability and enable the bacteria to tolerate high heat, desiccation, and hyperosmotic environments

[32,34]. In addition, peptidoglycans inhibit leukocyte migration and can activate complement [32,34]. Teichoic acid is species specific and allows staphylococci to adhere to keratinocytes via fibronectin [34,36]. This is especially important on mucosal surfaces, where the bacterial reservoir is believed to persist. Approximately 14% of *S intermedius* isolates possess clumping factor within the cell wall [10], whereas it is a constituent of the cell wall of *S aureus* [34]. This clumping factor, or coagulase, binds fibronectin, allowing the bacteria to form a clump that serves as protection against the host's defenses. Protein A was not initially associated with *S intermedius*, but its presence has since been demonstrated with increasingly sensitive assays and culture techniques [34]. The presence of protein A allows the bacteria to remain "masked," thus preventing antibody-mediated IgG clearance of coagulase-positive strains [36].

Exotoxins associated with staphylococci include cytolytic hemolysins, exfoliative toxins, enterotoxins, toxic shock toxins, and leukotoxins. Hemolysins cause damage to the cell walls of erythrocytes; to date, α toxin, β toxin, and δ toxin have been associated with *S aureus*, whereas a combination of β toxin and δ toxin seems to be associated with *S intermedius* [33,36]. Exfoliative toxins ETA and ETB have only been isolated from *S aureus*; however, a novel exfoliative toxin, SIET, has recently been isolated from *S intermedius* [37]. Enterotoxins A, B, C, and D have been associated with *S aureus* and can serve as superantigens, causing severe gastrointestinal disease. Currently the enterotoxins A, B, and C have been associated with *S intermedius*, albeit in significantly lower concentrations [33]. As a superantigen associated with *S aureus*, toxic shock syndrome toxin-1 (TSST-1) causes staphylococcal scalded syndrome in human beings but has also been reported in the literature in association with *S intermedius* [34,36,38]. *S aureus* produces Panton Valentine Leukocidin (PVL), which is analogous to Luk-I, the leukotoxin associated with *S intermedius*. Luk-I has been identified in staphylococcal strains isolated from normal dogs as well as from dogs with pyoderma or otitis and is cytotoxic to polymorphonuclear cells [39]. PVL has been associated with more severe forms of bacterial skin infections in human beings, such as furunculosis and tissue necrosis; however, in dogs, no difference between normal and affected groups was identified in regard to the amount of leukotoxin produced [39].

Similar to other *Staphylococcus* species, *S schleiferi* possesses a prominent glycocalyx [40], which contributes significantly to the production of a slime layer and the ability of *S schleiferi* to adhere to medical implant devices. In prior virulence studies, however, it was demonstrated that attachment to an implant is not required for lesion induction [41]. This was an unexpected finding, because *S schleiferi* has been presumed to be a less virulent strain in comparison to *S aureus* or *S intermedius*, requiring a foreign body as a site for attachment. Other components of the cell wall, such as peptidoglycans and teichoic acid, have not been specifically reported in regard to *S schleiferi*; however, because of the similarity between *Staphylococcus* species, it is assumed that these are shared features. A difference between the subspecies of *S schleiferi* exists, however, because protein A is only produced by *S schleiferi coagulans* [22]. Thus, in addition to the tube coagulase test, the presence or absence of protein A differentiates the subspecies of *S schleiferi* from one another.

Similar to *S aureus* and *S intermedius*, *S schleiferi* produces staphylococcal toxins. Several hemolysins (α, β, and δ) have been isolated and are associated with the production of cellular damage [22,40]. The production of a β hemolysin is unique among CoNS and helps to differentiate the coagulase-negative subspecies of *S schleiferi* from other CoNS. Only a few other *Staphylococcus* species produce β hemolysin, including *S aureus* and *S intermedius*, but they are coagulase-positive [42]. TSST-1 has not been associated with *S schleiferi* [43]. Additionally, *S schleiferi* does not seem to produce a leukotoxin similar to *S aureus* or *S intermedius*. Based on limited reports, *S schleiferi coagulans* does not possess PVL, as has been demonstrated in relation to *S aureus*, but only the coagulase-positive subspecies was evaluated [44]. The Luk-I leukotoxin currently has only been associated with *S intermedius*. Resembling *S aureus*, *S schleiferi* produces a fibronectin-binding protein [45], which may play a role in the pathogenesis of infections caused by this organism. Therefore, although *S schleiferi* does not seem to possess virulence markers to the extent of the other accepted pathogenic *Staphylococcus* species, *S schleiferi* is capable of causing severe infections in certain patients.

Staphylococcus Species Identification

Consistently, *S intermedius* has been reported as the most frequently isolated co-agulase-positive *Staphylococcus* species associated with canine pyoderma since it was reported in the 1970s. How do we know this is true? How can we be sure these isolates were actually *S intermedius*? Before the initial report differentiating *S intermedius* from *S aureus* [10], the literature reported all coagulase-positive isolates as *S aureus*. Since then, when referring to older publications, newer reports have assumed that isolates reported as *S aureus* were actually *S intermedius*. Now, with the newly reported *S schleiferi coagulans* also associated with pyoderma, it is likely that some of these isolates were misidentified previously as *S intermedius*, because most laboratories do not perform the extra steps required to differentiate between the species. Although the frequency of isolation of *S schleiferi coagulans* has been low in the human and veterinary literature, the true incidence is unknown.

S schleiferi is indistinguishable from *S intermedius* based on standard colony characteristics and biochemical tests (Fig. 2). Colonies typical of both species appear as opaque off-white colonies that are 1 mm or greater in diameter after 24 hours of incubation and are surrounded by a double zone of hemolysis on blood agar medium. In addition, both species display positive catalase and coagulase test results and no or delayed fermentation of maltose and mannitol [46]. Additional carbohydrate fermentation tests (see Fig. 2) are thus required to differentiate between the two species [21,46]. Although positive results are obtained from fermentation of trehalose and lactose for *S intermedius*, these tests are typically negative for *S schleiferi*. Also, when performing the Voges-Proskauer (VP) test, which is the production of acetoin from glucose or pyruvate, *S intermedius* typically gives a negative result and *S schleiferi* gives a positive result [46]. The

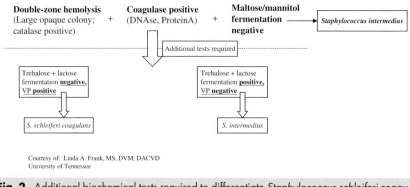

Fig. 2. Additional biochemical tests required to differentiate *Staphylococcus schleiferi* coagulans from *Staphylococcus intermedius*. VP, Voges-Proskauer test. (Courtesy of L.A. Frank, MS, DVM, Knoxville, TN.)

subspecies of *S schleiferi* are then differentiated based on the result of the tube coagulase test. *S schleiferi coagulans* is coagulase-positive, whereas *S schleiferi schleiferi* is coagulase-negative.

Adjustments in laboratory protocols are required for the future. New techniques to simplify the identification of CoNS are available and have been evaluated in the literature [17,47–49]. Laboratories must agree to adopt consistent methods of precise identification, such as accurate commercial test kits and additional carbohydrate fermentation tests, to reliably identify CoNS as well as the newer coagulase-positive species, which are similar to each other using conventional methods of identification.

BACTERIAL INFECTIONS

The more recent literature classifies bacterial skin infections based on the depth of skin involvement rather than on lesion distribution or underlying primary disease process. Because this article focuses on emerging pathogens, the diseases were classified based on the causative organism rather than on clinical presentation.

Staphylococcal Pyoderma

Staphylococcus species have been associated with surface, superficial, and deep pyoderma. Pyotraumatic dermatitis, skin-fold pyoderma (intertrigo), and mucocutaneous pyoderma are types of surface pyoderma with secondary *Staphylococcus* species involvement. These infections typically respond favorably to topical therapy, but recurrence is frequent if a primary disease process cannot be identified and controlled. Superficial infections are commonly diagnosed in clinical practice and include impetigo, superficial bacterial folliculitis (pyoderma), and superficial spreading pyoderma. Typically caused by *Staphylococcus* species, it is now recognized that other species of *Staphylococcus* can also serve as pathogens. Treatment is tailored for the expected organism as well as for the severity of the disease. Impetigo is recognized in young dogs and is characterized by subcorneal pustules that do not involve hair follicles. Skin that is thinly haired is more commonly affected, and the lesions are not typically pruritic. Antibiotics are rarely required, because the lesions often resolve without treatment; however, topical therapy with an appropriate dose and duration of oral antibiotic therapy may be required if concurrent superficial folliculitis is present. Superficial folliculitis is a common clinical presentation in dogs but is not common in cats. It is defined as inflammation of the superficial portion of the hair follicle, and inflammatory papules are the hallmark lesion [1]. Pruritus is routinely reported. Pyoderma is frequently secondary to an underlying primary process, and recurrence is likely without control of the predisposing disease. Empiric therapy is often chosen for treatment of uncomplicated cases of superficial folliculitis; however, with recurrence of lesions in the face of an appropriate dose and duration of therapy, culture and sensitivity testing should be considered and treatment adjustments made based on results. Deep bacterial infections are less commonly appreciated and are more serious in nature. Deep folliculitis, furunculosis, and cellulitis typically require longer courses of treatment, and scarring may complicate treatment. These lesions may be painful, and organisms in addition to *Staphylococcus* species, such as *Pseudomonas* spp, *Escherichia coli*, or *Proteus* spp may be involved. Culture of purulent material expressed from a nondraining lesion or macerated tissue culture obtained via sterile biopsy technique may be required to identify the causative agent or pattern of antibiotic resistance, especially if multiple abbreviated courses of treatment have failed previously.

Pseudomonas Pyoderma

Little information exists in the veterinary literature describing reports of bacterial skin infections associated with *Pseudomonas aeruginosa*. Recently, 15 cases of *Pseudomonas* pyoderma were described [50], with deep infections comprising most cases. Although less numerous, cases of superficial pyoderma were also reported. Folliculitis associated with *P aeruginosa* has been described in people in association with hot tubs or whirlpools [51–54], and similar cases of *P aeruginosa* have been anecdotally reported in association with self-service dog grooming facilities. Although these cases in people tend to be self-limiting and the veterinary cases respond to antibiotic therapy, it is important to recognize that unexpected organisms beyond the standard coagulase-positive *Staphylococcus* may serve as the causative agent in some instances.

TREATMENT

The antibiotics discussed in this section are those most commonly tested for susceptibility by veterinary microbiology laboratories on isolation of a gram-positive organism. Sources providing an excellent review of the mechanism of action of each drug are located elsewhere [55,56]. The recommended doses used in veterinary dermatology are listed in Table 2. A rational choice should be made when treating empirically, choosing the safest and potentially least

Table 2
Recommended antibiotics and doses for *Staphylococcus* infections

Name	Spectrum	Activity	Mechanism of action	Dose
Cephalexin	G+ G− (some) Some anaerobes	Bactericidal	Interference with bacterial cell wall synthesis	22–33 mg/kg q 12 h
Amoxicillin– clavulanic acid	G+ G− Anaerobes	Bactericidal	Interference with bacterial cell wall synthesis	22 mg/kg q 12 h
Trimethoprim- sulfamethoxazole	G+ G− Anaerobes	Bactericidal (if potentiated sulfa)	Inhibits bacterial cell folic acid metabolism	15 mg/kg q 12 h
Clindamycin	G+ Anaerobes	Bacteriostatic (bactericidal at higher concentrations)	Binds 50s subunit of bacterial ribosome	10 mg/kg q 12 h
Enrofloxacin, Marbofloxacin	G+ G−	Bactericidal	Interferes with bacterial DNA replication	10 mg/kg q 12 h (E) 5 mg/kg q 12 h (M)

Abbreviations: E, enrofloxacin; h, hours; M, marbofloxacin; q, every.

expensive drug that is effective against the expected pathogen. With recurrence of the infection or if new lesions are noted despite administration of an appropriate antibiotic, adjustments in antibiotic therapy should be made with culture and susceptibility data in hand. It is not uncommon for marked changes to occur in pathogenic bacterial strain composition during antibiotic therapy, and resistance patterns often change from susceptible to resistant as new strains are acquired [57]. As we gain additional information in regard to the role that CoNS and newly identified *Staphylococcus* species play as pathogens and as more laboratories begin to report identification of these species, our approach to antibiotic therapy regimens may change dramatically. Rather than selecting an antibiotic based on the next potent drug in the tier of antibiotics, anticipating the organism as well as its resistance pattern is a logical and valid approach to treating bacterial skin disease in small animals.

Aminoglycosides
Despite the fact that most microbiology laboratories report susceptibility data for aminoglycosides, their use in small animals for bacterial skin disease, such as pyoderma, is limited because of the parenteral rate of administration as well as the potential for nephrotoxicity and ototoxicity associated with repeated use. The primary mechanism of staphylococcal resistance is inactivation of the drug via bacterial enzymes [58], whereas altered porin size is responsible

for aerobic gram-negative bacterial resistance [55], such as that seen with *P aeruginosa*. Thus, although the aminoglycosides are bactericidal in behavior, they most likely play a larger role in treating life-threatening infections with limited antibiotic choices rather than those infections caused by staphylococcal species.

β-Lactam Antibiotics

Because of the high frequency with which *S intermedius* and *S aureus* produce β-lactamase, the penicillins are no longer a rational choice for the treatment of pyoderma; however, the empiric choice of a β-lactamase–stable antibiotic is often appropriate when treating staphylococcal skin infections. This class of drugs exhibits a broad spectrum of activity with low toxicity to the host. In addition, these drugs are typically given orally and remain affordable, improving ease of administration. They are effective against most *Staphylococcus* species because they are bactericidal and resistance to the β-lactamase–stable drugs has been slow in development [59]. To prevent recurrence or relapse of an infection, however, it is common practice to treat superficial skin infections for a minimum of 21 days, thus incorporating the concept of treating for 1 week beyond clinical remission when the medication is dispensed to the patient. Despite this recommendation, it is common to see prescriptions ranging from 7 to 10 or 14 days in the history of patients with recurrent bacterial skin infections. Although the β-lactamase–stable antibiotics remain effective when used appropriately, the practice of dosing for inappropriately brief periods should be discouraged, namely, because of the rise of incidence of CoNS infections that tend to be multidrug resistant and the emergence of methicillin-resistant strains.

As cases of methicillin-resistant staphylococcal infections increase, especially those from CoNS, a thorough consideration of previous treatments, including dose and duration of therapy, should be considered. Typically, drugs like cephalexin, cefadroxil, and amoxicillin–clavulanic acid are excellent choices when treating first-time infections or when a patient has previously been treated beyond the standard period of remission, because resistance to the β-lactamase–stable drugs occurs with low frequency [60], except with regard to methicillin-resistant isolates. With repeated exposure to subtherapeutic doses or durations of therapy, antibiotic pressure is applied, encouraging expression of the *mecA* gene for methicillin resistance. A recent study [61] demonstrated that methicillin-susceptible and methicillin-resistant strains of *S intermedius* and *S schleiferi* possess the *mecA* gene. Thus, the susceptible strains may only require upregulation of this genetic product, via antibiotic exposure, to display resistance to methicillin. In addition, it has been proposed that the widespread distribution of methicillin resistance within the CoNS may have begun with transfer of the *mecA* gene not only among CoNS but with *S aureus* as well [62].

Strains exhibiting methicillin resistance may seem to be susceptible to the β-lactam antibiotics in vitro but are actually resistant to the entire class of drugs in vivo. It is important to be aware of this, because most microbiology laboratories do not alter the report to reflect this; it is crucial to use the oxacillin or methicillin susceptibility result to guide interpretation of the results.

Fluorinated Quinolones

Fluoroquinolone antibiotics are commonly used to treat first-time and recurrent cases of pyoderma. These antibiotics, especially enrofloxacin, are widely used based on their broad-spectrum activity, ease of administration, and low toxicity [63]. They also are distributed to and easily penetrate most tissues, including scar tissue. In addition, they accumulate within white blood cells, increasing concentration at the target tissue site [55,63]. Finally, because of the extended half-life of these drugs and the postantibiotic effect reported, they can be given once daily, thus increasing compliance. It is crucial when using these drugs to consider their mechanism of action and the mechanisms with which organisms rapidly demonstrate resistance to this class of drugs. With increased use of fluoroquinolones in the past decade, the incidence of resistant isolates has increased as well [60,64,65].

The mechanisms of resistance described for the fluoroquinolone antibiotics are mutations and chromosomally mediated [55,63], targeting DNA gyrase or topoisomerase IV. An efflux pump has also been described in association with staphylococci resistance, which can grant resistance to other antimicrobials, including the cephalosporins [63]. This efflux pump may prove relevant in methicillin-resistant strains of *Staphylococcus*, because the few multidrug-resistant isolates recovered were from dogs receiving many antibiotics previously, including fluoroquinolones. Because the killing mechanism of this drug class is considered to be concentration dependent, or the amount of plasma drug concentration above the minimum inhibitory concentration (MIC) rather than time spent above the MIC, it is extremely important to select an appropriate dose targeting a peak plasma drug concentration 8 to 10 times the MIC for an organism [63] to discourage antibiotic resistance. Clinically, resistance has been noted to occur more rapidly when associated with underdosing or short durations of therapy [65,66]. Therefore when using fluoroquinolones for bacterial skin infections, it is essential to use culture and susceptibility data rather than blindly switching antibiotics when making adjustments to the regimen.

Poteniated Sulfonamides

The potentiated sulfonamides remain a reasonable choice for bacterial skin infections in small animals caused by *Staphylococcus* species. The CoNS as well as methicillin-resistant *Staphylococcus* species typically remain sensitive to this class of antibiotics. It is crucial to differentiate between sulfonamides and those that are potentiated, or combined with trimethoprim or ormetoprim, when choosing an antibiotic from this drug class, because resistance is frequent to the sulfonamides alone. In addition, the sulfonamides are bacteriostatic, whereas the potentiated sulfonamides are bactericidal and preferred when treating methicillin- or multidrug-resistant infections. The exact mechanisms of resistance to the sulfonamides and potentiated sulfonamides for *S intermedius* are not known;

however, for *S aureus*, they are considered to be chromosomally and plasmid mediated. The chromosomal mutation is associated with an overproduction of *p*-aminobenzoic acid and involves sulfonamide resistance, whereas the plasmid-mediated mechanism seems to reduce the affinity of dihydrofolate reductase for trimethoprim. Thus, one potential reason for the trend of continued potentiated sulfonamide susceptibility within *S intermedius* strains can be explained by the lack of plasmids found within this bacterial population [67]. Although plasmids are commonly found within strains of *S aureus*, this has not been demonstrated within strains of *S intermedius*.

Lincosamides and Macrolides

These classes of antibiotics share similar mechanisms of action, and their use is precluded most often by the frequency of resistance. Lincomycin and clindamycin represent the lincosamides most effective against *Staphylococcus* isolates. Lincomycin is used less commonly today because of an increase in resistance first noted in the late 1980s. Clindamycin is bacteriostatic at lower doses but is considered bactericidal when used at the dose indicated for osteomyelitis. Resistance via alteration in the drug-binding site on the 50s ribosome can limit successful use of this class of drugs, but the clinical benefit obtained as a result of their accumulation within white blood cells as well as distribution to fibrotic tissue and deep infections makes them an excellent choice when based on culture and susceptibility data.

Erythromycin and azithromycin are the macrolide antibiotics used most frequently. Their use is again limited by their bacteriostatic nature and the frequency of resistance. Erythromycin, when used for staphylococcal infections, is also known to induce resistance to multiple families of antibiotics, namely, the lincosamides. Less is known in regard to azithromycin and its use for bacterial skin diseases because it is relatively new to the market and few data exist regarding its use in veterinary dermatology. It is used most frequently for diseases of the respiratory tract; however, in human beings, a 5-day course of azithromycin was as effective as a 10-day course of cefadroxil for resolving skin infections [68].

Tetracyclines

Natural populations of *Staphylococcus* harbor tetracycline resistance. Despite decreasing use of this class of drugs in certain countries, the level of resistance remains near 50% in recent studies. Two mechanisms of resistance are currently recognized: an energy-dependent efflux pump and a ribosomal protection protein. The genes coding for the efflux pump are mainly found on plasmid DNA, whereas the genes coding for the ribosomal protection protein are typically associated with chromosomal DNA. In a recent study, 90% of the *S intermedius* isolates examined were resistant to tetracycline, with most isolates carrying chromosomal genes for the ribosomal protection protein [69]. These mechanisms, in combination with the bacteriostatic nature of this class of drugs, contribute to the infrequent recommendation for its use in bacterial skin diseases in animals today.

ZOONOTIC CONCERNS

Staphylococcus aureus and *Staphylococcus intermedius*

Evidence of zoonotic transmission between pets and owners has been described for *S aureus* and *S intermedius*. A methicillin-resistant strain of *S aureus* was isolated from a patient's wound as well as from the dog in the household with asymptomatic nasal carriage [70]. *S intermedius* was identified as the pathogenic organism in a healthy human patient with otitis externa and was also isolated from the ear, back, and chest of the dog in the household [71].

Staphylococcus schleiferi

Both subspecies of *S schleiferi* have been isolated from normal and diseased people and dogs [30,57,72]. *S schleiferi* has been reported as part of the normal human preaxillary flora [73], and carnivores have been implicated as the normal host [57]; however, this information is poorly documented in the literature. The true incidence of isolation of *S schleiferi* from people or dogs is unknown, and investigation into the role of this organism as a pathogen has only begun.

SUMMARY

The salient points posed by this article are as follows:

1. CoNS are capable of causing bacterial skin diseases in human beings and animals.
2. CoNS should be identified by human and veterinary microbiology laboratories, and susceptibility data should be reported.
3. Human and veterinary microbiology laboratories need to be aware of the newly identified *Staphylococcus* species and adjust their laboratory protocol to identify them properly.
4. Prudent use of antibiotics needs to be encouraged, based on culture and susceptibility data when indicated.
5. Evidence exists to support the communicable nature of *Staphylococcus* species between human beings and animals.

References

[1] Scott DW, Miller WH, Griffin CE. Bacterial skin diseases. In: Muller and Kirk's small animal dermatology. Philadelphia: WB Saunders; 2001. p. 274–335.
[2] Saijonmaa-Koulumies LE, Lloyd DH. Colonization of neonatal puppies by *Staphylococcus intermedius*. Vet Dermatol 2002;13:123–30.
[3] Somerville-Millar DA, Noble WC. Resident and transient bacteria of the skin. J Cutan Pathol 1974;1:260–4.
[4] Cox HU, Hoskins JD, Newman SS, et al. Temporal study of staphylococcal species on healthy dogs. Am J Vet Res 1988;49:747–51.
[5] White SD, Ihrke PJ, Stannard AA, et al. Occurrence of Staphylococcus aureus on the clinically normal canine hair coat. Am J Vet Res 1983;44:332–4.
[6] Noble WC. Skin carriage of the Micrococcaceae. J Clin Pathol 1969;22:249–53.
[7] Kloos WE, Zimmerman RJ, Smith RF. Preliminary studies on the characterization and distribution of Staphylococcus and Micrococcus species on animal skin. Appl Environ Microbiol 1976;31:53–9.
[8] White SD, Brown AE, Chapman PL, et al. Evaluation of aerobic bacteriologic culture of epidermal collarette specimens in dogs with superficial pyoderma. J Am Vet Med Assoc 2005;226:904–8.

[9] Allaker RP, Jensen L, Lloyd DH, et al. Colonization of neonatal puppies by staphylococci. Br Vet J 1992;148:523–8.

[10] Hájek V. *Staphylococcus intermedius*, a new species isolated from animals. Int J Syst Bacteriol 1976;26:401–8.

[11] Lloyd DH. Carriage of staphylococcus in dogs and other species. In: Harrison BA, editor. 20th Proceedings of the North American Veterinary Dermatology Forum. Sarasota, FL, 2005. p. 23–6.

[12] Harvey RG, Lloyd DH. The distribution of *Staphylococcus intermedius* and coagulase-negative staphylococci on the hair, skin surface, within the hair follicles and on the mucous membranes of dogs. Vet Dermatol 1994;5:75–82.

[13] Saijonmaa-Koulumies LEM, Myllys V, Lloyd DH. Diversity and stability of the *Staphylococcus intermedius* flora in three bitches and their puppies. Epidemiol Infect 2003;131:931–7.

[14] Lloyd DH. Staphylococcus as a pathogen. In: Harrison BA, editor. 20th Proceedings of the North American Veterinary Dermatology Forum. Sarasota, FL, 2005. p. 28–31.

[15] Lloyd DH. Antimicrobial resistance. In: Harrison BA, editor. 20th Proceedings of the North American Veterinary Dermatology Forum. Sarasota, FL, 2005. p. 33–6.

[16] Kloos WE, Bannerman TL. Update on clinical significance of coagulase-negative staphylococci. Clin Microbiol Rev 1994;7:117–40.

[17] Ieven M, Verhoeven J, Pattyn SR, et al. Rapid and economical method for species identification of clinically significant coagulase-negative staphylococci. J Clin Microbiol 1995;33:1060–3.

[18] Bannerman TL, Kleeman KT, Kloos WE. Evaluation of the Vitek Systems Gram-Positive Identification card for species identification of coagulase-negative staphylococci. J Clin Microbiol 1993;31:1322–5.

[19] Kleeman KT, Bannerman TL, Kloos WE. Species distribution of coagulase-negative staphylococci isolates at a community hospital and implications for selection of staphylococcal identification procedures. J Clin Microbiol 1993;31:1318–21.

[20] Freney J, Brun Y, Bes M, et al. *Staphylococcus lugdunensis* sp. nov. and *Staphyloccocus schleiferi* sp. nov., two species from human clinical specimens. Int J Syst Bacteriol 1988;38:168–72.

[21] Igimi S, Takahashi E, Mitsuoka T. Staphylococcus schleiferi subsp. coagulans subsp. nov., isolated from the external auditory meatus of dogs with external ear otitis. Int J Syst Bacteriol 1990;40:409–11.

[22] Vandenesch F, Lebeau C, Bes M, et al. Clotting activity in Staphylococcus schleiferi subspecies from human patients. J Clin Microbiol 1994;32:388–92.

[23] Kluytmans J, Berg H, Steegh P, et al. Outbreak of Staphylococcus schleiferi wound infections: strain characterization by randomly amplified polymorphic DNA analysis, PCR ribotyping, conventional ribotyping, and pulsed-field gel electrophoresis. J Clin Microbiol 1998;36:2214–9.

[24] Jean-Pierre H, Darbas H, Jean-Roussenq A, et al. Pathogenicity in two cases of Staphylococcus schleiferi, a recently described species. J Clin Microbiol 1989;27:2110–1.

[25] Leung MJ, Nuttall N, Mazur M, et al. Case of Staphylococcus schleiferi endocarditis and a simple scheme to identify clumping factor-positive staphylococci. J Clin Microbiol 1999;37:3353–6.

[26] Calvo J, Hernández JL, Fariñas MC, et al. Osteomyelitis caused by *Staphylococcus schleiferi* and evidence of misidentification of this staphylococcus species by an automated bacterial identification system. J Clin Microbiol 2000;38:3887–9.

[27] Öztürkeri H, Kocabeyoglu Ö, Yergök YZ, et al. Distribution of coagulase-negative staphylococci, including the newly described species *Staphylococcus schleiferi*, in nosocomial and community acquired urinary tract infections. Eur J Clin Microbiol Infect Dis 1994;13:1076–9.

[28] Hernandez JL, Calvo J, Sota R, et al. Clinical and microbiological characteristics of 28 patients with *Staphylococcus schleiferi* infection. Eur J Clin Microbiol Infect Dis 2001;20:153–8.

[29] Bès M, Guérin-Faublée V, Freney J, et al. Isolation of *Staphylococcus schleiferi* subspecies *coagulans* from two cases of canine pyoderma. Vet Rec 2002;150:487–8.

[30] Frank LA, Kania SA, Hnilica KA, et al. Isolation of *Staphylococcus schleiferi* from dogs with pyoderma. J Am Vet Med Assoc 2003;222:451–4.

[31] Holm BR, Petersson U, Mörner A, et al. Antimicrobial resistance in staphylococci from canine pyoderma: a prospective study of first-time and recurrent cases in Sweden. Vet Rec 2002;151:600–5.

[32] Kloos WE. Staphylococcus. In: Collier L, Balows A, Sussman M, editors. Topley and Wilson's microbiology and microbial infections. 9th edition. New York: Oxford University Press; 1998. p. 577–632.

[33] Greene RT, Lammler C. *Staphylococcus intermedius*: current knowledge on a pathogen of veterinary importance. J Vet Med B Infect Dis Vet Public Health 1993;40:206–14.

[34] Mason IS, Mason KV, Lloyd DH. A review of the biology of canine skin with respect to the commensals *Staphylococcus intermedius*, *Demodex canis* and *Malassezia pachydermatis*. Vet Dermatol 1996;7:119–32.

[35] Keane KA, Taylor DJ. Slime-producing *Staphylococcus* species in canine pyoderma. Vet Rec 1992;130:75.

[36] Murray PR. Staphylococcus and related organisms. In: Murray PR, Rosenthal KS, Kobayashi GS, et al, editors. Medical microbiology. 4th edition. St. Louis (MO): Mosby; 2002. p. 202–16.

[37] Terauchi R, Sato H, Hasegawa T, et al. Isolation of exfoliative toxin from *Staphylococcus intermedius* and its local toxicity in dogs. Vet Microbiol 2003;94:19–29.

[38] Sasaki A, Shimizu A, Kawano J, et al. Characteristics of *Staphylococcus intermedius* isolates from diseased and healthy dogs. J Vet Med Sci 2005;67:103–6.

[39] Futagawa-Saito K, Sugiyama T, Karube S, et al. Prevalence and characterization of leukotoxin-producing Staphylococcus intermedius in isolates from dogs and pigeons. J Clin Microbiol 2004;42:5324–6.

[40] Lambe DW Jr, Ferguson KP, Keplinger JL. Pathogenicity of *Staphylococcus lugdunensis*, *Staphylococcus schleiferi*, and three other coagulase-negative staphylococci in a mouse model and possible virulence factors. Can J Microbiol 1990;36:455–63.

[41] Ferguson KP, Lambe DW Jr, Keplinger JL. Comparison of the pathogenicity of three species of coagulase-negative *Staphylococcus* in a mouse model with and without a foreign body. Can J Microbiol 1991;37:722–4.

[42] Hébert GA. Hemolysins and other characteristics that help differentiate and biotype Staphylococcus lugdunensis and Staphylococcus schleiferi. J Clin Microbiol 1990;28: 2425–31.

[43] Fleurette J, Bes M, Brun Y, et al. Clinical isolates of *Staphylococcus lugdunensis* and S. *schleiferi*: bacteriological characteristics and susceptibility to antimicrobial agents. Res Microbiol 1989;140:107–18.

[44] Roberts S, O'Shea K, Morris D, et al. A real-time PCR assay to detect the Panton Valentine Leukocidin toxin in staphylococci: screening *Staphylococcus schleiferi* subspecies *coagulans* strains from companion animals. Vet Microbiol 2005;107:139–144.

[45] Peacock SJ, Lina G, Etienne J, et al. *Staphylococcus schleiferi* subsp. *schleiferi* expresses a fibronectin-binding protein. Infect Immun 1999;67:4272–5.

[46] Kloos WE, Bannerman TL. Staphylococcus and micrococcus. In: Murray PR, Baron EJ, Pfaller MA, et al, editors. Manual of clinical microbiology. Washington (DC): ASM Press; 1999. p. 264–82.

[47] Zdovc I, Ocepek M, Pirs T, et al. Microbiological features of *Staphylococcus schleiferi* subsp. *coagulans*, isolated from dogs and possible misidentification with other canine coagulase-positive staphylococci. J Vet Med B Infect Dis Vet Public Health 2004;51: 449–54.

[48] Couto I, Pereira S, Miragaia M, et al. Identification of clinical staphylococcal isolates from humans by internal transcribed spacer PCR. J Clin Microbiol 2001;39:3099–103.

[49] Carretto E, Barbarini D, Couto I, et al. Identification of coagulase-negative staphylococci other than Staphylococcus epidermidis by automated ribotyping. Clin Microbiol Infect 2005;11:177–84.

[50] Hillier A, Alcorn JR, Cole LK, et al. Pyoderma due to *Pseudomonas aeruginosa* infection in dogs: 15 cases [abstract]. In: Miller EP, editor. 18th Proceedings of the American Academy of Veterinary Dermatology and American College of Veterinary Dermatology. Monterey, CA, 2003. p. 222.

[51] McCausland WJ, Cox PJ. Pseudomonas infection traced to motel whirlpool. J Environ Health 1975;37:455–9.

[52] Washburn J, Jacobson JA, Marston E, et al. Pseudomonas aeruginosa rash associated with a whirlpool. JAMA 1976;235:2205–7.

[53] Hopkins RS, Abbott DO, Wallace LE. Follicular dermatitis outbreak caused by Pseudomonas aeruginosa associated with a motel's indoor swimming pool. Public Health Rep 1981;96: 246–9.

[54] Tate D, Mawer S, Newton A. Outbreak of Pseudomonas aeruginosa folliculitis associated with a swimming pool inflatable. Epidemiol Infect 2003;130:187–92.

[55] Boothe DM. Antimicrobial drugs. In: Small animal clinical pharmacology and therapeutics. Philadelphia: WB Saunders; 2001. p. 150–73.

[56] Prescott JF. Beta-lactam antibiotics: cephalosporins and cephamycins. In: Prescott JF, Baggot JD, Walker RD, editors. Antimicrobial therapy in veterinary medicine. Ames (IA): Iowa State University Press; 2000. p. 134–59.

[57] Kloos WE. Taxonomy and systematics of staphylococci indigenous to humans. In: Crossley KB, Archer G, editors. The staphylococci in human disease. Philadelphia: Churchill Livingstone; 1997. p. 113–37.

[58] Ganiere J-P, Medaille C, Mangion C. Antimicrobial drug susceptibility of *Staphylococcus intermedius* clinical isolates from canine pyoderma. J Vet Med B Infect Dis Vet Public Health 2005;52:25–31.

[59] Mason IS, Kietzmann M. Cephalosporins—pharmacological basis of clinical use in veterinary dermatology. Vet Dermatol 1999;10:187–92.

[60] Prescott JF, Hanna WJB, Reid-Smith R, et al. Antimicrobial drug use and resistance in dogs. Can Vet J 2002;43:107–16.

[61] Kania SA, Williamson NL, Frank LA, et al. Methicillin resistance of staphylococci isolated from the skin of dogs with pyoderma. Am J Vet Res 2004;65:1265–8.

[62] Wu SW, de Lencastre H, Tomasz A. Recruitment of the mecA gene homologue of Staphylococcus sciuri into a resistance determinant and expression of the resistant phenotype in Staphylococcus aureus. J Bacteriol 2001;183:2417–24.

[63] Walker RD. Fluoroquinolones. In: Prescott JF, Baggot JD, Walker RD, editors. Antimicrobial therapy in veterinary medicine. Ames (IA): Iowa State University Press; 2000. p. 315–38.

[64] Ihrke PJ, Papich MG, DeManuelle TC. The use of fluoroquinolones in veterinary dermatology. Vet Dermatol 1999;10:193–204.

[65] Ganiere J-P, Medaille C, Limet A, et al. Antimicrobial activity of enrofloxacin against *Staphylococcus intermedius* strains isolated from canine pyodermas. Vet Dermatol 2001;12: 171–5.

[66] Lloyd D, Lamport AI, Noble WC, et al. Fluoroquinolone resistance in *Staphylococcus intermedius*. Vet Dermatol 1999;10:193–204.

[67] Kloos WE, Orban BS, Walker DD. Plasmid composition of Staphylococcus species. Can J Microbiol 1981;27:271–8.

[68] Jennings MB, McCarty JM, Scheffler NM, et al. Comparison of azithromycin and cefadroxil for the treatment of uncomplicated skin and skin structure infections. Cutis 2003;72:240–4.

[69] Kim TJ, Na YR, Lee JI. Investigations into the basis of chloramphenicol and tetracycline resistance in Staphylococcus intermedius isolates from cases of pyoderma in dogs. J Vet Med B Infect Dis Vet Public Health 2005;52:119–24.

[70] Manian FA. Asymptomatic nasal carriage of mupirocin-resistant, methicillin-resistant *Staphylococcus aureus* (MRSA) in a pet dog associated with MRSA infection in household contacts. Clin Infect Dis 2003;36:26–8.

[71] Tanner MA, Everett CL, Youvan DC. Molecular phylogenetic evidence for noninvasive zoonotic transmission of Staphylococcus intermedius from a canine pet to a human. J Clin Microbiol 2000;38:1628–31.

[72] Hnilica KA, May ER. Staphylococcal pyoderma: an emerging problem. Compend Contin Educ Pract Vet 2004;26:560–8.

[73] Celard M, Vandenesch F, Darbas H, et al. Pacemaker infection caused by *Staphylococcus schleiferi*, a member of the human preaxillary flora: four case reports. Clin Infect Dis 1997;24:1014–5.

German Shepherd Dog Pyoderma

Edmund J. Rosser, Jr, DVM

Department of Small Animal Clinical Sciences, Michigan State University College of Veterinary Medicine, East Lansing, MI 48824-1314, USA

An often frustrating and somewhat unique recurrent or refractory deep pyoderma has been described in the German Shepherd Dog [1,2]. The disease is characterized by pruritus (the chief complaint), with deep pyoderma typically beginning over the lumbosacral region. The condition may progress to affect multiple regions of the body and become a generalized skin disease. Several studies have attempted to define the pathophysiology of this distinctive disorder [3–15]. These studies have been unable to specify a unifactorial defect to account for the development of this condition in all cases. A prospective study conducted over a 5-year period examined several parameters in 12 German Shepherd Dogs affected by German Shepherd Dog pyoderma (GSP) [16]. The results of this study revealed that GSP should be considered a disease caused by multiple underlying disease conditions and should not be considered a skin disease caused by any one specific defect in any given case of GSP. Similarly, other authors have suggested that rather than looking at GSP as a disease of multifactorial etiology, it may be more useful to view it as a characteristic clinical syndrome triggered by a variety of other diseases in susceptible individuals [17].

PATHOPHYSIOLOGY

The underlying disease processes that may be involved in the development of GSP include flea allergy dermatitis, atopic dermatitis, cutaneous adverse food reactions (food allergy), hypothyroidism, ehrlichiosis, and T- and B-lymphocyte and neutrophil abnormalities [1,2,5,7,8,10,13–15,17]. With regard to the immune system abnormalities observed in dogs with GSP, some of the lymphocyte changes may only be occurring as a consequence of the disease process rather than as its cause, because suppression of lymphocytes observed during in vitro lymphocyte stimulation testing (mitogen stimulation testing) has also been reported in dogs of other breeds with chronic staphylococcal pyoderma [18]. It has also been reported that dogs with GSP may have some specific lymphocyte subset abnormalities, specifically a relative increase in CD8+

E-mail address: rosser@cvm.msu.edu

0195-5616/06/$ – see front matter
doi:10.1016/j.cvsm.2005.09.008

T lymphocytes, a relative decrease in CD4+ T lymphocytes, and a relative decrease in CD21+ B lymphocytes when compared with normal German Shepherd Dogs [10,15]. More recently, however, it has been shown that normal German Shepherd Dogs have the lowest absolute counts of individual lymphocyte subpopulations as well as a relative increase in CD8+ T lymphocytes and a relative decrease in CD21+ B lymphocytes when compared with other breeds of normal dogs [19]. It has also been suggested that GSP may have a genetically inherited component [4]. In a number of instances, the disease seems to be idiopathic in nature [1,2,12,15,16]. A systematic approach that can be used to help establish the underlying disease (or multiple diseases) involved in any given case of GSP is discussed further in the section on diagnosis.

The most common bacteria isolated from dogs with GSP is *Staphylococcus intermedius* [1,2,6,15,16]. This organism may be present as the only bacterial pathogen or in combination with other bacteria, including β-hemolytic streptococci, *Proteus mirabilis*, or *Corynebacterium* spp.

HISTORY AND SIGNALMENT

The initial chief complaint of the owners of dogs affected by GSP is pruritus. The most commonly affected areas are the lumbosacral region, abdominal and/or inguinal region, and posterior and/or medial thigh region. The initial onset of pruritus may be a warm-weather seasonal problem (ie, the condition would initially resolve spontaneously during the winter months) or a persistent and nonseasonal problem. Dogs that have an initial warm-weather problem tend to develop a more persistent and nonseasonal problem after several years, however. The distribution pattern of pruritus often changes as the disease progresses and may involve various regions of the body, including the periorbital and/or facial region, axillary region, pinnae, lateral stifle region, lateral thorax, neck, and feet, or become a generalized disease problem [16].

The age of onset for dogs affected by GSP is extremely variable and ranges from 3 months to 13 years of age [1,2,15,16]. The sex predisposition regarding the development of this disease varies between studies, with none being reported [1,2,16] or a possible increased incidence in male dogs [15,17]. Obviously, purebred German Shepherd Dogs are predisposed to the development of this disease, but it is important to note that a similar condition may occur in German Shepherd crossbred dogs and other herding breeds of dogs (ie, Belgian Malinois, Belgian Sheepdog, Belgian Tervuren) as well as in Dalmatians and Bull Terrier breeds [8,9,11,12,17,20].

CLINICAL SIGNS

The most common lesion initially observed in cases of GSP is clinically similar to that of a "hot spot" and is usually first noticed in the lumbosacral region, lateral hip, or lateral thigh region (Fig. 1). As the disease progresses, several additional lesions may be observed, including areas of posttraumatic alopecia, hyperpigmentation, papules, pustules, hemorrhagic bullae, ulcers, crusts, and draining tracts (usually with a hemopurulent discharge) with surrounding

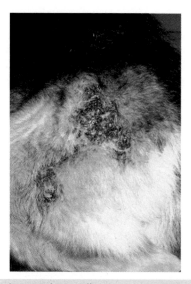

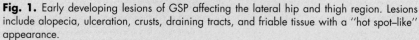

Fig. 1. Early developing lesions of GSP affecting the lateral hip and thigh region. Lesions include alopecia, ulceration, crusts, draining tracts, and friable tissue with a "hot spot–like" appearance.

friable tissue. The disease ultimately takes on the appearance of chronic deep pyoderma or cellulitis, and there is frequently an associated regional lymphadenopathy. Less commonly observed clinical signs may include a purulent otitis externa, perianal fistulas, focal metatarsal fistulas (sterile pedal panniculitis), and fever with signs of systemic illness [15–17].

DIAGNOSIS

In the evaluation of a German Shepherd Dog presented to you with pruritus and deep pyoderma, several deep skin scrapings should initially be performed to examine for the possibility of *Demodex canis* mites. Canine demodicosis should be considered an important and early rule out for any breed of dog presenting with deep pyoderma. If deep skin scrapings are negative, numerous superficial skin scrapings and transparent cellulose adhesive tape preparations should be taken and examined for the presence of *Sarcoptes* or *Cheyletiella* mites, because these ectoparasites should be considered as possible underlying causes of pruritus for all dogs.

Results of a complete blood cell count (CBC) and serum chemistry profile are usually normal or reveal evidence of the chronic nature of the bacterial infection associated with GSP, including mild to moderate leukocytosis with neutrophilia and lymphopenia and increased serum globulins. In addition, the CBC and serum chemistry profile should be examined for any abnormalities suggestive of an underlying metabolic disease process (ie, hyperadrenocorticism, hypothyroidism, diabetes mellitus), because these may cause chronic or recurrent deep pyoderma in any breed of dog. Results of urinalysis may indicate the presence of proteinuria [1,16], suggesting the possibility of immune complex deposition glomerulonephritis secondary to the chronic exposure to the bacterial antigens causing the deep pyoderma. In cases in which this finding has been observed, treatment of these dogs with an appropriate systemic antibiotic may result in the resolution of proteinuria [16].

Culture and Susceptibility Testing

Bacterial culture and susceptibility testing should always be performed in dogs suspected of having GSP to aid in the definitive selection of the most appropriate antibiotic to use in the adjunctive treatment of this disease. The reasons for this are threefold and include the following: (1) many of these dogs have previously been on an antibiotic, and antibiotic resistance often develops; (2) the infection in these cases is deep, and there is the potential for the development of bacteremia and septicemia; and (3) the duration of antibiotic therapy in the initial treatment of this disease is usually 6 to 8 weeks, and the clinician needs to be certain that the optimum antibiotic has been selected when trying to eliminate the bacterial component to this disease complex. The samples for culture should be taken using a sterile swab placed deep within an aseptically prepared draining tract or a core of tissue taken by surgical biopsy (usually a 6-mm punch biopsy sample, which is then submitted for macerated tissue culture). The clinician should request that the samples be cultured to examine for the presence of aerobic bacteria, anaerobic bacteria, and fungi. Anaerobic bacteria or a deep fungal organism (especially sporotrichosis, blastomycosis, histoplasmosis, and coccidioidomycosis) may mimic the clinical appearance of deep pyoderma caused by aerobic bacteria.

Histopathologic Examination

The histopathologic examination of skin biopsies most commonly reveals the presence of a pyogranulomatous inflammatory reaction, folliculitis, and furunculosis [2,16,21]. The biopsies may also be examined using special stains to look for the presence of bacteria or fungi within the affected tissues.

DIAGNOSTIC APPROACH AND TREATMENT

As you can see, the diagnosis of GSP is initially a diagnosis of exclusion by eliminating the several other possible causes of chronic and deep pyoderma that could affect any breed of dog. Once these have been excluded, the diagnosis of GSP is established by the characteristic clinical appearance, skin biopsy results (deep pyoderma consistent with that of GSP), and cultures indicating the presence of *S intermedius*, with or without the growth of additional aerobic or anaerobic bacteria.

Systemic Antibiotic and Topical Treatment and Re-Evaluation of Treatment Responses

At this stage in the diagnostic workup, the dog should be treated with a systemic antibiotic, which is selected based on the results of culture and susceptibility testing. It is critical that the antibiotic be given at the appropriate dose and frequency of administration (Table 1). Cephalexin and enrofloxacin have been suggested as appropriate systemic antibiotics for use in the management of dogs with GSP [16,17]. The author's preference is to initiate systemic antibiotic treatment using cephalexin at a dose of 22 mg/kg administered every 8 hours, pending the results of bacterial susceptibility testing. Concurrently, the dog should also be bathed twice weekly with a medicated shampoo, such as a 2.5% to 3.0% benzoyl peroxide shampoo (Pyoben, Virbac Animal Health, Fort Worth, Texas; OxyDex, DVM Pharmaceuticals, Miami, Florida; or Benzoyl-Plus, Evsco Pharmaceuticals, Buena, New Jersey) or a 3% to 4% chlorhexidine shampoo (Maximum ChlorhexiDerm, DVM Pharmaceuticals; or Hexadene, Virbac Animal Health). The shampoo should be lathered and then left on the skin for 10 minutes before rinsing. The initial duration of treatment is a minimum of 4 weeks; at that time, the dog is re-examined. The guideline to be used for the total duration of systemic antibiotic treatment is to treat the dog for 2 weeks beyond apparent complete clinical remission. In general, this usually requires a total of 8 weeks of continuous systemic antibiotic and topical treatment. Most commonly, the recheck examination after 4 weeks of treatment reveals a noticeable improvement in the severity of the deep pyoderma; however, as the pyoderma has improved, some degree of pruritus persists. The degree of pruritus is usually noticeably decreased compared with the initial evaluation. It is critical that this remaining pruritus not be masked by the use of any antipruritic drugs (especially glucocorticoids), because the distribution pattern of the persisting pruritus can be used as an aid to establishing the underlying disease process. The dog is then sent home on an additional 4 weeks of therapy using the systemic antibiotic and twice-weekly bathing. If the persisting pruritus is intolerable at this stage, additional diagnostic testing may be

Table 1
Systemic antibiotics recommended in the treatment of staphylococcal pyodermas in cases of German Shepherd Dog pyoderma

Antibiotic	Recommended oral dose
Clindamycin	5.5 mg/kg q 12 h or 11 mg/kg q 24 h
Erythromycin	15 mg/kg q 8 h
Cephalexin	22 mg/kg q 8 h or 33 mg/kg q 12 h
Cefadroxil	22 mg/kg q 12 h
Cefpodoxime	5–10 mg/kg q 24 h
Trimethoprim/sulfadiazine	15–30 mg/kg q 12 h
Ormetoprim/sulfadimethoxine	55 mg/kg on day 1, then 27.5 mg/kg q 24 h
Amoxicillin/clavulanate	13.75 mg/kg q 12 h
Enrofloxacin[a]	5–20 mg/kg q 24 h

Abbreviations: h, hours; q, every.
[a] Only recommended in instances of recurrent pyodermas when culture and susceptibility testing indicate its required use.

considered or the dog may be treated with an antihistamine to minimize but not eliminate the pruritus.

The clinician can then use the dog's response to treatment as an aid to establishing any likely underlying diseases that may be present. Most commonly, the recheck examination after 8 weeks of treatment reveals resolution of the deep pyoderma; however, as the pyoderma has improved, the pruritus persists. If the most prevalent areas of pruritus are the lumbosacral region, abdominal and/or inguinal region, posterior and/or medial thigh region, lateral hip, or lateral thigh region, an underlying flea allergy dermatitis reaction is most likely one of the dog's problems. At this point, an aggressive flea treatment protocol should be added to the treatment regimen. You can also consider performing an intradermal test (IDT) using flea antigen only (along with a positive control and a negative control) to document the presence of a type I or type IV hypersensitivity reaction to fleas.

If the recheck examination after 8 weeks of therapy indicates that the most prevalent areas of pruritus are some combination of the face, ear pinnae, inguinal region, axillary region, feet, and proximal anterior foreleg region, an underlying food allergy or atopic dermatitis is the likely problem. When the initial history indicates that the pruritus and pyoderma started as a warm-weather seasonal problem, further examination for the presence of atopic dermatitis needs to be considered. This can be done by recommending an IDT or in vitro serologic allergy test (eg, enzyme-linked immunosorbent assay [ELISA], radioallergosorbent test [RAST]) for aeroallergens. If the results of such tests fit the history of the dog's pruritus, lending support to the diagnosis of atopic dermatitis, allergen-specific immunotherapy (ASIT) with aqueous allergens should be added to the treatment regimen. When the initial history indicates that the pruritus and pyoderma started as a nonseasonal problem, a food allergy or atopic dermatitis area is the likely problem. At this point, a home-cooked elimination diet trial of 8 to 12 weeks' duration should be recommended to examine for the presence of a food allergy component [22]. If the dog's pruritus resolves, the dog can be rechallenged with its previous dog food to evaluate for the return of the pruritus (which most specifically confirms the presence of a food allergy) or can be fed a commercially prepared hypoallergenic diet that contains ingredients similar to those used in the home-cooked elimination diet. If the dog's pruritus is nonresponsive to the elimination diet trial, the clinician should recommend an IDT or in vitro serologic allergy test (eg, ELISA, RAST) for aeroallergens to examine for the presence of a nonseasonal atopic dermatitis component to the dog's pruritus. Once again, if the results of such tests fit the history of the dog's pruritus, lending support to the diagnosis of atopic dermatitis, ASIT with aqueous allergens should be added to the treatment regimen.

In some instances, the recheck examination after 4 to 8 weeks of treatment on systemic antibiotics and topical shampoo therapy reveals complete resolution of the deep pyoderma; as the pyoderma has resolved, the pruritus has vanished. Once again, the total treatment time for such cases is 2 weeks beyond apparent complete clinical remission, usually requiring a total of 8 weeks of therapy. In some instances, this therapy results in permanent remission of the previously recurrent pyoderma. This would suggest that the initial insult to the skin was only transient in nature and that the aggressive treatment protocol for the deep pyoderma eliminated the infection. This type of observation emphasizes the need for the use of an appropriate systemic antibiotic based on the results of culture and susceptibility testing and an adequate duration of treatment in all cases of deep pyoderma. In some instances, however, the pyoderma still has the audacity to recur after this aggressive treatment protocol, and such diseases as hypothyroidism or a cell-mediated immunodeficiency need to be considered. It should be emphasized that although these two diseases may be the underlying problems in dogs with GSP, these diseases tend to be much less commonly encountered than the diseases discussed to this point. Hypothyroidism should be evaluated by submitting serum for a thyroid profile, which preferably measures total thyroxine (T_4), free T_4 (via equilibrium dialysis), endogenous thyroid-stimulating hormone (TSH), triiodothyronine (T_3) and T_4 autoantibodies, and thyroglobulin autoantibodies. If hypothyroidism is confirmed, sodium levothyroxine replacement therapy should be added to the treatment regimen. Cell-mediated immunodeficiency can be further investigated by performing an in vitro lymphocyte stimulation test (mitogen stimulation test) [7,14,16]. Unfortunately, this test is not currently commercially available and is usually only performed at academic and research institutions. If cell-mediated immunodeficiency is suspected, immunostimulation using a commercially available bacterin (staphage lysate) may be added to the treatment regimen [16,23]. The staphage lysate injections may be given using the following protocol: 0.25 mL administered subcutaneously on week 1, 0.50 mL on week 2, 0.75 mL on week 3, 1.0 mL on week 4, and then 1 mL every 3 to 21 days as needed to prevent the recurrence of the pyoderma [24,25]. It is important to remember that the patient should also be given an appropriate systemic antibiotic and topical shampoo therapy for the first 4 to 8 weeks of treatment (until the infection has resolved).

Maintenance Antibiotics

In instances in which an underlying disease process cannot be identified (so-called "idiopathic GSP"), the clinician may need to consider a maintenance antibiotic treatment protocol. Before this recommendation is offered, make certain that the owner is aware of the possible risk of developing a resistant bacterial infection in the skin or elsewhere in the body. There are several treatment protocols published, but the author's preference is use of the antibiotic on a continuous basis at a suboptimal dose. As an example, if the initial appropriate dose of the antibiotic is 500 mg administered every 8 hours, give the antibiotic at that dose until clinical remission of the pyoderma has been re-established. Then, gradually decrease the dose over several weeks to 500 mg administered every 12 hours and, finally, to 250 to 500 mg administered every 24 to 48 hours. Bactericidal antibiotics with a low potential for development of resistance and minimal side effects have been most effective, such as cephalexin. In cases of relapse of the pyoderma, perform bacterial culture and susceptibility testing to examine for possible bacterial resistance to the antibiotic.

SUMMARY

Although dogs with GSP may have clinically similar presentations, the underlying causes of the disease process can be multifactorial in etiology. The combination of diseases present for a given dog with GSP varies from case to case. The management of GSP requires a thorough and systematic approach to investigate each dog for possible triggering disease processes. As each disease is identified, the specific treatment for that disease needs to be initiated, along with aggressive concurrent medical therapy using systemic antibiotics and medicated baths. If the patient's response to treatment is only partial, the investigation for additional underlying diseases should continue. In using this approach, the clinician should be better able to control the recurrent or refractory nature of GSP.

References

[1] Wisselink MA, Willemse A, Koeman JP. Deep pyoderma in the German shepherd dog. J Am Anim Hosp Assoc 1985;21:773–6.
[2] Krick SA, Scott DW. Bacterial folliculitis, furunculosis, and cellulitis in the German shepherd dog: a retrospective analysis of 17 cases. J Am Anim Hosp Assoc 1989;26:23–30.
[3] Wisselink MA, Bernadina WE, Willemse A, et al. Immunologic aspects of German shepherd dog pyoderma (GSP). Vet Immunol Immunopathol 1988;19:67–77.
[4] Wisselink MA, Bouw J, der Weduwen SA, et al. German shepherd dog pyoderma: a genetic disorder. Vet Q 1989;11:161–4.
[5] Wisselink MA, Koeman JP, van den Ingh TSGAM, et al. Investigations on the role of flea antigen in the pathogenesis of German shepherd dog pyoderma (GSP). Vet Q 1990;12:21–8.
[6] Wisselink MA, Koeman JP, van den Ingh TSGAM, et al. Investigations on the role of staphylococci in the pathogenesis of German shepherd dog pyoderma (GSP). Vet Q 1990;12: 29–34.
[7] Miller WH. Deep pyoderma in two German Shepherd dogs associated with a cell-mediated immunodeficiency. J Am Anim Hosp Assoc 1991;27:513–7.
[8] Day MJ. An immunopathological study of deep pyoderma in the dog. Res Vet Sci 1994;56: 18–23.
[9] Day MJ, Mazza G. Tissue immunoglobulin G subclasses observed in immune-mediated dermatopathy, deep pyoderma and hypersensitivity dermatitis in dogs. Res Vet Sci 1995;58: 82–9.
[10] Chabanne L, Marchal T, Denerolle P, et al. Lymphocyte subset abnormalities in German Shepherd dog pyoderma. Vet Immunol Immunopathol 1995;49:189–98.
[11] Wisselink MA, van Kessel KPM, Willemse T. Leukocyte mobilization to skin lesions, determination of cell surface receptors (CD11b/CD18) and phagocytic capacities of neutrophils in dogs with chronic deep pyoderma. 1997;57:179–86.
[12] Shearer DH, Day MJ. Aspects of the humoral immune response to Staphylococcus intermedius in dogs with superficial pyoderma, deep pyoderma and anal furunculosis. 1997; 58:107–20.
[13] Cerundolo R, de Caprariis D, Manna L, et al. Recurrent deep pyoderma in German Shepherd dogs with concurrent ehrlichiosis. In: Kwochka KW, Willemse T, von Tscharner C, editors. Advances in veterinary dermatology, vol. 3. Oxford, United Kingdom: Butterworth Heinemann; 1998. p. 556–7.

[14] Toman M, Svoboda M, Rybnicek J, et al. Secondary immunodeficiency in dogs with enteric, dermatologic, infectious or parasitic diseases. J Vet Med B Infect Dis Vet Public Health 1998;45:321–34.

[15] Denerolle P, Bourdoiseau G, Magnol J, et al. German Shepherd dog pyoderma: a prospective study of 23 cases. Vet Dermatol 1998;9:243–8.

[16] Rosser EJ. German shepherd dog pyoderma: a prospective study of 12 dogs. J Am Anim Hosp Assoc 1997;33:355–63.

[17] Ihrke PJ, DeManuelle TC. German Shepherd dog pyoderma: an overview and antimicrobial management. Supplement to the Compend Contin Educ Pract Vet 1999;21:44–9.

[18] Barta O. Serum's lymphocyte immunoregulatory factors (SLIF). Vet Immunol Immunopathol 1983;4:279–306.

[19] Faldyna M, Leva L, Knotigova P, et al. Lymphocyte subsets in peripheral blood of dogs—a flow cytometric study. Vet Immunol Immunopathol 2001;82:23–37.

[20] Rosser EJ. German Shepherd dog pyoderma. Compend Contin Educ Pract Vet 1998;20(7): 831–40.

[21] Gross TL, Ihrke PJ, Walder EJ. Veterinary dermatopathology. A macroscopic and microscopic evaluation of canine and feline skin disease. St. Louis (MO): Mosby–Year Book; 1992. p. 252–5.

[22] Rosser EJ. Diagnosis of food allergy in dogs. J Am Vet Med Assoc 1993;203:259–62.

[23] Foster AP. Immunomodulation and immunodeficiency. Vet Dermatol 2004;15(2):115–26.

[24] Rosser EJ. Bacterial antigens. In: Muller GH, Kirk RW, Scott DW, editors. Small animal dermatology. 3rd edition. Philadelphia: WB Saunders; 1983. p. 164.

[25] Rosser EJ. Pyoderma. In: Birchard SJ, Sherding RG, editors. Saunders manual of small animal practice. 2nd edition. Philadelphia: WB Saunders; 2000. p. 305–12.

Updates on the Management of Canine Epitheliotropic Cutaneous T-Cell Lymphoma

Louis-Philippe de Lorimier, DVM

Department of Veterinary Clinical Medicine, College of Veterinary Medicine, University of Illinois at Urbana-Champaign, 1008 West Hazelwood Drive, Urbana, IL 61802, USA

E pitheliotropic cutaneous T-cell lymphoma (CTCL), including mycosis fungoides, Sézary syndrome, and pagetoid reticulosis, is the most common form of cutaneous lymphoma in dogs [1,2]. Although lymphoma is a common cancer in dogs, the cutaneous variant is relatively uncommon, accounting only for approximately 5% of all canine lymphomas [3–5]. In dogs, CTCL is generally a disease of CD8+ cytotoxic T cells, contrary to the human form, in which mature CD4+ helper T cells predominate [1,3,6–8]. In that respect, canine CTCL may better model uncommon human CD8+ subtypes of CTCL, including certain variants chiefly developing before 20 years of age [9–12]. Canine CTCL is generally considered a low-grade malignancy predominantly affecting older dogs, with a mean age around 9 to 12 years [2–6]. Various clinical presentations are described with CTCL in dogs and human beings, all of which usually include some form of erythroderma, with the typical progression going from the patch stage, to the plaque stage, to the tumor stage, and, finally, to the disseminated stage with nodal involvement and, occasionally, circulating Sézary cells (leukemic stage) [1,4–8,13,14]. Although the skin is the most common primary site of canine CTCL, lesions are also commonly found in the oral cavity and at mucocutaneous junctions [1,4,5,14]. The true prognosis of canine CTCL remains difficult to determine because it may vary according to the stage of the disease at diagnosis and the therapeutic response. This review focuses on advances in the therapeutic management of canine CTCL.

SKIN-DIRECTED THERAPY

For localized, superficial, or early disease, skin-directed therapy may be indicated and remains the mainstay of therapy in human beings with patch- or

E-mail address: delorimi@uiuc.edu

0195-5616/06/$ – see front matter
doi:10.1016/j.cvsm.2005.09.013

plaque-stage CTCL [8,15,16]. Skin-directed therapy includes surgery, topical therapies, phototherapy, photodynamic therapy (PDT), and radiation therapy.

Surgery

Surgery may occasionally be recommended for solitary lesions of canine CTCL only after additional lesions or dissemination of the disease has been ruled out via thorough clinical staging of the patient. Because lymphoma should always be considered a potentially systemic disorder, surgical resection of a solitary lesion of CTCL, should it be chosen as the initial therapy for a case of canine CTCL, is often followed by adjuvant systemic chemotherapy. Nonetheless, occasional patients with solitary lesions of CTCL treated with surgery alone live to see long relapse-free intervals (Fig. 1) [5,17–19].

Topical Therapies

Topical drugs are the mainstay of therapy for CTCL in human patients and may be valuable as well for a subset of canine patients with the condition. Factors limiting more widespread use of topically applied therapeutic agents to dogs include exposure to the drug by the caretaker, advanced-stage disease in many dogs at diagnosis, local or systemic side effects of certain topical agents, high cost with newer agents, and the cleaning habits of dogs limiting the duration of exposure to the drug and crucial time-dependent cytotoxicity.

Topical corticosteroids

Although poorly described in the veterinary literature, topical corticosteroids are commonly used for the early superficial stages of CTCL in people, with reported response rates as high as 82% to 94% with patch-stage disease [15,16,20]. Many human patients treated with topical corticosteroids receive benefit of that therapy before a definitive diagnosis, and the same is likely true of dogs with CTCL [15]. Despite the lack of reports on efficacy, it is plausible that many canine patients with superficial or early CTCL may profit from topical corticosteroid therapy, if not with clinical remission, at least with some

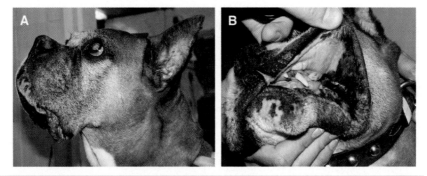

Fig. 1. Solitary nodular CTCL lesion of the lip in an 11-year-old male castrated Boxer before (A) and 3 weeks after (B) surgical resection. This dog did not receive systemic chemotherapy and died of unrelated causes (head trauma) 4 months after surgery, without evidence of local recurrence or dissemination.

degree of symptomatic relief. Veterinary-approved shampoos, lotions, or sprays containing 1% hydrocortisone, sometimes with lidocaine, could benefit a certain number of CTCL patients with patch- or plaque-stage disease. More potent and longer acting corticosteroids, such as topical triamcinolone (0.015% topical spray), may be more beneficial to other patients.

Topical mechlorethamine

Mechlorethamine, a bifunctional alkylating agent of the nitrogen mustard family, is the best described topical therapy for CTCL in dogs and people [5,7,8,14–16,18,21]. Good responses have been described in dogs with patch- or plaque-stage disease, and a complete response rate approaching 75% is reported for human patients with early disease [5,15,16,18,20]. The main advantages of topical mechlorethamine are the lack of significant systemic absorption and absence of significant side effects in the patient [16]. Because canine CTCL is frequently diagnosed in later or disseminated stages, however, and because of the carcinogenic potential and other adverse skin reactions to long-term exposure by the owner or veterinary staff, most veterinary oncologists do not routinely recommend topical mechlorethamine for the treatment of canine CTCL [8,14].

Topical carmustine

A bifunctional alkylating agent of the nitrosourea family, carmustine (1,3′-bis-(2-chloroethyl)-1-nitrosurea ([BCNU]) is also occasionally used in human patients with early-stage CTCL [7,8,14,16]. Response rates similar to those achieved with topical mechlorethamine are obtained with early-stage disease [7,16]. The main advantage of carmustine over mechlorethamine is the absence of significant cutaneous toxicity, whereas the main disadvantage is systemic absorption resulting in myelotoxicity [7,8,16]. The use of topical carmustine for canine CTCL remains to be reported.

Topical retinoids

A synthetic retinoid selectively activating retinoid X receptors (RXRs), bexarotene (1% gel) is available in a gel formulation for the topical treatment of early-stage CTCL in people [15,16]. Overall response rates greater than 60% have been reported, and the main toxicity is mild to moderate irritation at the site of application in up to 70% of patients [15,16]. No report on the use of topical bexarotene exists in the veterinary literature, and the expense of the drug is a definite limitation for its more common use [16].

A naturally occurring all-*trans*-retinoic acid with relative selectivity for retinoic acid receptors (RARs), tretinoin is available as a cream for topical use. Although the topical use of tretinoin is not reported in the published veterinary literature, it has shown to be useful in a few dogs with early-stage CTCL. The 0.1% tretinoin cream can be applied over half of the body once a day, alternating between sides of the body daily to avoid severe cutaneous reactions (K.L. Campbell, DVM, MS, personal communication, 2005).

Topical bexarotene or tretinoin may be used in combination with topical corticosteroids when treating CTCL, possibly with additive effects.

Imiquimod

A topical immunomodulator of the imidazoquinoline family approved for the treatment of genital warts in people, imiquimod was recently reported for the treatment of the patch and plaque stages of CTCL in people [16,22]. In a pilot study on 6 patients, 3 showed histologic clearance of the treated lesions and topical reactions were limited to the patients responding to therapy [22]. The use of imiquimod for canine cutaneous malignancies is not reported in the veterinary literature, but the drug holds promise for the treatment of such conditions as CTCL, dermal hemangiosarcoma, and squamous cell carcinoma [23].

Phototherapy

Phototherapy involves the use of ultraviolet (UV) radiation, generally UVA or UVB wavelengths. The long-wave UVA radiation has the advantage of deeper penetration compared with UVB radiation and is often used in combination with psoralen, a photosensitizer (psoralen plus UVA [PUVA]) [7,8,15,16]. Therapy with PUVA involves the ingestion of psoralen, followed by exposure of the skin to UVA radiation [16]. For early (patch and plaque stages) CTCL in human patients, PUVA has a complete response rate of 74% and an overall response rate of 95%, with a median time to complete clearing of approximately 3 months and responses that are often long lasting in such patients [15]. Reported side effects include dose-related acute burning and erythema, accelerated photoaging, and a long-term increased risk of nonmelanoma skin cancers [15]. Therapy with PUVA has yet to be reported in the veterinary literature.

Photodynamic Therapy

There are a few reports on the use of PDT with topically applied 5-aminolevulinic acid (5-ALA) in people with CTCL [16]. A preferential uptake of 5-ALA by activated and malignant T cells is reported, and exposure to 630 ± 15-nm light activates 5-ALA, resulting in the destruction of malignant T cells [16]. The main role of PDT for CTCL has been in the management of localized lesions that did not respond to more traditional therapies, and further studies are required [16]. Although PDT has not been reported for the treatment of canine CTCL, its use for other tumors of companion animals has been described, with favorable responses and toxicity profiles [24,25].

Radiation Therapy

Lymphocytes, whether normal or malignant, are known to be exquisitely radiosensitive [7,8]. The use of radiation therapy for select CTCL cases is thus a reasonable option when available. Total skin electron beam therapy (TSEBT) is commonly used for early stages of CTCL in people, and overall response rates approach 100% in that setting, with only mild to moderate skin toxicity [7,8,15,16]. The total dose applied to the skin surface is generally in the range of 30 to 36 Gy in small daily fractions, over 3 to 4 weeks [7,8]. Despite excellent response rates, patients with more advanced disease stages are prone to relapse [15]. In addition, this treatment modality requires complex planning and specialized equipment. Nevertheless, an ongoing study is evaluating the potential of modified TSEBT for canine CTCL, and preliminary results in four dogs reveal that it is well tolerated, with one patient having tumor control for more than 20 months [26]. Furthermore, a case report describing the use of orthovoltage radiation to treat the entire skin of a dog with CTCL supports the applicability of that skin-directed therapy [27]. Finally, radiation therapy can be successfully used to treat localized CTCL or to palliate the signs of painful or otherwise troublesome lesions, often leading to long-term local control even with bulky tumor-stage lesions (Fig. 2) [7,8].

DISEASE-MODIFYING AGENTS
Systemic Retinoids
Retinoids are natural or synthetic analogues of vitamin A that exert profound effects on the growth, maturation, and differentiation of many normal cell types in vitro and in vivo [28]. The systemic use of retinoids for CTCL in human patients, specifically the newer RXR-selective bexarotene, results in response rates approaching 45%, with a 20% complete response rate [7,8,15,16]. As a result of its favorable toxicity profile, bexarotene is often combined with other therapies in people, permitting superior response rates [15]. The main toxicities observed with bexarotene in human beings are hypertriglyceridemia, hypercholesterolemia, and hypothyroidism [15,16]. There are no published reports on the use of bexarotene in dogs with CTCL. First-generation retinoids generally bind to RARs and RXRs, occasionally with relative RAR selectivity [28]. The use of mixed synthetic retinoids, such as etretinate and isotretinoin, has been described in the veterinary literature, and an encouraging response rate

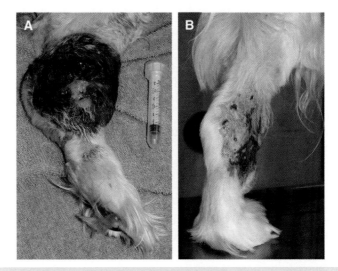

Fig. 2. Ulcerated and painful nodular CTCL lesion on the left hock of a 6-year-old female spayed Cocker Spaniel before (A) and 1 month after (B) three coarse fractions of megavoltage radiation therapy. This dog had disseminated tumor-stage CTCL treated with systemic drugs, and radiation therapy was successfully used on that lesion for palliative purposes only.

of 42% was reported in a study on 14 dogs with cutaneous lymphoma [4,5,20,28–31,32]. In addition, an unpublished study evaluated all known RAR and RXR isoforms (α, β, and γ) via immunohistochemistry and found all CTCL samples to be positive for various combinations, supporting the rationale use of retinoids for canine CTCL cases [33]. Retinoids remain an interesting option for canine CTCL, especially in light of nonoverlapping toxicity with standard cytotoxic chemotherapy. The two main disadvantages of retinoid therapy are the time lapse between initiation of therapy and observation of a clinical response when used alone (weeks to months) and the relatively high cost of the drug. When used to treat CTCL in dogs, isotretinoin is generally administered at 3 mg/kg orally in one daily dose or divided twice daily.

Denileukin Diftitox

A fusion toxin protein consisting of the interleukin (IL)-2 coding sequences combined with those for diphtheria toxin, denileukin diftitox ingeniously combines the T-cell targeting activity of IL-2 with the cytotoxic properties of diphtheria toxin A chain, leading to apoptosis of the target cell population [15]. In heavily treated human patients with intermediate- to advanced-stage CTCL, denileukin diftitox provided an overall response rate of 30%, with a 10% complete response rate [7,8,15,16]. The main toxicity of denileukin diftitox in people is a dose-dependent vascular leak syndrome, occurring to severe levels in up to 20% of treated patients [7,8,15,16]. IL-2 receptors have been identified on canine CTCL cells and may support the use of such targeted therapy in that species [34,35]. Nevertheless, this author is aware of anecdotal reports of severe and lethal systemic toxicity in two dogs with T-cell malignancies after denileukin diftitox infusions and cannot recommend its use until further research is conducted.

Fatty Acids

Supplementation with Ω-3 and Ω-6 fatty acids is not reported as an effective treatment modality for human CTCL. Clinical remissions were reported in 7 of 10 dogs after high-dose linoleate administration, however, specifically in the form of safflower oil [36,37]. This interesting low-toxicity approach awaits further larger prospective investigations alone and combined with other treatment modalities.

Cyclosporine

Although it seems conceivable that cyclosporine, a specific inhibitor of T-cell activation and intracellular signaling, may have activity against neoplastic T cells, limited studies have shown it to be ineffective in achieving clinical remission in human and canine patients with CTCL [38,39].

Interferons

Interferons (IFNs), including IFNα, IFNβ, and IFNγ, are biologic response modifiers with antiproliferative, cytotoxic, and immunomodulatory effects [15]. Of them, the use of recombinant IFNα has been best described, mainly for the palliative management of advanced or refractory CTCL in human beings, with complete response rates in the range of 10% to 25% [7,8,15,16]. Sporadic anecdotal reports point toward some efficacy of IFNα in the treatment of canine CTCL at a dosage of 1 to 1.5 million U/m^2 administered subcutaneously three times per week, but further controlled studies are warranted [40].

SYSTEMIC CHEMOTHERAPY

Canine CTCL is often diagnosed at a relatively late stage of the disease, with multifocal or disseminated plaque- or tumor-stage lesions. Consequently, the use of systemic chemotherapy has been most commonly recommended and described in the veterinary literature.

Single Agent
Corticosteroids

Because normal and neoplastic lymphocytes are sensitive to corticosteroids, with apoptosis resulting from their binding to nuclear receptors, this class of drugs has often been reported to provide some clinical improvement in canine CTCL patients in the form of palliative relief if not remission as such [4,5,14,17–19,21,32]. With corticosteroids as monotherapy, typically oral prednisone (0.5–2.0 mg/kg/d, generally starting higher and tapering), long-lived clinical responses are infrequent. Therefore, corticosteroids are most typically used in combination with cytotoxic chemotherapy agents.

Lomustine

Lomustine, also known as CCNU [1-(2-chloroethyl)-3-cyclohexyl-1-nitroso-urea], is a monofunctional alkylating agent of the nitrosourea family [41]. Growing interest in using lomustine for various canine and feline cancers has emerged in the last decade, fueled by relative low cost when compared with other systemic chemotherapy agents, good oral bioavailability, reasonable clinical efficacy, and relatively predictable toxicity. A study using lomustine monotherapy to treat resistant canine lymphoma described an overall response rate of 27%, which is comparable to that of other rescue chemotherapy protocols [41]. The main reported toxicity of lomustine chemotherapy is myelosuppression, especially in the form of neutropenia and thrombocytopenia, which can be severe at the higher end of the dose range [41]. Another reported side effect is hepatotoxicity. A study on 179 dogs receiving lomustine for various cancers reported an incidence of hepatotoxicity of 6.1%, with 7 of 11 dogs with hepatotoxicity dying of progressive liver failure [42]. In a study on 45 dogs with various cancers treated with lomustine by another group, liver toxicity, as defined by marked elevations in alanine aminotransferase levels after therapy, was observed in 51% of dogs [43]. Independent of the true incidence of liver toxicity or dose used, it is recommend to perform liver profiles and complete blood cell counts before every administration of lomustine in cancer-bearing dogs.

An initial pilot study describing the use of lomustine in seven dogs with cutaneous lymphoma, including five dogs with epitheliotropic lymphoma, reported that all dogs achieved complete remission, with durations ranging from 2 to 15 months [44]. The dosage used in that initial study was 50 mg/m^2 administered every 21 days until relapse. Two dogs with surgically resected lesions of epitheliotropic CTCL and treated with adjuvant lomustine had the longest remissions in that small study (7 and 15 months), whereas the two dogs with nonepitheliotropic cutaneous lymphoma had the shortest remissions (2 and 3 months) [44].

After the encouraging results of this pilot study, lomustine therapy has been used nearly routinely by veterinary oncologists and dermatologists to treat canine CTCL in recent years (Figs. 3 and 4). A retrospective study described 36 dogs with CTCL treated with lomustine, 19 of which had received other chemotherapeutic agents for their disease before lomustine therapy [45]. In that report, the median starting dose of lomustine was 70 mg/m^2 (7 dogs required dose reduction) and the median number of treatments administered was three. Twenty-eight (78%) of the 36 dogs achieved a measurable response, with 6 of them (16%) achieving complete remission, for an overall median duration of 106 days [45]. The main toxicities reported in this group of dogs included myelosuppression in 29% of dogs and liver enzyme elevations in 86% of dogs. Another recent retrospective study reported on the use of lomustine to treat CTCL in 46 dogs [46]. In that study, which included 2 dogs with Sézary syndrome and at least 7 dogs with confirmed nodal involvement, 32 dogs had received some form of therapy before lomustine, leaving 14 dogs with

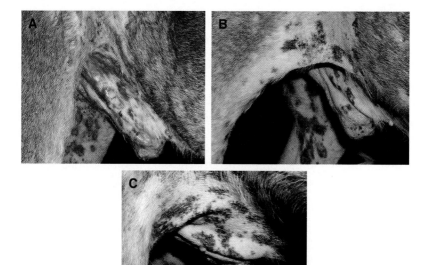

Fig. 3. Diffuse plaque-stage CTCL in a 10-year-old male castrated English Bulldog. Inguinal area lesions before (A) and after 21 days (B) and 42 days (C) of lomustine therapy. This dog achieved a complete clinical remission with disappearance of the active lesions, followed by hyperpigmentation and, eventually, hair regrowth.

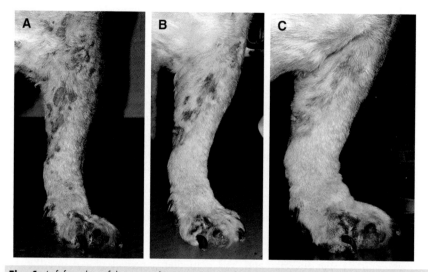

Fig. 4. Left front leg of the same dog as in Fig. 3, showing gradual improvement in the lesions from day 0 (A) to day 21 (B) and day 42 (C) after lomustine therapy.

chemonaive CTCL. The median dose of lomustine was 60 mg/m^2, and the median number of treatments administered was four [46]. Thirty-eight (83%) of the 46 dogs achieved a measurable response, with 15 of them (33%) achieving complete remission, for an overall median response duration of 86 days. Myelosuppression was reported in 21% of dogs, and liver enzyme elevation was reported in 42% of dogs [46]. In both studies, a number of dogs were concurrently receiving corticosteroids and, rarely, other chemotherapy drugs or disease-modifying agents. Collectively, the two recent retrospective studies on a total of 82 dogs with CTCL treated with lomustine at 60 to 70 mg/m^2 suggest an overall response rate of 80%, with 26% achieving complete remission, and a median response duration approaching 95 days [45,46]. These results demonstrate activity of lomustine chemotherapy for canine CTCL, but further research is warranted to evaluate combination protocols, standardize an optimal dosage, and evaluate efficacy when used for previously untreated CTCL.

Interestingly, although oral lomustine is used mainly for brain tumors and Hodgkin's disease in human beings, a search of the medical literature in English fails to reveal reports discussing its use in the management of CTCL, with the exception of an early study describing successful treatment with topical lomustine [47]. This comes as a relative surprise, because it is known that topical carmustine provides favorable response rates in early-stage disease, but a possible explanation may lie in the myelosuppressive properties of systemic lomustine in human beings [7,16]. Furthermore, a study demonstrated that neoplastic T lymphocytes of CTCL cell lines or collected from 26 human patients with clinical disease generally had low to undetectable levels of O^6-alkylguanine-DNA alkyltransferase (AGT), the main DNA repair enzyme responsible for cell resistance to certain alkylating agents, including lomustine [48,49]. A similar study evaluating AGT expression in canine cancers is underway and will attempt to predict the response of various cancers to drugs such as lomustine [50].

L-asparaginase

L-asparaginase (L-ASP) is an enzyme-purified from *Escherichia coli* that degrades circulating pools of L-asparagine. A nonessential amino acid, L-asparagine is synthesized by transamination of L-aspartic acid, with the amine group donated by glutamine and the reaction catalyzed by L-asparagine synthetase. The latter enzyme is constitutive in most tissues, but chemonaive malignant cells of lymphocytic lineage typically do not express it, making them susceptible to apoptosis when circulating pools of L-asparagine are depleted. A study evaluating pegylated L-ASP, a form of L-ASP encapsulated in polyethylene glycol for more favorable pharmacokinetic and toxicity profiles, reported that all 7 treated dogs with CTCL initially responded to the therapy, with improved clinical signs and appearance of the cutaneous lesions [51]. Although the dogs benefited from that therapy and had a median survival of 9.0 months, responses were partial and often short lived [51]. In that study, the dosage of pegylated L-ASP was 30 IU/kg of body weight (BW) administered intramuscularly or intraperitoneally once to twice weekly. Pegylated L-ASP is expensive, but free (nonpegylated) L-ASP, being generally well tolerated and not myelosuppressive per se, is often used in combination with other cytotoxic chemotherapy agents and remains a reasonable option to consider for patients with advanced disease or discomfort. In a recent retrospective study evaluating lomustine for canine CTCL, 5 of 46 dogs received at least one dose of L-ASP, generally at initiation of lomustine therapy [46]. The dose of nonpegylated L-ASP is 10,000 IU/m^2 or 400 IU/kg administered intramuscularly or subcutaneously 15 minutes after a 1-mg/kg intramuscular injection of diphenhydramine. The drug can be administered every 7 to 14 days or as needed to reinduce remission. The risk of allergic or anaphylactic reactions may increase with the number of doses previously administered and is highest when given via the intravenous route, which should be avoided.

Dacarbazine

Dacarbazine, or DTIC [(dimethyltriazeno) imidazole-carboxamide] is a nonclassic alkylating agent used mainly for the treatment of malignant melanoma, Hodgkin's disease, and sarcoma in human patients. A case report described durable complete clinical remission after three cycles of dacarbazine at 1000 mg/m^2 in a dog with CTCL and nodal involvement, supporting its potential role in the treatment of this condition [52]. Because low or undetectable AGT expression was demonstrated in human CTCL cells, and because that enzyme also confers resistance to dacarbazine and temozolomide, these drugs stand out as reasonable options for the disease [48,49]. Although the use of dacarbazine for people with CTCL is poorly described, temozolomide, an oral analogue of DTIC, has demonstrated activity in a few patients with advanced CTCL in initial trials, and further studies are ongoing [15].

Pegylated doxorubicin

Doxorubicin, an antitumor antibiotic, acts mainly by inhibiting topoisomerase II and is arguably the most versatile cytotoxic chemotherapy agent used, with known activity on a multitude of different cancers. A pegylated liposomal form of doxorubicin exists and has shown encouraging efficacy in pretreated or refractory advanced-stage CTCL in human beings [53–55]. Overall response rates as high as 88% have been reported in such patients, including a 44% complete response rate, with a tolerable toxicity profile, making pegylated doxorubicin an attractive therapeutic option in human patients with CTCL when compared with other systemic chemotherapeutic options [53–55]. Pegylated doxorubicin has been evaluated in dogs with various cancers, and of nine dogs with CTCL, there were three complete responses (median remission length of 90 days) and one partial response, for an overall response rate of 44% in that small group [56]. The average dose of pegylated doxorubicin for cancer-bearing dogs in that study was 1 mg/kg administered intravenously over 5 to 10 minutes every 3 weeks. Pegylated doxorubicin has the advantages of better pharmacokinetics, lower cardiac toxicity, and enhanced cytotoxicity to certain tumor cells [56]. Palmar-plantar erythrodysesthesia (PPES), also known as hand-foot syndrome, is a cutaneous reaction observed with pegylated doxorubicin administration in nearly 25% of treated dogs and can be dose limiting for many patients receiving the drug [56,57]. Concurrent administration of high doses of pyridoxine (vitamin B_6) helps to decrease the incidence and severity of PPES markedly, thereby limiting treatment delays or discontinuations [57]. The other main disadvantage impeding more common use of that drug is a hefty price tag, with the cost of pegylated doxorubicin per milligram currently approaching 30 times that of native doxorubicin.

Other single agents

Other single-agent chemotherapy drugs with reported efficacy in human patients with late-stage CTCL have included methotrexate, etoposide, bleomycin, vincristine, vinblastine, chlorambucil, cyclophosphamide, and native doxorubicin [7,8]. Complete responses are obtained in 15% to 30% of patients, and response durations are often short [7,8]. There are isolated reports of single-agent chemotherapy alone or combined with corticosteroids for the treatment of canine CTCL in the veterinary literature, but convincing evidence supporting specific agents is lacking [5,17,18,58]. Newer drugs with promising activity in people include temozolomide, purine analogues (fludarabine, pentostatin, and cladribine), and the pyrimidine analogue gemcitabine, with overall response rates of 20% to 60% [7,8,15]. Other than a recently published study on gemcitabine in dogs, the use of these novel chemotherapy agents remains to be reported in dogs with naturally occurring cancer [59].

Combination Chemotherapy Protocols

In human beings with advanced-stage CTCL, combination chemotherapy protocols do not seem to offer any advantage over single-agent therapy, with complete remission rates approaching 30% to 50% and responses often being short lived [7,8,15,16]. The most commonly reported combination protocols are cyclophosphamide, doxorubicin, vincristine, and prednisone (CHOP) and cyclophosphamide, vincristine, and prednisone (COP) [7,8,15]. Various combinations of prednisone, vincristine, and cyclophosphamide with or without doxorubicin have been reported in small series of canine CTCL cases, usually with moderate success and survival times averaging between 2 and 6 months [5,17,18,58,60,61]. Anecdotally, we have observed partial and complete responses at our institution on a few dogs with CTCL treated with CHOP, some of which had previously failed lomustine therapy (Fig. 5). Published observations from one investigator regarding a protocol combining cyclophosphamide, vincristine, cytosine arabinoside, and prednisone (COAP) described five of six dogs obtaining partial or complete remission lasting longer than 12 months on average and with a median survival greater than 399 days [62]. The same author reported on some dogs failing COAP but responding to doxorubicin-based protocols, such as CHOP [62]. Such observations are useful and should be a prelude to larger prospective studies using standardized protocols to define better the role of combination chemotherapy for specific disease stages of canine CTCL.

MULTIMODALITY AND SUPPORTIVE THERAPY

In general, combined modality therapy in human patients with CTCL does not seem to provide better overall survival times, although complete response rates are higher [15]. Nevertheless, it seems rational to consider combining various treatment modalities with nonoverlapping toxicities and to focus on improving or maintaining quality of life in patients with a chronic condition that is generally not curable. An example would be the combination of surgery or radiation therapy on localized lesions, followed by systemic therapy. Another example for advanced disseminated disease would be to consider skin-directed therapy (electron beam or topical drugs) together with systemic therapy in the form of

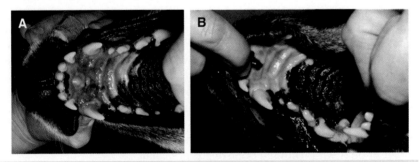

Fig. 5. Oral CTCL lesion in a 14-year-old male castrated German Shepherd Dog before (A) and 3 months after (B) institution of a CHOP-like protocol. This dog had previously failed lomustine therapy and lived 13 months after initial diagnosis, eventually progressing to disseminated cutaneous nodular disease with lymph node involvement.

chemotherapy (including corticosteroids), retinoids, and essential fatty acid supplements. Prospective studies evaluating various combinations on large numbers of dogs with CTCL could be difficult to conduct, however, because of the relative rarity of the condition in the first place.

Supportive and symptomatic therapy is also important and includes the use of antibiotics when secondary bacterial infection is suspected or confirmed [63] and the use of analgesics as needed when pain or discomfort is suspected or identified [64,65].

OTHER THERAPIES IN HUMAN BEINGS

Various other therapies are in clinical trials or currently being used for human patients with CTCL. Extracorporeal photophoresis involves the delivering of PUVA on the patient's white blood cells with an extracorporeal technique after collection through leukapheresis [7,8,15,16]. Various monoclonal antibodies (mAbs), such as the T101 Y 90 conjugate (murine mAb targeting the CD5 surface antigen, coupled to the isotope yttrium-90), a chimeric anti-CD4 mAb, and alemtuzumab (humanized mAb targeting the CD52 surface antigen), are being investigated and have shown some efficacy, although more research is clearly needed [15]. Humanized or chimeric mAbs have limited potential for application in dogs because of the formation of neutralizing canine antihuman antibodies. Additionally, certain cytokines, including IL-2 and IL-12, have demonstrated efficacy, although the side-effect profile, especially with systemic IL-2 administration, precludes more widespread use in human patients [15,16]. Finally, autologous and allogeneic stem cell transplantation has been used for advanced CTCL unresponsive to standard therapy in human patients [15,16]. Allogeneic transplantation carries more risk of complications, including graft-versus-host disease, but generally provides longer lasting remissions [15,16].

SUMMARY

Canine CTCL is an uncommon variant of lymphoma that may benefit from a variety of therapies. Recent advances in the veterinary oncology field support the use of the oral alkylator lomustine as one of the therapeutic tools benefiting canine CTCL patients, whereas ongoing and future clinical research should aim to expand and optimize treatment options. It is our experience that the overall prognosis of dogs with CTCL is difficult to establish and likely depends on the stage of disease at diagnosis, therapeutic choice, and response to therapy, with survival times varying from a few weeks to longer than 18 months. Dogs diagnosed with early disease (patch or plaque stage) may survive for more than 8 to 12 months with appropriate treatment, whereas dogs with more advanced disease (tumor or disseminated stage) may only live 3 to 6 months despite good initial responses to therapy. The key to better management of CTCL, and possibly improved prognosis, therefore lies in early definitive diagnosis through the biopsy of any suspect lesions unresponsive to empiric therapy, the implementation of a therapy with proven value and acceptable toxicity, and adequate supportive care to maintain or improve the patient's quality of life.

References

[1] Moore PF, Olivry T, Naydan D. Canine cutaneous epitheliotropic lymphoma (mycosis fungoides) is a proliferative disorder of CD8+ T cells. Am J Pathol 1994;144(2):421–9.

[2] Fournel-Fleury C, Magnol JP, Bricaire P, et al. Cytohistological and immunological classification of canine malignant lymphomas: comparison with human non-Hodgkin's lymphomas. J Comp Pathol 1997;117(1):35–59.

[3] Fournel Fleury C, Ponce F, Felman P, et al. Canine T-cell lymphomas: a morphological, immunological, and clinical study of 46 new cases. Vet Pathol 2002;39:92–109.

[4] Moore PF, Olivry T. Cutaneous lymphomas in companion animals. Clin Dermatol 1994;12: 499–505.

[5] Beale KM, Bolon B. Canine cutaneous lymphosarcoma: epitheliotropic and non-epitheliotropic, a retrospective study. In: Ihrke PJ, Mason IS, White SD, editors. Advances in veterinary dermatology, vol. 2. New York: Pergamon Press; 1993. p. 273–84.

[6] Valli VE, Jacobs RM, Parodi AL, et al. Cutaneous epitheliotropic lymphoma. In: Histological classification of hematopoietic tumors of domestic animals. Washington (DC): Armed Forces Institute of Pathology; 2002. p. 42–3.

[7] Hoppe RT, Harvell JD, Kim YH. Mycosis fungoides. In: Mauch PM, Armitage JO, Harris NL, et al, editors. Non-Hodgkin's lymphomas. Philadelphia: Lippincott Williams & Wilkins; 2004. p. 307–31.

[8] Wilson LD, Jones GW, Kacinski BM, et al. Cutaneous T-cell lymphomas. In: DeVita VT Jr, Hellman S, Rosenberg SA, editors. Cancer: principles and practice of oncology. 6th edition. Philadelphia: JB Lippincott; 2001. p. 2316–30.

[9] El Shabrawi-Caelen L, Cerroni L, Medeiros LJ, et al. Hypopigmented mycosis fungoides: frequent expression of a CD8+ T-cell phenotype. Am J Surg Pathol 2002;26(4):450–7.

[10] Whittam LR, Calonje E, Orchard G, et al. CD8-positive juvenile onset mycosis fungoides: an immunohistochemical and genotypic analysis of six cases. Br J Dermatol 2000;143(6): 1199–204.

[11] Ben-Amitai D, Michael D, Feinmesser M, et al. Juvenile mycosis fungoides diagnosed before 18 years of age. Acta Derm Venereol 2003;83(6):451–6.

[12] Berti E, Tomasini D, Vermeer MH, et al. Primary cutaneous CD8-positive epidermotropic T cell lymphomas: a distinct clinicopathological entity with an aggressive clinical behavior. Am J Pathol 1999;155(2):483–92.

[13] Goldschmidt MH, Shofer FS. Cutaneous lymphosarcoma. In: Skin tumors of the dog and cat. Oxford: Butterworth-Heinmann; 1992. p. 252–64.

[14] Angus JC, de Lorimier LP. Lymphohistiocytic neoplasms. In: Campbell KL, editor. Small animal dermatology secrets. Philadelphia: Hanley & Belfus; 2004. p. 425–42.

[15] Apisarnthanarax N, Talpur R, Duvic M. Treatment of cutaneous T-cell lymphoma. Am J Clin Dermatol 2002;3(3):193–215.

[16] Knobler E. Current management strategies for cutaneous T-cell lymphoma. Clin Dermatol 2004;22:197–208.

[17] Wilcock BP, Yager JA. The behavior or epidermotropic lymphoma in twenty-five dogs. Can Vet J 1989;30(9):754–6.

[18] Walton DK. Canine epidermotropic lymphoma (mycosis fungoides and pagetoid reticulosis). In: Kirk RW, editor. Current veterinary therapy IX. Philadelphia: WB Saunders; 1986. p. 609–14.

[19] Rosenthal RC, MacEwen EG. Treatment of lymphoma in dogs. J Am Vet Med Assoc 1990;196(5):774–81.

[20] Donaldson D, Day MJ. Epitheliotropic lymphoma (mycosis fungoides) presenting as blepharoconjunctivitis in an Irish setter. J Small Anim Pract 2000;41(7):317–20.

[21] Miller WH Jr. Canine cutaneous lymphoma. In: Kirk RW, editor. Current veterinary therapy VII. Philadelphia: WB Saunders; 1980. p. 493–5.

[22] Deeths MJ, Chapman JT, Dellavalle RP, et al. Treatment of patch and plaque stage mycosis fungoides with imiquimod 5% cream. J Am Acad Dermatol 2005;52:275–80.

[23] Barber LG. Imidazoquinolines: immunotherapy for cutaneous viral and neoplastic lesions. Vet Cancer Soc Newsletter 2005;29(3):7–11.

[24] Lucroy MD. Photodynamic therapy for companion animals with cancer. Vet Clin North Am Small Anim Pract 2002;32(3):693–702.

[25] Frimberger AE, Moore AS, Cincotta L, et al. Photodynamic therapy of naturally occurring tumors in animals using a novel benzophenothiazine photosensitizer. Clin Cancer Res 1998;4(9):2207–18.

[26] Prescott DM, Gordon J. Total skin electron beam irradiation for generalized cutaneous lymphoma [abstract]. In: Proceedings of the 24th Annual Conference of the Veterinary Cancer Society. Kansas City (MO); 2004. p. 50.

[27] DeBoer DJ, Turrel JM, Moore PF. Mycosis fungoides in a dog: demonstration of T-cell specificity and response to radiotherapy. J Am Anim Hosp Assoc 1990;26(6):566–72.

[28] Souza CHM, Kitchell BE. The role of retinoids in cancer therapy: a literature review. Vet Cancer Soc Newsletter 2002;26(4):6–8.

[29] White SD, Rosychuk RAW, Scott KV, et al. Use of isotretinoin and etretinate for the treatment of benign cutaneous neoplasia and cutaneous lymphoma in dogs. J Am Vet Med Assoc 1993;202(3):387–91.

[30] Power HT, Ihrke PJ. Synthetic retinoids in veterinary dermatology. Vet Clin North Am Small Anim Pract 1990;20:1525–39.

[31] Kwochka KW. Retinoids in dermatology. In: Kirk RW, editor. Current veterinary therapy X. Philadelphia: WB Saunders; 1989. p. 553–9.

[32] Bouchard H. Epitheliotropic lymphoma in a dog. Can Vet J 2000;41(8):628–30.

[33] Souza CHM, Valli VE, Toledo-Piza E, et al. Detection of retinoid receptors in canine cutaneous lymphoma [abstract]. In: Proceedings of the 23rd Annual Conference of the Veterinary Cancer Society. Madison (WI): 2003. p. 1.

[34] Helfand SC, Modiano JF, Moore PF, et al. Functional interleukin-2 receptors are expressed on natural killer-like leukemic cells from a dog with cutaneous lymphoma. Blood 1995;86(2):636–45.

[35] Dickerson EB, Fosmire S, Padilla ML, et al. Potential to target dysregulated interleukin-2 receptor expression in canine lymphoid and hematopoietic malignancies as a model for human cancer. J Immunother 2002;25(1):36–45.

[36] Iwamoto KS, Bennett LR, Norman A, et al. Linoleate produces remission in canine mycosis fungoides. Cancer Lett 1992;64:17–22.

[37] Petersen A, Wood S, Rosser E. The use of safflower oil for the treatment of mycosis fungoides in two dogs [abstract]. In: Proceedings of the 15th Annual Meeting of the American Academy of Veterinary Dermatology (concurrent sessions). Maui (HI):1999. p. 49–50.

[38] Cooper DL, Braverman IM, Sarris AH, et al. Cyclosporine treatment of refractory T-cell lymphomas. Cancer 1993;71(7):2335–41.

[39] Rosenkrantz WS, Griffin CE, Barr RJ. Clinical evaluation of cyclosporine in animal models with cutaneous immune-mediated disease and epitheliotropic lymphoma. J Am Anim Hosp Assoc 1989;25(4):377–84.

[40] White SD. Newly introduced drugs in veterinary dermatology [abstract]. In: Proceedings of the Third World Congress of Veterinary Dermatology. Edinburgh (UK); 1996. p. 84.

[41] Moore AS, London CA, Wood CA, et al. Lomustine (CCNU) for the treatment of resistant lymphoma in dogs. J Vet Intern Med 1999;13(5):395–8.

[42] Kristal O, Rassnick KM, Gliatto JM, et al. Hepatotoxicity associated with CCNU (lomustine) chemotherapy in dogs. J Vet Intern Med 2004;18(1):75–80.

[43] Lara A, Kisseberth WC, Couto CG. Hepatotoxicity associated with lomustine treatment in dogs with cancer [abstract]. In: Proceedings of the 24th Annual Conference of the Veterinary Cancer Society. Kansas City (MO): 2004. p. 14.

[44] Graham JC, Myers RK. Pilot study on the use of lomustine (CCNU) for the treatment of cutaneous lymphoma in dogs [abstract 125]. In: Proceedings of the 17th Annual Forum of the College of Veterinary Internal Medicine. Chicago: 1999. p. 723.

[45] Williams LE, Rassnick KM, Power HT, et al. CCNU in the treatment of canine epitheliotropic lymphoma. J Vet Intern Med 2006, in press.

[46] Risbon RE, Burgess K, Skorupski K, et.al. CCNU (lomustine) for cutaneous epitheliotropic lymphoma: a retrospective study of 46 dogs (1999–2004) [abstract]. In: Proceedings of the 24th Annual Conference of the Veterinary Cancer Society. Kansas City (MO): 2004. p. 15.

[47] Zackheim HS, Epstein EH. Treatment of mycosis fungoides with topical nitrosourea compounds: further studies. Arch Dermatol 1975;111(12):1564–70.

[48] Dolan ME, McRae BL, Ferries-Rowe E, et al. O^6-alkylguanine-DNA alkyltransferase in cutaneous T-cell lymphoma: implication for treatment with alkylating agents. Clin Cancer Res 1999;5:2059–64.

[49] Baer JC, Freeman AA, Newlands ES, et al. Depletion of O6-alkylguanine-DNA alkyltransferase correlates with potentiation of temozolomide and CCNU toxicity in human tumour cells. Br J Cancer 1993;67(6):1299–302.

[50] Skorupski K, Casal M, O'Malley T, et al. Identification of canine O^6-alkylguanine-DNA alkyltransferase for prediction of response to nitrosourea chemotherapy [abstract]. In: Proceedings of the 24th Annual Conference of the Veterinary Cancer Society. Kansas City (MO): 2004. p. 34.

[51] Moriello KA, MacEwen EG, Schultz KT. PEG-L-asparaginase in the treatment of canine epitheliotropic lymphoma and histiocytic proliferation dermatitis. In: Ihrke PJ, Mason IS, White SD, editors. Advances in veterinary dermatology, vol. 2. Oxford, United Kingdom: Pergamon Press; 1993. p. 293–9.

[52] Lemarié SL, Eddlestone SM. Treatment of cutaneous T-cell lymphoma with dacarbazine in a dog. Vet Dermatol 1997;8:41–6.

[53] Wollina U, Graefe T, Karte K. Treatment of relapsing or recalcitrant cutaneous T-cell lymphoma with pegylated liposomal doxorubicin. J Am Acad Dermatol 2000;42:40–6.

[54] Wollina U, Dummer R, Brockmeyer NH, et al. Multicenter study of pegylated liposomal doxorubicin in patients with cutaneous T-cell lymphoma. Cancer 2003;98:993–1001.

[55] Di Lorenzo G, Di Trolio R, Delfino M, et al. Pegylated liposomal doxorubicin in stage IVB mycosis fungoides. Br J Dermatol 2005;153:183–5.

[56] Vail DM, Kravis LD, Cooley AJ, et al. Preclinical trial of doxorubicin entrapped in sterically stabilized liposomes in dogs with spontaneously arising malignant tumors. Cancer Chemother Pharmacol 1997;39(5):410–6.

[57] Vail DM, Chun R, Thamm DH, et al. Efficacy of pyridoxine to ameliorate the cutaneous toxicity associated with doxorubicin containing pegylated (Stealth) liposomes: a randomized, double-blind clinical trial using a canine model. Clin Cancer Res 1998;4:1567–71.

[58] McKeever PJ, Grindem CB, Stevens JB, et al. Canine cutaneous lymphoma. J Am Vet Med Assoc 1982;180(5):531–6.

[59] Kosarek CE, Kisseberth WC, Gallant SL, et al. Clinical evaluation of gemcitabine in dogs with spontaneously occurring malignancies. J Vet Intern Med 2005;19(1):81–6.

[60] Brown NO, Nesbitt GB, Patnaik AK, et al. Cutaneous lymphosarcoma in the dog: a disease with variable clinical and histologic manifestations. J Am Anim Hosp Assoc 1980;16: 565–72.

[61] Hamilton TA, Cook JR Jr, Braund KG, et al. Vincristine-induced peripheral neuropathy in a dog. J Am Vet Med Assoc 1991;198(4):635–8.

[62] Couto GC. Cutaneous lymphoma. In: Campfield WW, editor. Proceedings of the 11th Kal Kan Symposium. Vernon (CA): Kal Kan Foods, Inc., 1987. p. 71–7.

[63] Tsambiras PE, Patel S, Greene JN, et al. Infectious complications of cutaneous T-cell lymphoma. Cancer Control 2001;8(2):185–8.

[64] Devulder J, Lambert J, Naeyaert JM. Gabapentin for pain control in cancer patients' wound dressing care. J Pain Symptom Manage 2001;22(1):622–6.

[65] Hata T, Aikoh T, Hirokawa M, et al. Mycosis fungoides with involvement of the oral mucosa. Int J Oral Maxillofac Surg 1998;27(2):127–8.

Update on Canine Demodicosis

Kinga Gortel, DVM, MS

Animal Dermatology Clinic, 13286 Fiji Way, Marina del Rey, CA 90292, USA

D
emodicosis is a common and often serious skin disease of the dog. The understanding of demodicosis, the inflammatory skin disease caused by the presence of larger than normal numbers of *Demodex* mites in the skin, has changed in recent years. The prognosis for patients with generalized disease has improved in the past decade. Furthermore, mites other than *Demodex canis* have been demonstrated in canine demodicosis. Advances in clarifying the role of the immune system in the disease have also been made. Perhaps the most important progress, however, has been made in the treatment of demodicosis in dogs.

DEMODEX MITES

Most healthy dogs are thought to possess *D canis* mites as part of their normal cutaneous flora. The mites are transmitted to neonates from the bitch within 2 to 3 days of birth. They feed on skin cells, sebum, and epidermal debris and spend their entire life cycle on the host. Mite numbers are kept at relatively low numbers by the host, and it is difficult to demonstrate *Demodex* mites in the skin of most healthy dogs [1]. The life cycle of *D canis* consists of four stages: a fusiform egg, a six-legged larva, an eight-legged nymph, and an eight-legged adult [1].

In addition to *D canis*, two less common species of *Demodex* mites have been reported in the dog. This is not surprising, because many mammals harbor more than one species of *Demodex* mite.

A short-bodied "stubby" *Demodex* mite has been reported to coinfect the skin of some dogs with *D canis*. It measures approximately 50% the length of the *D canis* female mite and may reside in the stratum corneum rather than within hair follicles [2–4]. There are no distinguishing features of the history or clinical signs specific to this mite [2]. It is likely that this mite may be missed on routine skin scrapings because it is found with the more ubiquitous *D canis*.

Demodex injai is a large-bodied mite whose adults, nymphs, larvae, and eggs are of greater size than those of *D canis*. Adult male *D injai* mites (361 µm long) are more than two times the length of *D canis* male mites (168 µm long), and the

E-mail address: kgortel@hotmail.com

0195-5616/06/$ – see front matter
doi:10.1016/j.cvsm.2005.09.003

adult female mites (334 μm long) are approximately 50% longer than the *D canis* female mites (224 μm long) [5]. This mite seems to show a preference for the dorsal trunk of adult dogs and histologically seems to inhabit the hair follicles and sebaceous ducts. Terrier breeds and their crosses, particularly West Highland White terriers, were overrepresented in one study [6]. Excessive greasiness in affected skin is a common clinical sign [6]. This mite can be found alone [7], although coinfection with *D canis* is possible [5]. *D injai* may be underdiagnosed because of its unusual presentation and the potential for low numbers of mites to be found on skin scrapings. In one report of eight cases, none were suspected of having demodicosis at referral [6].

CLINICAL DISEASE

Infection with *Demodex* mites is typically described as localized or generalized demodicosis. Although there are no uniformly accepted criteria for differentiating one form from the other, generalized demodicosis usually refers to infection of an entire body region, complete involvement of two or more feet, or more than six lesions [1,8].

Localized demodicosis usually consists of one to several small, erythematous, scaly, and often hyperpigmented areas of alopecia, most commonly on the face and forelegs (Fig. 1). Pruritus in demodicosis is variable but is more severe when secondary pyoderma is present. Most cases occur in young dogs (3–6 months of age) and resolve without treatment [1]. Progression to generalized disease is rare. A less common form of localized disease is demodicosis limited to the ear canals, which is associated with a ceruminous otitis externa and usually requires therapy [1].

Generalized demodicosis usually starts in dogs less than 18 months of age. Adult dogs (older than 4 years of age) develop the disease less frequently. The lesions may be similar to those of localized demodicosis, but they are usually more severe and are complicated by secondary pyoderma. Cutaneous changes in young and older patients include comedones, papules, pustules,

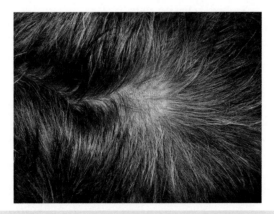

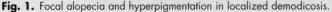

Fig. 1. Focal alopecia and hyperpigmentation in localized demodicosis.

follicular casts, plaques, crusts, edema, and deep folliculitis and furunculosis [8]. Peripheral lymphadenopathy is common. Pain, pruritus, and malaise may be present and can be severe enough for owners to elect to euthanize affected dogs. Secondary infection, often with *Staphylococcus intermedius*, is usually present and variably severe. In juvenile- (Figs. 2 and 3) and adult-onset generalized demodicosis (Fig. 4), involvement of the feet (pododemodicosis) is common and requires longer treatment periods to resolve [9]. It is suspected that in the adult-onset patients, concurrent immunosuppressive factors may be present to allow the previously controlled mites to proliferate excessively. Identification and control of these factors, which include hyperadrenocorticism (spontaneous or iatrogenic), hypothyroidism, heartworm disease, leishmaniasis, and neoplasia, are beneficial but not always critical to the successful treatment of the disease [1,9,10]. Administration of corticosteroids before the onset of generalized demodicosis was identified most often as an underlying cause for demodicosis in one study [9]. The role of these potentially immunosuppressive factors, and whether they are truly underlying the development of the disease or simply existing concurrently with it, is not well understood.

PATHOGENESIS

Purebred dogs seem to be at increased risk of developing the juvenile- and adult-onset forms of the disease. The breeds listed to be predisposed vary among reports. A hereditary predisposition is likely, with certain litters containing most or all puppies affected. An autosomal recessive mode of inheritance has been proposed based on limited numbers of kennels [1]. In addition to breed, other factors predisposing to demodicosis include age, poor nutrition, estrus, parturition, stress, endoparasites, and debilitating diseases [1].

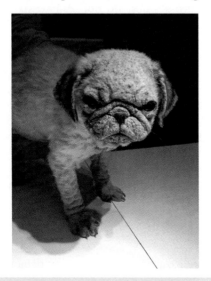

Fig. 2. Young pug with juvenile-onset generalized demodicosis.
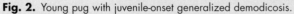

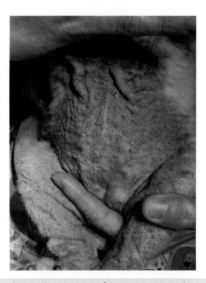

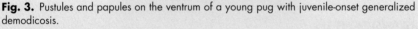

Fig. 3. Pustules and papules on the ventrum of a young pug with juvenile-onset generalized demodicosis.

Although it seems that the immune system is crucial in keeping mite numbers low in normal dogs, the contribution of the immune system in allowing the development of demodicosis is still poorly understood. Puppies that exhibit demodicosis do not seem to suffer from other symptoms of immune dysfunction. Furthermore, although some dogs treated with immunosuppressive agents develop demodicosis, most do not. A mite-specific immunoincompetence of variable severity may explain these differences [1]. Dogs with chronic generalized demodicosis are believed to possess a mite-specific deficiency of T-lymphocyte function. The deficiency may be exaggerated by humoral factors associated with concurrent pyoderma and increased mite numbers. Several studies have demonstrated decreased in vitro lymphocyte blastogenesis responses in dogs with generalized demodicosis compared with normal dogs. A decreased interleukin-2 response seen in dogs with juvenile-onset generalized demodicosis may indicate that the abnormal immune response in these patients is related to an irregularity in T helper cell function [11]. Our understanding of the immune factors involved in this disease is far from complete.

Because genetic factors are strongly suspected to play a major role in the disease, dogs with generalized demodicosis, their siblings, and their parents should not be bred.

DIAGNOSIS

The diagnosis of demodicosis is usually made by demonstrating the mites on deep skin scrapings. Although *Demodex* mites are part of the normal flora of the canine skin, their numbers are low and it is rare to find mites unless

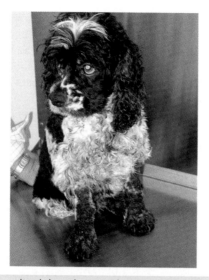

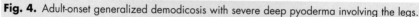

Fig. 4. Adult-onset generalized demodicosis with severe deep pyoderma involving the legs.

they are excessively proliferating. The finding of low numbers of mites on a skin scraping should not be ignored; rather, additional scrapings should be collected. The diagnosis of demodicosis is supported by the presence of large numbers of mites or a large proportion of immature forms of the mite [1].

Skin scrapings require a microscope, a microscope slide, mineral oil, and a scraping instrument. Scraping instruments include number 10 scalpel blades and curets. A dull scalpel blade or curet can be reused for scrapings to reduce the chance of injury to the operator or patient. Skin scrapings can be performed quickly and easily on most dogs, although some patients require sedation for this procedure. Affected skin is squeezed before or during the scraping to extrude the mites from the hair follicles, and skin scrapings must be deep enough to cause capillary bleeding. A small amount of mineral oil may be dropped on the skin or on the scraping instrument to trap the material for examination. The number of sites to be scraped depends on the patient, ranging from one site if only one lesion is present to three or more sites for the diagnosis and monitoring of generalized disease.

The examination of scraped material should be thorough and methodic. Several scrapings may be combined on one slide for ease of examination. If droplets of blood are not observed within the scraped material, the scrapings may not have been of adequate depth. A coverslip placed over the scraped material greatly eases examination of the scraping, and lowering the condenser makes the mites easier to find as a result of increased contrast.

Skin scrapings should be evaluated for the approximate numbers of mites, which may be assigned a value (eg, 0–4+). An approximation of the proportion of immature forms to adult mites is also useful, particularly for monitoring during therapy. The approximate proportion of mites that seem to be alive (moving) should also be recorded. Most patients present with a high proportion of immature and live mites at initial presentation. Continuing to find a high proportion of live immature mites during therapy should warrant a change in the type or intensity of treatment. Finding dead mites or even parts of mites on skin scrapings should be considered a positive scraping for the purposes of monitoring therapy and indicates the need for continuing treatment of the patient.

An additional technique that is useful for the diagnosis of some patients with demodicosis is microscopic examination of plucked hairs. This technique is particularly well suited to sensitive or delicate areas, such as the feet and periocular skin, or to patients that are difficult to restrain (Fig. 5). Hair plucks should also be examined before sedation in patients that do not allow skin scrapings because of temperament or pain. With this technique, hair is plucked from affected skin and examined under mineral oil and a coverslip. Mites can often be seen within the follicular keratin. Because this technique is likely less sensitive than skin scrapings, it should not be used to rule out the diagnosis of demodicosis or to assess an end point of therapy.

It is not uncommon for veterinary dermatologists to examine patients with demodicosis in which the diagnosis has not been made before referral. Most commonly, skin scrapings have not been performed on these patients. It is imperative not to overlook this simple diagnostic test, particularly in patients with chronic skin disease.

Demodicosis is occasionally diagnosed by histopathologic examination. If a skin scraping has not been performed before a biopsy, this more invasive diagnostic procedure may be unnecessary. Histopathologic examination is an appropriate diagnostic test, however, if demodicosis is suspected but skin scrapings have been negative. This is particularly common in patients with chronic

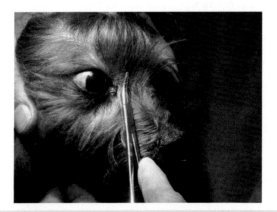

Fig. 5. Hair plucks may be used to demonstrate *Demodex* mites in areas that are difficult to skin scrape.

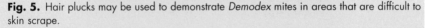

scarred lesions, such as those of pododemodicosis. A biopsy is also appropriate if the demodicosis has been diagnosed but the appearance of the skin suggests a concurrent dermatopathy, such as calcinosis cutis or cutaneous lymphoma. Shar Pei dogs are also reported to be more difficult to skin scrape successfully and may require a biopsy to make a diagnosis [1].

Owners of dogs with juvenile-onset generalized demodicosis should be questioned about recent or ongoing stressors, including inadequate nutrition, surgery and anesthesia, boarding, estrus (female dogs), and internal or external parasitism. Routine clinical laboratory testing is not useful in most young dogs with demodicosis but should be considered in patients with severe disease. In older dogs, a search for concurrent or underlying sources of immune suppression may be more fruitful. Identification and elimination of these factors are helpful for the eventual resolution of the disease. Particular emphasis should be placed on a thorough drug history, including any possible oral, topical, or injectable corticosteroids. Routine clinical laboratory testing, including thyroid hormone evaluation, should be performed. It is important to consider that thyroid hormone concentrations may be suppressed by the presence of severe inflammatory disease, various medications, or other potentially immunosuppressive conditions (eg, hyperadrenocorticism). The possibility of hyperadrenocorticism and neoplasia should be considered in adult dogs with generalized demodicosis. Some veterinarians recommend repeating diagnostic testing periodically in case demodicosis is an early symptom of yet undiagnosed disease.

TREATMENT
Localized Demodicosis
Localized demodicosis does not require treatment because it can be expected to resolve spontaneously within 6 to 8 weeks [1]. The application of miticidal treatment in cases of localized disease does not allow a determination of which patients may progress to generalized disease, and this determination is important for dogs who originate from breeding programs. There is also no evidence that treatment actually prevents the disease from becoming generalized [1]. Topical therapy with an antimicrobial agent, such as mupirocin ointment or benzoyl peroxide gel, may be prescribed. Owners should be informed that lesions can be expected to worsen before improving. The general health of the dog should also be assessed at this time to ensure that any factors capable of suppressing the immune system are controlled.

Generalized Demodicosis
Generalized demodicosis is a serious disease that can sometimes be life threatening. Owners should know that treatment of this condition can be lengthy and expensive. Premature discontinuation of therapy is a leading cause of treatment failure; thus, owners must be informed that continuation of treatment for a period past the resolution of clinical signs is critical to ensuring success. Not all patients with generalized demodicosis require miticidal therapy. Because

dogs less than 1 year of age may recover spontaneously, observation with repeated skin scrapings over 4 to 6 weeks is a reasonable approach to young dogs with mild generalized disease. If mite numbers increase or the condition worsens, miticidal therapy should be initiated [1].

The general health of the patient should be assessed and addressed when generalized demodicosis is diagnosed. This is particularly critical for patients with adult-onset disease. Any concurrent or suspected underlying diseases should be treated. Immunosuppressive medications should be stopped whenever possible.

Most dogs with generalized demodicosis suffer from secondary superficial or deep pyoderma. The bacterial infection, particularly if it is deep, increases the pruritus, pain, and malaise of affected patients. Long courses of oral antibiotics, often 6 weeks or more, are needed. Impression smears from the affected skin usually confirm the presence of bacteria. *S intermedius* is the most common bacterium involved; thus, good antistaphylococcal antibiotics are almost always appropriate. If rods predominate, however, culture and susceptibility testing is indicated to guide antimicrobial therapy.

Therapy for generalized demodicosis must be monitored by the clinical and parasitologic responses. Skin scrapings are usually repeated every 2 to 4 weeks. A parasitologic cure means skin scrapings that are negative for mites of any stage, including dead mites or mite segments. At least four scrapings should be collected from previously affected areas to declare a parasitologic cure [1]. Treatment should be continued until two consecutive skin scrapings are negative. In chronic cases, it is prudent to continue therapy for an additional 4 weeks past the two negative scrapings. A patient can be declared cured of the disease if there has been no relapse within 12 months of the cessation of therapy.

Anesthesia and surgery are potent stressors and may exacerbate or precipitate relapses of the demodicosis. Unfortunately, many patients with generalized disease are young dogs in need of surgical sterilization. Elective surgery should be postponed until secondary pyoderma is well controlled so as to avoid surgical complications. Waiting until skin scrapings are negative for mites, however, may not prudent. Timely sterilization prevents exacerbation of demodicosis associated with estrus. It also ensures that affected dogs are not inadvertently or deliberately bred. Finally, sterilization after therapy is complete may result in a relapse, because the patient is not protected by miticidal treatment.

Numerous studies have been published evaluating miticidal treatment protocols for generalized demodicosis. A recent evidence-based review of these studies has been published [8]. The efficacy of various treatments varies tremendously among studies, and this variability is increased by the inclusion of juvenile- and adult-onset cases as well as by inadequate follow-up in some studies. The evidence-based review found good evidence for recommending the following treatments for generalized demodicosis: amitraz (0.025%–0.05% dips every 7–14 days), ivermectin (300–600 µg/kg orally daily), milbemycin oxime (2 mg/kg orally daily), and moxidectin (400 µg/kg orally daily) [8].

Amitraz

Amitraz is the only product currently licensed in the United States and Canada for the treatment of generalized demodicosis. Amitraz is an acaricide and insecticide that inhibits monoamine oxidase and prostaglandin synthesis. It is also an α_2-adrenergic agonist [12]. It is licensed for use as a 0.025% dip every 14 days in dogs older than 4 months of age [13]. Some dogs cannot be cured with this protocol, so a number of variations using a higher concentration or dipping frequency have been studied. Because amitraz is an Environmental Protection Agency (EPA)–registered pesticide, however, it is a violation of federal law to use it in a manner inconsistent with its labeling. Although using the product more frequently or at higher concentrations can increase the likelihood of a cure, the other treatment options, such as the use of macrocyclic lactones, may be preferable to the extralabel use of amitraz [1].

Amitraz is applied as a dip to normal and affected skin. For best results, the hair should be clipped in medium- and long-haired dogs. Skin contact is improved by shampooing immediately before the dip or the day before administration. Benzoyl peroxide shampoo is used for its follicular-flushing activity. Crusts should be removed whenever possible. The patient must not get wet between applications of the dip. In patients with severe deep pyoderma, treatment of the bacterial infection using antibiotics and shampoos is advisable before the use of the dip [13]. The manufacturer recommends dips every 14 days until two successive skin scrapings demonstrate no live mites. It is imperative, however, that the dips be continued until the skin scrapings are negative for all mites as outlined previously.

Because amitraz is a monoamine oxidase inhibitor and an α_2-adrenergic agonist [12], there is concern for toxicity in the patient and the handler. It is not uncommon for owners to report depression and sleepiness in their pet for 24 to 48 hours after a dip. Close observation of the dog for several hours after a dip is recommended to observe for signs of toxicity, which are usually attributable to its α_2-adrenergic activity and include marked sedation, bradycardia, decreased temperature, and hyperglycemia [14]. Toxicity can be counteracted by the use of the α_2 antagonists atipamezole or yohimbine, and patients with a history of adverse reactions may be premedicated with these drugs. Low doses of atipamezole (50 µg/kg administered intramuscularly) were found to reverse symptoms of toxicity within 10 minutes of intramuscular injection [14]. Small dogs are thought to be at greater risk for development of side effects, and it has been recommended that they be dipped with a half-strength solution. Diabetic dogs are also a concern because of the potential for hyperglycemia [13].

Studies reporting the efficacy of amitraz treatment vary widely in the reported success rates. An evidence-based review of a number of studies of the use of amitraz for generalized demodicosis showed treatment success ranging from 0% to 100% but, overall, found good evidence for recommending amitraz (0.025%–0.05% every 7–14 days). Increasing the concentration and frequency is associated with a higher success rate [15] and may be effective in patients that fail conventional therapy. These off-label protocols include the use of amitraz at 0.05% to 0.1% once weekly, 0.125% amitraz on alternating halves of the body, and even 1.25% amitraz weekly with premedication [8]. Amitraz may also be mixed in mineral oil (1:9 ratio) for treatment of pododemodicosis and demodectic otitis [1].

Amitraz may interact with other drugs, including other monoamine oxidase inhibitors and sedatives. The safety of not only the patient but the handler should be considered. Drugs capable of monoamine oxidase inhibition, including some antidepressants and deprenyl/selegiline, should be avoided in these dogs. Handlers applying the dips should also be made aware of these potential interactions, although the likelihood of toxicity is not known. People using monoamine oxidase inhibitors or those with diabetes, Parkinson's disease, or respiratory diseases probably should not handle amitraz. The dip must be applied in a well-ventilated space using protective clothing and gloves. Because monoamine oxidase inhibitors have traditionally been stopped 2 weeks before anesthesia [16] in human patients, it may be prudent not to administer anesthesia shortly after amitraz administration.

Macrocyclic Lactones

An alternative to the use of amitraz in patients with generalized demodicosis is the use of the macrocyclic lactones. This group includes the avermectins (ivermectin and doramectin) and the milbemycins (milbemycin oxime and moxidectin). Macrocyclic lactones potentiate glutamate-gated chloride channels or gamma-aminobutyric acid (GABA)–gated chloride channels of the mite's nervous system, resulting in increased cell permeability to chloride ions. This causes neuromuscular blocking, which paralyzes and kills the parasite [17]. Mammals lack glutamate-gated chloride channels in the peripheral nervous system, and GABA is found in the central nervous system. Because these drugs do not cross the blood-brain barrier, they are generally not toxic to mammals [8,17].

Macrocyclic lactones are now often the first choice for treating generalized demodicosis by many veterinarians. They have several advantages over amitraz and are gaining favor as a first line of therapy. The oral route of administration is preferable to dipping for many clients. Furthermore, treatment can be initiated even if severe secondary pyoderma is present, and frequent bathing does not interfere with therapy. There is less potential for sedation and less risk for the person administering the treatment. Unfortunately, one of the major disadvantages of using the macrocyclic lactones for the treatment of this disease is the off-label use of the drugs when a licensed treatment is available. The side effects with the avermectins, although rare, can be extremely serious, and no specific reversal agent exists. Finally, the cost of treating large dogs is considerable.

Ivermectin

Ivermectin is usually dosed at 300 to 600 µg/kg/d orally for treatment of generalized canine demodicosis [18–20]. Most often, an injectable form of the medication is administered orally. An evidence-based review of studies showed good evidence of recommending ivermectin at this dose range for the treatment of generalized demodicosis [8]. Adverse effects are rare and usually include lethargy, mydriasis, and ataxia. These side effects may sometimes occur after several weeks of therapy. The most worrisome aspect of treatment, however, is the potential for acute severe neurologic toxicity. It can occur in any dog but is common in Collies and less so in other herding breeds. In general, the drug should not be used in Collies and other herding breeds at the doses needed to treat demodicosis. Ivermectin sensitivity in Collies has been traced to a mutation of the multidrug resistance (mdr1) gene. This gene encodes for P-glycoprotein, an integral part of the blood-brain barrier, which transports drugs from the brain back into the blood. Dogs that are homozygous for the mutation show the ivermectin-sensitive phenotype [17]. A commercial test is available for detecting the mutation in dogs and should be considered if ivermectin must be used in a herding breed dog. Information is available at the Washington State University Veterinary Clinical Pathology Laboratory web site [21]. It should be noted that a number of drugs, including cyclosporines, calcium channel antagonists, and various antimicrobial agents, are capable of P-glycoprotein inhibition and thus could be expected to precipitate neurotoxicity in patients receiving ivermectin.

Safety in administering daily oral ivermectin may be improved but not ensured by gradually increasing the amount administered over several days until the desired dose is reached. For example, if a daily dose of 400 μg/kg is desired, the patient may be given only 50 μg/kg on the first day, with an additional 50 μg/kg added daily until the full dose is reached on the eighth day. The owners should be instructed to observe the pet closely over this period and to stop administration and contact the veterinarian if any symptoms, such as lethargy, incoordination, or mydriasis, are noted.

The dose of ivermectin required to treat dogs with generalized demodicosis varies among patients. Although some veterinarians prefer to treat all patients with 600 μg/kg/d, another approach to reduce cost and side effects is to use a lower dose, such as 400 μg/kg/d, and to increase the dose by 100 μg/kg on a monthly basis if needed. The decision to increase the dose can be made on the basis of the clinical and parasitologic response.

Milbemycin Oxime

A number of studies have evaluated the use of daily oral milbemycin oxime for treatment of generalized demodicosis. Milbemycin oxime is available as an oral heartworm preventative and is available in four tablet sizes ranging from 2.3 to 23 mg. The doses used to treat generalized disease have ranged from 0.5 to 2 mg/kg/d up to 3.1 mg/kg/d [8,22,23]. Cure rates are highly variable, but an evidence-based review of the literature found good evidence for recommending treatment with milbemycin oxime at 2 mg/kg/d [8]. This dose is generally well tolerated even by ivermectin-sensitive dogs [1], and this is the major advantage of the drug. A major disadvantage of milbemycin oxime, however, is its expense.

Moxidectin

Moxidectin is another milbemycin that has been evaluated for treatment of canine generalized demodicosis. There are few studies available, but there is good evidence for recommending moxidectin at a dose of 400 μg/kg/d administered orally [8,24,25]. Side effects, such as ataxia and lethargy, have been seen. Moxidectin is available in a large-animal formulation oral and pour-on formulation as well as an oral monthly canine heartworm preventative. It is also available as a topical 1% solution combined with imidacloprid, which is marketed in several countries for monthly parasite control in dogs. It is not yet known whether topical application of moxidectin is helpful in canine generalized demodicosis.

Doramectin

Doramectin is another macrocyclic lactone that has been investigated for the treatment of generalized demodicosis. It has been used at weekly subcutaneous injections of 600 μg/kg without adverse effects and with apparent efficacy [26]. This drug is not safe for use in ivermectin-sensitive patients and thus should be avoided in Collies and other herding breeds. It is available as an injectable solution for cattle and swine. Based on this study, there is fair evidence for the use of doramectin [8].

SUMMARY

Demodicosis continues to be a common and important skin disease of the dog. Deep skin scrapings should routinely be performed on dogs with dermatologic conditions to ensure the timely diagnosis of this disease. Fortunately, the prognosis for the disease has improved in recent years. In part, this is attributable to a better understanding of the factors that contribute to generalized demodicosis. The greatest progress, however, has been made in the options for treatment of this disease.

References

[1] Scott DW, Miller WH, Griffin CE. Muller and Kirk's small animal dermatology. 6th edition. Philadelphia: WB Saunders; 2001.
[2] Chesney CJ. Short form of Demodex species mite in the dog: occurrence and measurements. J Small Anim Pract 1999;40:58–61.
[3] Chen C. A short-tailed demodectic mite and Demodex canis infestation in a Chihuahua dog. Vet Dermatol 1995;6(4):227–9.
[4] Tamura Y, Kawamura Y, Inoue I, et al. Scanning electron microscopy description of a new species of Demodex canis spp. Vet Dermatol 2001;12:275–8.
[5] Desch CE, Hillier A. Demodex injai: a new species of hair follicle mite (Acari: Demodecidae) from the domestic dog (Canidae). J Med Entomol 2003;40(2):146–9.
[6] Robson DC, Burton GG, Bassett R, et al. Eight cases of demodicosis cased by a long-bodied Demodex species (1997–2002). Aust Vet Pract 2003;33:64–74.
[7] Hillier A, Desch CE. Large-bodied Demodex mite infestation in 4 dogs. J Am Vet Med Assoc 2002;220(5):623–7.
[8] Mueller RS. Treatment protocols for demodicosis: an evidence-based review. Vet Dermatol 2004;15:75–89.
[9] Lemarie SL, Hosgood G, Foil CS. A retrospective study of juvenile- and adult-onset generalized demodicosis in dogs (1986–91). Vet Dermatol 1996;7:3–10.

[10] Duclos DD, Jeffers JG, Schanley KJ. Prognosis for treatment of adult-onset demodicosis in dogs: 34 cases (1979–1990). J Am Vet Med Assoc 1994;204(4):616–9.

[11] Lemarié SL, Horohov DW. Evaluation of interleukin-2 production and interleukin-2 receptor expression in dogs with generalized demodicosis. Vet Dermatol 1996;7:213–9.

[12] Gursoy S, Kunt N, Kayagusuz K, et al. Intravenous amitraz poisoning. Clin Toxicol 2005;43:113–6.

[13] Plumb DC. Veterinary drug handbook. 4th edition. Ames (IA): Iowa State Press; 2002.

[14] Hugnet C, Buronfosse F, Pineau X, et al. Toxicity and kinetics of amitraz in dogs. Am J Vet Res 1996;57:1506–10.

[15] Kwochka KW, Kunkle GA. The efficacy of amitraz for generalized demodicosis in dogs: a study of two concentrations and frequencies of application. Compend Contin Educ Pract Vet 1985;7:8–17.

[16] Hill S, Yau K, Whitwam J. MAOIs to RIMAs in anaesthesia—a literature review. Psychopharmacology (Berl) 1992;106(Suppl):S43–5.

[17] Mealey KL, Bentjen SA, Gay JM, et al. Ivermectin sensitivity in collies is associated with a deletion mutation of the mdr1 gene. Pharmacogenetics 2001;11:727–33.

[18] Fondati A. Efficacy of daily oral ivermectin in the treatment of 10 cases of generalized demodicosis in adult dogs. Vet Dermatol 1996;7:99–104.

[19] Medleau L, Ristic Z, McElveen DR. Daily ivermectin for treatment of generalized demodicosis in dogs. Vet Dermatol 1996;7:209–12.

[20] Ristic Z, Medleau L, Paradis M, et al. Ivermectin for the treatment of generalized demodicosis in dogs. J Am Anim Hosp Assoc 1995;207:1308–10.

[21] Washington State University Veterinary Clinical Pathology Laboratory. Available at: www.vetmed.wsu.edu/depts-vcpl/test.asp. Accessed November 16, 2005.

[22] Miller WH, Scott DW, Wellington JR, et al. Clinical efficacy of milbemycin oxime in the treatment of generalized demodicosis in adult dogs. J Am Vet Med Assoc 1993;2003:1426–9.

[23] Holm BR. Efficacy of milbemycin oxime in the treatment of canine generalized demodicosis: a retrospective study of 99 dogs (1995–2000). Vet Dermatol 2003;14:189–95.

[24] Bensignor E, Carlotti D, eds. Moxidectin in the treatment of generalized demodicosis in dogs. A pilot study: 8 cases. In: Kwochka KW, Willemse T, Tscharner CV, editors. Advances in veterinary dermatology. Oxford, United Kingdom: Butterworth-Heinemann; 1998.

[25] Wagner R, Wendlberger U. Field efficacy of moxidectin in dogs and rabbits naturally infested with Sarcoptes spp., Demodex spp. and Psoroptes spp. mites. Vet Parasitol 2000;93:149–58.

[26] Johnstone IP. Doramectin as a treatment for canine and feline demodicosis. Aust Vet Pract 2002;32:98–103.

Sebaceous Adenitis

Candace A. Sousa, DVM

Veterinary Specialty Team, Pfizer Animal Health, 4588 Echo Springs Circle,
El Dorado Hills, CA 95762, USA

S
ebaceous adenitis is a rare idiopathic dermatosis that has been described
most often in dogs but has been reported to occur in other mammals.
The disease seems to represent an inflammatory disorder directed
against or centered on the sebaceous glands.

SEBACEOUS GLANDS

Sebaceous glands are simple or branched alveolar glands that are distributed
throughout the haired skin of mammals. They connect to the hair follicle
through a duct at the infundibulum. The glands produce an oily secretion
that forms a surface emulsion, along with sweat and epidermal lipids, that
spreads over the surface of the skin and hairs. This emulsion functions to retain
moisture and maintain proper hydration of the skin and acts as a physical barrier as well as a chemical barrier against potential pathogens. The emulsion
contains inorganic salts and proteins that inhibit microorganisms; the antiviral
glycoprotein interferon; and immunoglobulins, particularly IgA. Within the
stratum corneum, terminally differentiated corneocytes are suspended in this
extracellular lipid matrix similar to a wall of bricks and mortar.

Sebum is composed predominantly of triglycerides and wax esters. The surface lipids of dogs and cats contains more sterol esters, free cholesterol, cholesterol esters, and wax diesters than in human beings and fewer triglycerides, free
fatty acids, and squalene. Once the sebum enters the hair follicle, it becomes
contaminated with lipase-producing bacteria (*Propionibacterium* spp, *Staphylococcus*
spp), which results in the production of free fatty acids. Many of these fatty
acids (linoleic, myristic, oleic, and palmitic acid) have antimicrobial actions [1].

ETIOLOGY

Sebaceous adenitis was first described in three dogs in 1985 [2] and then in
1987 in the Standard Poodle [3]. It is an uncommon inflammatory disease process that is centered on the sebaceous glands and typically leads to their complete destruction. The etiology is unknown. Because the disease is diagnosed

E-mail address: candace.sousa@pfizer.com

0195-5616/06/$ – see front matter
doi:10.1016/j.cvsm.2005.09.009

more commonly in certain breeds, there seems to be a genetic predisposition. In the Standard Poodle, the disease seems to be inherited as an autosomal recessive trait with variable expression [4]. Recently, an autosomal recessive mode of inheritance has been suggested for the Akita [5]. The Orthopedic Foundation of America (OFA) has developed a registry for affected dogs [6]. Pedigree information on these dogs as well as on nonaffected dogs is kept to be used by breeders in an effort to decrease the number of affected dogs.

Other proposed causes included an autoimmune attack against the sebaceous glands, destruction of the glands with loss resulting in a loss of intercellular lipids and hyperkeratosis, a defect of lipid metabolism, a defect in keratinization, a paired genetic defect of sebaceous gland and epidermal alterations, and a hypersensitivity reaction [7].

SIGNALMENT
Sebaceous adenitis has been reported most commonly in the Standard Poodle, Akita, Samoyed, Chow Chow, and Vizsla, although the disease has been reported in more than 50 other pure and mixed breeds of dogs, in cats [8], and in rabbits [9]. Young adult to middle-aged dogs are most commonly affected, and no sex predilection has been noted.

CLINICAL SIGNS
Sebaceous adenitis in dogs is nonpruritic unless there is a secondary staphylococcal skin infection. The clinical disease differs in short-coated versus long-coated or plush-coated breeds of dogs. In the former, the lesions tend to be nodular with multifocal annular and serpiginous areas of alopecia and fine white scaling. The head and pinnae are usually the first areas involved, and the condition often progresses to involve the trunk. The condition tends to give the dogs a "moth-eaten" appearance [10,11]. There is speculation that the disease in some dogs, such as the Vizsla, may actually not be a primary sebaceous adenitis but a sterile granulomatous disease in which the sebaceous glands are destroyed as "innocent bystanders" (Thelma Gross, DVM, Peter Ihrke, VMD, personal communication, 2004).

Early clinical disease in the long- or plush-coated breeds may be subtle, with the appearance of clumps of adherent scales, many adhering to the hair shafts, and minimal alopecia. The hairs are often dull and brittle and can develop a brown to red tint [4,5]. In more chronic cases, the hair coat may become thin. The alopecia may be patchy but is usually more generalized, and the degree of scaling is pronounced. When the remaining hairs are epilated from the follicles, they tend to have an adherent cast of follicular debris around the root. Affected areas usually initially involve the head and pinnae, followed by the trunk, tail, and legs (Figs. 1–3).

Scaling and follicular plugging are most likely the result of the lack of sebum. Because sebum has antibacterial properties, secondary staphylococcal folliculitis and even furunculosis may develop. These dogs often have papules,

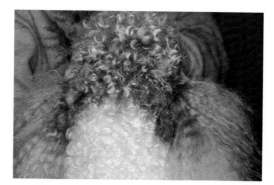

Fig. 1. White Standard Poodle, 5 years old, female, spayed, with sebaceous adenitis affecting the head only. Note the darker hair coat of the head onto the pinnae.

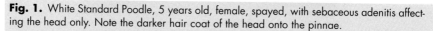

pustules, or nodules on the skin and an odor. Occasionally, dogs may be pruritic secondary to the bacterial colonization.

One report describes two cats with sebaceous adenitis that presented with generalized heavy adherent scales, partial alopecia, and distinctive rims of dark brown to black thick adherent scales along the margins of the eyelids [8].

Another report described the condition in domestic rabbits. The animals developed clinical lesions from 2.5 to 6 years of age. Lesions first appeared around the face and neck and became generalized after several months. All reported cases eventually developed a generalized nonpruritic exfoliative dermatitis with patchy to coalescing areas of alopecia [9].

DIAGNOSIS

The diagnosis of sebaceous adenitis can be suspected based on the signalment of the patient, history, and physical examination. The differential diagnosis

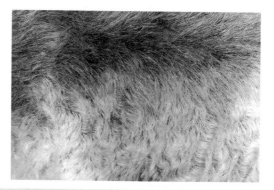

Fig. 2. White standard poodle, 3 years old, male, castrated, with patchy area of sebaceous adenitis on the trunk. Note that the affected hairs are darker, straighter, and coarser than the nonaffected hairs.

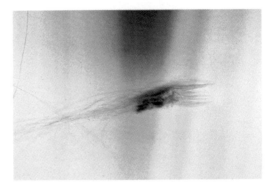

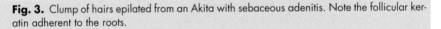

Fig. 3. Clump of hairs epilated from an Akita with sebaceous adenitis. Note the follicular keratin adherent to the roots.

includes infectious conditions, such as demodicosis, dermatophytosis, or staphylococcal folliculitis and pyoderma; endocrinopathies, especially hypothyroidism; nutritional deficiencies of zinc or fatty acids or nutritionally responsive conditions, such as zinc-responsive dermatosis or vitamin A–responsive dermatosis; congenital or hereditary conditions, such as ichthyosis; and autoimmune dermatoses, such as pemphigus foliaceus and systemic lupus erythematosus. The definitive diagnosis of sebaceous adenitis is confirmed by a histopathologic examination of the skin.

HISTOPATHOLOGY

The histopathologic findings in skin biopsy samples taken from the dog vary during the course of the disease [3]. The primary histopathologic pattern seen is often a distinctly nodular granulomatous to pyogranulomatous inflammatory reaction centered in a middermal perifollicular location. The cellular infiltrate is composed of histiocytes, lymphocytes, neutrophils, and plasma cells. Often, there are no remnants of sebaceous glands. In late cases, the lesion may be restricted to a mild hypercellularity in the region of the sebaceous glands or even to merely an absence of glands. In extremely advanced cases, follicular atrophy or dysplasia may be seen with focal perifollicular fibrosis (Figs. 4 and 5). In contrast to classic sebaceous adenitis, the disease in short-coated dogs, such as the Vizsla, is characterized by discrete nodular inflammation that is centered on the isthmus of hair follicles. Although this inflammation is often "lop-sided," suggesting targeting of the sebaceous glands, some cases have symmetric lesions or larger foci of inflammation that occasionally track along the entire hair follicle.

The epidermis typically demonstrates marked orthokeratotic hyperkeratosis and irregular epidermal hyperplasia. Follicular keratosis is prominent in some forms of the disease. Vertically oriented keratin lamellae may seem to "erupt" from the follicular ostia.

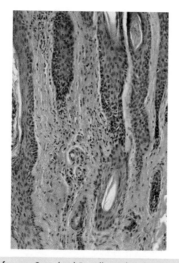

Fig. 4. Histologic section from a Standard Poodle with sebaceous adenitis. Note the periadnexal fibrosis at the site of previous sebaceous glands. (Courtesy of T.L. Gross, DVM, Sacramento, CA)

Immunohistologic examination of skin samples from dogs shows that there are a large number of dendritic antigen-presenting cells and T cells focused on the middle portion of the hair follicle and extending into the sebaceous duct early in the course of the disease. This suggests an immune-mediated pathogenesis for sebaceous adenitis [10].

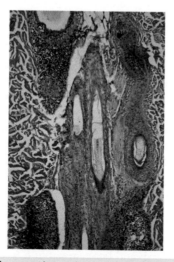

Fig. 5. Histologic section from an Akita with sebaceous adenitis. Note the mural folliculitis in the area where the sebaceous glands usually enter the follicle. (Courtesy of T.L. Gross, DVM, Sacramento, CA)

In cats, a moderate to severe lymphocytic infiltrate is often present in place of the sebaceous glands. There is a severe diffuse orthokeratotic hyperkeratosis of the epidermis without significant follicular hyperkeratosis. The epidermis contains mild lymphocytic exocytosis, patchy foci of hydropic degeneration, and rare dyskeratotic keratinocytes [8].

TREATMENT

There is no known way to stop the inflammatory process or to make the sebaceous glands regrow. Sebaceous adenitis is commonly unresponsive to treatment with anti-inflammatory or immunosuppressive doses of glucocorticoids or various nutritional supplements (eg, zinc, vitamin A, vitamin E, vegetable and animal fats.) Instead, treatment is focused on palliation of the clinical symptoms. The goals of treatment include removal of the excess scales, improvement in the quality of the hair coat, and possible regrowth of hair. Because the disease cannot be cured, some level of maintenance therapy is usually required for the life of the animal [11].

Successful treatment has been reported with the regular use of antiseborrheic shampoos, conditioners, topical oil or humectant sprays or soaks, oral vitamin A, synthetic retinoids, oral fatty acids, and cyclosporine. If there is a concurrent bacterial colonization or infection, oral antibiotic therapy is of use in controlling the odor and pruritus.

Shampoos that contain a combination of sulfur and salicylic acid can be used as often as three times per week. After leaving the shampoo on for a minimum of 10 minutes, a significant amount of the scales can be removed from the coat. Often, a soft brush is used to help loosen and remove the scales. This may accelerate the regrowth of hair. After the shampoo is rinsed off, a final application of a conditioning cream rinse or a mixture of propylene glycol and water (final concentration of 50%–75% propylene glycol), which acts as a humectant, can be used.

Some owners of severely affected Standard Poodles have resorted to using a bath oil treatment. Any light mineral oil–containing bath oil (eg, generic baby oil, Alpha Keri Bath Oil [Westwood Pharmaceuticals, Buffalo, NY]) is rubbed well into the hair coat and allowed to soak into the coat for approximately 1 hour. The oil is then removed with several bathings using liquid dishwashing liquid. This can be repeated as needed every 7 to 30 days.

When topical treatment alone has been ineffective, oral vitamin A (retinol) at 10,000 IU administered orally twice daily up to 20,000 to 30,000 IU twice daily can be tried. It has been estimated to result in approximately 80% to 90% clinical improvement within 3 months [12]. Isotretinoin has been shown to be effective in the treatment of sebaceous adenitis in Vizslas and other breeds of dogs [13,14]. The dose recommended is 1 mg/kg administered orally once to twice daily. Improvement should be seen within 6 weeks; at that time, the frequency of administration can be decreased to every other day or the dose lowered to 0.5 mg/kg administered once daily. Other synthetic retinoids have also been shown to be an effective treatment in some cases.

There are anecdotal reports of dogs that respond to treatment with a combination of oral tetracycline and niacinamide. For dogs that weigh less than 25 kg, both medications are administered at 250 mg every 8 hours. Dogs that weigh more than 25 kg are treated with 500 mg of each every 8 hours. There are also anecdotal reports of clinical improvement when dogs were treated with doxycycline in combination with vitamin A.

Finally, for dogs with sebaceous adenitis that have not responded to treatment with oral retinoids, cyclosporinecan be used at a dose of 5 mg/kg administered orally twice daily [15,16].

References

[1] Scott DW, Miller WH Jr, Griffin CE. Structure and function. In: Muller and Kirk's small animal dermatology. 6th edition. Philadelphia: WB Saunders; 2001. p. 48–51.

[2] Scott DW. Granulomatous sebaceous adenitis in dogs. J Am Anim Hosp Assoc 1986;22: 631–4.

[3] Rosser EJ, Dunstan RW, Breen PT, et al. Sebaceous adenitis with hyperkeratosis in the standard poodle: a discussion of 10 cases. J Am Anim Hosp Assoc 1987;23:341–5.

[4] Dunstan RW, Hargis AM. The diagnosis of sebaceous adenitis in standard poodle dogs. In: Bonagura JD, editor. Kirk's current veterinary therapy XII. Philadelphia: WB Saunders; 1995. p. 619–22.

[5] Reichler IM, Hauser B, Schiller I, et al. Sebaceous adenitis in the Akita: clinical observations, histopathology and hereditary. Vet Dermatol 2001;12(5):243–53.

[6] Orthopedic Foundation of America. Available at: http://www.offa.org/sainfo.html.

[7] Scott DW, Miller WH Jr, Griffin CE. Sebaceous adenitis. In: Muller and Kirk's small animal dermatology. 6th edition. Philadelphia: WB Saunders; 2001. p. 1140–6.

[8] Baer K, Shoulberg N, Helton K. Sebaceous adenitis-like disease in two cats. Vet Pathol 1993;30:437.

[9] White SD, Linder K, Schultheiss P, et al. Sebaceous adenitis in four domestic rabbits (Oryctatagus cuniculus). Vet Dermatol 2000;11(1):53–9.

[10] Rybnicek J, Affolter VK, Moore PF. Sebaceous adenitis: an immunohistological examination. In: Kwochka KW, Willemse T, von Tscharner C, editors. Advances in veterinary dermatology, vol. 3. Oxford, United Kingdom: Butterworth Heinemann; 1998. p. 539–40.

[11] Rosser EJ. Therapy for sebaceous adenitis. In: Bonagura JD, editor. Kirk's current veterinary therapy XIII. Philadelphia: WB Saunders; 2000. p. 572–3.

[12] DeManuelle T, Rothstein E. Food allergy and nutritionally related skin disease. In: Thoday KL, Foil CS, Bond R, editors. Advances in veterinary dermatology, vol. 4. Oxford, United Kingdom: Blackwell Science; 2002. p. 224–30.

[13] Stewart LJ, White SD, Carpenter JL. Isotretinoin in the treatment of sebaceous adenitis in two Vizslas. J Am Anim Hosp Assoc 1991;27:65–71.

[14] White SD, Rosychuk RAW, Scott KV, et al. Sebaceous adenitis in dogs and results of treatment with isotretinoin and etretinate: 30 cases (1990–1994). J Am Vet Med Assoc 1995;207(2):197–200.

[15] Carothers MA, Kwochka KW, Rojko JL. Cyclosporine-responsive granulomatous sebaceous adenitis in a dog. J Am Vet Med Assoc 1991;198(9):1645–8.

[16] Linek M, Boss C, Haemmerling R, et al. Effects of cyclosporine A on clinical and histologic abnormalities in dogs with sebaceous adenitis. J Am Vet Med Assoc 2005;226(1):59–64.

Vesicular Cutaneous Lupus

Hilary A. Jackson, BVMS, DVD, MRCVS

North Carolina State University, College of Veterinary Medicine, 4700 Hillsborough Street,
Raleigh, NC 27606, USA

In the late 1960s and early 1970s, an erosive skin disease of the Rough Collie and Shetland Sheepdog was first reported as hidradenitis suppurativa [1,2]. Later, an identical condition in the same breeds was characterized as bullous pemphigoid (BP) based on the histologic finding of dermoepidermal separation [3,4]. The phenotype exhibited by these patients seems to be markedly different from that of dogs now known to be affected with the canine homologue of human BP [5]. In 1995, the disease was described as an idiopathic ulcerative disease of Rough Collies and Shetland Sheepdogs, and it was suggested that this disease may be a variant of familial canine dermatomyositis, a hereditary condition in these breeds [6].

In 2001, Jackson and Olivry [7] compared the historical, clinical, and histologic features of idiopathic ulcerative dermatosis and familial canine dermatomyositis. They found many distinctions between the two diseases and furthermore suggested that the ulcerative dermatosis was a form of cutaneous lupus erythematosus. This led to further publications substantiating this claim [8,9]. In this review, the author presents the historical and clinical features characteristic of this disease, the evidence supporting its characterization as cutaneous lupus, and, finally, a review of current treatment recommendations.

HISTORICAL AND CLINICAL FINDINGS

Vesicular cutaneous lupus erythematosus (VCLE) is a rare disease of the Rough Collie, Shetland Sheepdog, and their crosses. A clinically and histologically indistinguishable disease has occasionally been noted in unrelated breeds by this author.

This disease typically affects adult dogs. In a case series of 17 dogs, the age of onset ranged from 3 to 11 years, with a median age of 6 years. The female/male ratio was 2.4:1 [9]. Although Shetland Sheepdogs and their crosses represented 70% of these cases, it is possible that this may only reflect the relative popularity of this breed. No comparison could be made with the general canine population, because case material was drawn from throughout the United States.

E-mail address: hilary_jackson@ncsu.edu

0195-5616/06/$ – see front matter
doi:10.1016/j.cvsm.2005.09.005

One interesting feature of VCLE is that the disease usually occurs in the spring and summer months and has been noted to relapse at the same time in subsequent years. This, and the fact that the less well-haired areas of the skin are affected, suggests a role for sunlight in the pathogenesis of the disease.

The primary lesion is a transient vesicle or bulla that may only be appreciated in histologic sections of early lesions because they rupture readily to manifest as annular, polycyclic, or serpiginous ulceration (Figs. 1 and 2). The lesions are typically distributed over the groin, axillae, and ventral abdomen and often involve the mucocutaneous junctions and concave aspects of the pinnae. Lesions can be advanced at clinical presentation, because the dense hair coat in these dogs can mask the advent of early lesions. Extensive involvement can lead to secondary complications, such as bacteremia and septicemia [7].

CLINICAL AND SURGICAL PATHOLOGIC FINDINGS

There are no specific routine laboratory findings in VCLE, although granular casts were found in the urine of some affected dogs [7].

Diagnosis of VCLE is based on breed specificity, history, and clinical presentation supported by characteristic histopathologic findings. Multiple skin biopsies should be collected from affected dogs. Vesicles and bulla are ideal; however, as previously mentioned, these are rarely present because of their fragile nature. Collecting multiple wedge biopsies at right angles to the margin of freshly ulcerated and normal skin is optimal. Wedge biopsies are usually sectioned longitudinally, thus profiling the leading edge of the ulcer.

VCLE is characterized by a lymphocyte-rich interface dermatitis and folliculitis. Multifocal areas of vesiculation at the dermoepidermal junction may be appreciated, resulting from the coalescence of vacuolated basal keratinocytes.

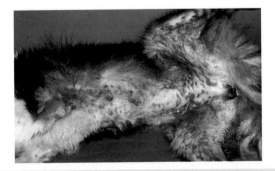

Fig. 1. Ventral distribution of ulceration in a Rough Collie with VCLE (*From* Jackson HA, Olivry T. Ulscerative dermatosis of the Shetland sheepdog and rough collie dog may represent a novel vesicular variant of cutaneous lupus erythematosus. Veterinary Dermatology 2001;12:20; with permission.)

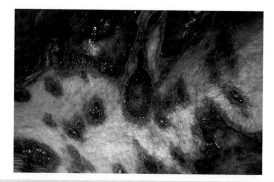

Fig. 2. Polycyclic and serpiginous pattern of ulcerations in VCLE. (*From* Jackson HA, Olivry T. Ulscerative dermatosis of the Shetland sheepdog and rough collie dog may represent a novel vesicular variant of cutaneous lupus erythematosus. Veterinary Dermatology 2001;12:21; with permission.)

IMMUNOPATHOLOGIC FINDINGS

Clinical and histologic features of canine VCLE resemble those of subacute cutaneous lupus erythematosus (SCLE) in man. In people, this disease is characterized by a photosensitive polymorphic inflammatory eruption that occurs over sun-exposed skin. Histologic features of SCLE include epidermal atrophy, individual keratinocyte apoptosis, and a lymphocytic interface dermatitis that affects surface and adnexal epithelium. Focal dermal-epidermal separation can also occur [10]. Forty percent to 70% of human patients with SCLE have circulating autoantibodies directed against the extractable (ie, soluble) nuclear antigens (ENAs) Ro/SSA and La/SSB [11].

Lesional skin of Collies and Shetland Sheepdogs with VCLE is characterized by a lymphocyte-rich interface dermatitis [7]. Using immunohistochemical techniques, apoptosis of basal keratinocytes associated with epidermotropism and dermal infiltration of T lymphocytes and antigen-presenting dendritic cells was demonstrated in the skin of affected dogs [9].

Using a direct immunofluorescence method, immunoglobulin deposition could be demonstrated in all the cases examined in this series. The immunoglobulins were present in the cytoplasm of basal and suprabasal keratinocytes (43%), in the blood vessel endothelium (93%) and at the dermoepidermal junction (50%). This last location resembles the "lupus-band" seen in human beings with cutaneous lupus.

Circulating autoantibodies to ENAs were detected by enzyme-linked immunosorbent assay (ELISA) in 9 (82%) of the 11 cases tested by immunoblotting or ELISA, and autoantibodies to Ro/SSA or La/SSB were found most commonly (in 55% of all cases tested or in 75% of anti-ENA autoantibody-positive dogs). In contrast to these observations, antibodies to Ro/SSA have been detected only rarely in canine sera in previous surveys [12–14].

TREATMENT

Given that this disease is uncommonly seen, it is difficult to make sound treatment recommendations based on large numbers of cases. Before 2004, it was suggested that prednisone administered at a dose of 1 to 2 mg kg^{-1} twice daily should be used in the acute stages of the disease. Additionally, pentoxifylline at a dose of 400 mg administered once daily and vitamin E supplementation were suggested to be beneficial [6]. In a retrospective study published in 2004, Jackson [8] reported the clinical outcome of a series of 11 cases of VCLE. In this series, the best long-term therapeutic outcome was achieved with oral administration of immunosuppressive doses of prednisone or methylprednisolone alone or in combination with azathioprine. Both drugs were tapered over time according to the clinical response. Complete remission was not achieved in all cases, and long-term adverse effects of systemic glucocorticoids were reported in all dogs receiving this treatment modality. Of note was one dog with mild disease localized on the abdomen that responded completely to topical fluocinolone. Four dogs in this series were treated with pentoxifylline, and the total dose given in a 24-hour period ranged from 9 to 30 mg kg^{-1}. A poor response was seen with this therapy. It is noteworthy, however, that the dosing recommendations for pentoxifylline in the dog have changed over the years; a recent pharmokinetic study suggests that an oral dose of 15 mg kg^{-1} administered three times daily achieves plasma concentrations similar to therapeutic levels in human beings [15]. Only one of four dogs in this series received a similar dose; however, this dog died after 3 months of therapy. There are anecdotal reports of oral cyclosporine at a dose of 5 mg kg^{-1} administered once daily as being an effective alternative therapeutic option for VCLE (Ann Mattise, DVM, Thierry Olivry, DVM, North Carolina State University College of Veterinary Medicine, personal communication, 2005). Investigation into the treatment of VCLE with antimalarials, such as hydroxychloroquine sulfate, quinacrine, or chloroquine phosphate, is warranted because this is an effective therapeutic approach for patients with SCLE [16].

Three dogs in the previous series were euthanized for reasons directly related to the disease.

In all cases in that series, an oral bacteriocidal antibiotic and topical antibacterial shampooing were prescribed at initial presentation. Many dogs required intermittent courses of oral antibiotics throughout the course of their disease or regular shampoo therapy.

Although the exact role of sunlight in the pathogenesis of VCLE is currently unknown, sun avoidance or the use of a sunscreen is recommended for affected dogs.

SUMMARY

VCLE is a specific disease of middle-aged Rough Collies and Shetland Sheepdogs and is distinct from familial canine dermatomyositis seen in the same breeds. Female dogs may be predisposed. The presentation is clinically distinct, but a definitive diagnosis relies on the demonstration of a cell-rich interface dermatitis in skin biopsies taken from affected areas. This can be a debilitating skin disease, and aggressive immunosuppressive therapy is warranted in severe cases. Sun avoidance is also recommended.

References
[1] Reedy LM, Mallett R, Freeman RG. Hidradenitis suppurativa in a female Shetland sheepdog. Vet Med Small Anim Clin 1973;68:1262.

[2] Schwartman RM, Maguire HG. Staphylococcal apocrine gland infections in the dog (canine hidradenitis suppurativa). Br Vet J 1969;125:121–6.

[3] Scott D, Manning T, Lewis R. Linear IgA dermatoses in the dog: bullous pemphigoid, discoid lupus erythematosus and a subcorneal pustular dermatitis. Cornell Vet 1982;72:394–402.

[4] White SD, Rosser EJ, Ihrke PJ, et al. Bullous pemphigoid in a dog: treatment with six-mercaptopurine. J Am Vet Med Assoc 1981;185:683–5.

[5] Olivry T, Fine J-D, Dunston SM. Canine epidermolysis bullosa acquisita; circulating autoantibodies target the aminoterminal noncollagenous (NC1) domain of collagen VII in anchoring fibrils. Vet Dermatol 1998;9:19–31.

[6] Ihrke PJ, Gross TL. Ulcerative dermatosis of Shetland sheepdogs and collies. In: Bonagura JD, editor. Kirk's current veterinary therapy XII (small animal practice). Philadelphia: WB Saunders; 1995. p. 639–40.

[7] Jackson HA, Olivry T. Ulcerative dermatosis of the Shetland sheepdog and rough collie dog may represent a novel vesicular variant of cutaneous lupus erythematosus. Vet Dermatol 2001;12:19–27.

[8] Jackson HA. Eleven cases of vesicular cutaneous lupus erythematosus in Shetland sheepdogs and rough collies: clinical management and prognosis. Vet Dermatol 2004;15:37–41.

[9] Jackson HA, Olivry T, Berget F, et al. Immunopathology of vesicular cutaneous lupus erythematosus in the rough collie and Shetland sheepdog: a canine homologue of subacute cutaneous lupus erythematosus in humans. Vet Dermatol 2004;15:230–9.

[10] David-Bajaar KM, Davis BM. Pathology, immunopathology and immunohistochemistry in cutaneous lupus erythematosus. Lupus 1997;6:145–57.

[11] Wenzel J, Gerdsen R, Uerlich M, et al. Antibodies targeting extractable nuclear antigens: historical development and current knowledge. Br J Dermatol 2001;145:859–67.

[12] Costa O, Fournel C, Lotchouang E, et al. Specificities of antinuclear antibodies detected in dogs with systemic lupus erythematosus. Vet Immunol Immunopathol 1984;7:369–82.

[13] Monier J, Fournel C, Lapras M, et al. Systemic lupus erythematosus in a colony of dogs. Am J Vet Res 1988;49:46–51.

[14] White SD, Rosychuk RAW, Schur PH. Investigation of antibodies to extractable nuclear antigens in dogs. Am J Vet Res 1992;53(6):1019–21.

[15] Marsella R, Nicklin DF, Munson JW, et al. Pharmokinetics of pentoxifylline in dogs after oral and intravenous administration. Am J Vet Res 2000;61:631–7.

[16] Patel P, Werth V. Cutaneous lupus erythematosus: a review. Dermatol Clin 2002;20:373–85.

INDEX

A

Abscess(es)
    cat bite, 121

Acetaminophen
    in veterinary dermatology management,
      5–6

Acid(s)
    fatty
      for epitheliotropic canine CTCL,
        218

Acne
    chin, 131
    feline, 131

Acquired pinnal folding, 133

Acral lick dermatitis (ALD)
    carbon dioxide lasers for, 34–35

Actinic in situ carcinoma
    carbon dioxide lasers for, 25–27

Actinomycosis, 123

Acupuncture
    in veterinary dermatology management,
      9

AD. See *Atopic dermatitis (AD)*.

Adenitis
    sebaceous, **243–249.** See also *Sebaceous
      adenitis*.

Age
    as factor in GSP, 204
    α_2-Agonists
    in veterinary dermatology management,
      7

ALD. See *Acral lick dermatitis (ALD)*.

Algae, 121

Allergen-specific immunotherapy
    for atopy and AD, 164–166

Allergic reactions
    feline, 126

Allergy testing
    intradermal
      anesthesia for, 10–12

Alopecia
    preauricular, 132

Alternative therapies
    in veterinary dermatology management,
      9–10

Amantadine
    in veterinary dermatology management,
      8

Aminoglycoside(s)
    for bacterial skin diseases, 194–195

Amitraz
    for canine demodicosis, 237–238

Analgesia/analgesics
    in veterinary dermatology management,
      7

Anesthesia/anesthetics
    for intradermal allergy testing, 10–12
    local
      in veterinary dermatology, 2–4

Animal shelters
    dermatophytosis in
      management of, **89–114.** See also
        *Dermatophytosis, in animal
        shelters, management of*.

Animals in shelters
    skin diseases of, **59–88.** See also *Skin
      diseases, of animals in shelters*.

Antibacterial agents
    for dermatologic conditions, 49–51

Antibiotic(s)
    ß-lactam
      for bacterial skin diseases, 195–196
    maintenance
      for GSP, 209–210
    systemic
      for GSP, 206–209

Anticytokine therapy
    for atopy and AD, 167–168

Antifungal agents
    for dermatologic conditions, 47–49
    for dermatophytosis in animal shelters,
      108–110

Anti-inflammatory drugs
    nonsteroidal (NSAIDs)
      in veterinary dermatology
        management, 6

Note: Page numbers of article titles are in **boldface** type.

0195-5616/06/$ – see front matter
doi:10.1016/S0195-5616(05)00172-5